Quality of Life Issues in Dermatology

Guest Editor

SUEPHY C. CHEN, MD, MS

DERMATOLOGIC CLINICS

www.derm.theclinics.com

Consulting Editor
BRUCE H. THIERS, MD

April 2012 • Volume 30 • Number 2

SAUNDERS an imprint of ELSEVIER, Inc.

W.B. SAUNDERS COMPANY
A Division of Elsevier Inc.

1600 John F. Kennedy Boulevard • Suite 1800 • Philadelphia, PA 19103-2899

http://www.theclinics.com

DERMATOLOGIC CLINICS Volume 30, Number 2
April 2012 ISSN 0733-8635, ISBN-13: 978-1-4557-3852-6

Editor: Stephanie Donley
Developmental Editor: Teia Stone

Dermatologic Clinics (ISSN 0733-8635) is published quarterly by Elsevier Inc., 360 Park Avenue South, New York, NY 10010-1710. Months of publication are January, April, July, and October. Business and editorial offices: 1600 John F. Kennedy Blvd., Suite 1800, Philadelphia, PA 19103-2899. Customer service office: 11830 Westline Drive, St. Louis, MO 63146. Periodicals postage paid at New York, NY, and additional mailing offices. Subscription prices are USD 346.00 per year for US individuals, USD 512.00 per year for US institutions, USD 404.00 per year for Canadian individuals, USD 613.00 per year for Canadian institutions, USD 473.00 per year for international individuals, USD 613.00 per year for international institutions, USD 161.00 per year for US students/residents, and USD 233.00 per year for Canadian and international students/residents. International air speed delivery is included in all *Clinics* subscription prices. All prices are subject to change without notice. **POSTMASTER:** Send address changes to *Dermatologic Clinics*, Elsevier Health Sciences Division, Subscription Customer Service, 3251 Riverport Lane, Maryland Heights, MO 63043. **Customer Service: 1-800-654-2452 (U.S. and Canada); 314-447-8871 (outside U.S. and Canada). Fax: 314-447-8029. E-mail: journalscustomerservice-usa@elsevier.com (for print support); journalsonlinesupport-usa@elsevier.com (for online support).**

Reprints. For copies of 100 or more, of articles in this publication, please contact the Commercial Reprints Department, Elsevier Inc., 360 Park Avenue South, New York, New York 10010-1710. Tel.: (212) 633-3813; Fax: (212) 462-1935; Email: reprints@elsevier.com.

The *Dermatologic Clinics* is covered in *MEDLINE/PubMed (Index Medicus), Current Contents/Clinical Medicine, Excerpta Medica, Chemical Abstracts,* and *ISI/BIOMED.*

Printed and bound by CPI Group (UK) Ltd, Croydon, CR0 4YY

Transferred to digital print 2012

Contributors

CONSULTING EDITOR

BRUCE H. THIERS, MD
Professor and Chairman, Department of
Dermatology and Dermatologic Surgery,
Medical University of South Carolina,
Charleston, South Carolina

GUEST EDITOR

SUEPHY C. CHEN, MD, MS
Associate Professor, Division of Dermatology,
Atlanta Veterans Affairs Medical Center,
Decatur; Department of Dermatology,
Emory University, Atlanta, Georgia

AUTHORS

LAUREN E. BARNES, BS
Medical Student, Department of Dermatology,
Center for Dermatology Research, Wake
Forest School of Medicine, Winston-Salem,
North Carolina

MOHAMMAD K.A. BASRA, DDSc, MD
Department of Dermatology and Wound
Healing, Cardiff University School of Medicine,
Heath Park, Cardiff, Wales, United Kingdom

SULOCHANA S. BHANDARKAR, MD
Assistant Professor of Dermatology,
Department of Dermatology, School of
Medicine, Emory University, Atlanta, Georgia

TINA BHUTANI, MD
Clinical Research Fellow, Department of
Dermatology, Psoriasis and Skin Treatment
Center, University of California San Francisco
Medical Center, San Francisco, California

SUEPHY C. CHEN, MD, MS
Associate Professor, Division of Dermatology,
Atlanta Veterans Affairs Medical Center,
Decatur; Department of Dermatology,
Emory University, Atlanta, Georgia

MAHBUB M.U. CHOWDHURY, FRCP
Department of Dermatology, Welsh Institute
of Dermatology, University Hospital
of Wales, Heath Park, Cardiff, Wales,
United Kingdom

MARY-MARGARET CHREN, MD
Professor, Department of Dermatology,
University of California at San Francisco,
San Francisco, California

JANICE N. CORMIER, MD, MPH
Department of Surgical Oncology, The
University of Texas MD Anderson Cancer
Center, Houston, Texas

KATE D. CROMWELL, MS
Department of Surgical Oncology, The
University of Texas MD Anderson Cancer
Center, Houston, Texas

FEREYDOUN DAVATCHI, MD
Chief, Department of Rheumatology
Research Center, Shariati Hospital,
Tehran University for Medical Sciences,
Tehran, Iran

J. de KORTE, MA, PhD
Department of Dermatology, Aquamarine
Foundation, Academic Medical Center,
University of Amsterdam, Amsterdam,
The Netherlands

LAURA K. DELONG, MD, MPH
Assistant Professor, Department of
Dermatology, Emory University School of
Medicine, Emory Clinic, Atlanta; Division of
Dermatology, Atlanta Veterans Affairs Medical
Center, Decatur, Georgia

STEVEN R. FELDMAN, MD, PhD
Professor, Departments of Dermatology,
Pathology, and Public Health Sciences,
Center for Dermatology Research, Wake
Forest School of Medicine, Winston-Salem,
North Carolina

ALAN B. FLEISCHER JR, MD
Professor, Department of Dermatology,
Center for Dermatology Research, Wake
Forest School of Medicine, Winston-Salem,
North Carolina

NICK FREEMANTLE, PhD
Professor, Department of Primary Care and
Population Health, University College London
Medical School, London, United Kingdom

**JOHN W. FREW, MBBS (Hons),
MMed (Clin Epi)**
Resident Medical Officer, Department of
Dermatology, St George Hospital; Research
Student, Faculty of Medicine, University
of New South Wales, Sydney, New South
Wales, Australia

MISHA M. HELLER, BA
Clinical Research Investigator, Department
of Dermatology, Psoriasis and Skin Treatment
Center, University of California San Francisco
Medical Center, San Francisco; Medical
Student, Keck School of Medicine,
University of Southern California,
Los Angeles, California

SEEMA P. KINI, MD, MS
Resident Physician, Department of
Dermatology, Emory University School of
Medicine, Emory Clinic, Atlanta, Georgia

JOHN Y.M. KOO, MD
Professor and Vice Chairman, Department
of Dermatology; Director, Psoriasis and Skin
Treatment Center, University of California
San Francisco Medical Center,
San Francisco, California

ROOPAL V. KUNDU, MD
Assistant Professor of Dermatology,
Department of Dermatology; Director,
Northwestern Center for Ethnic Skin,
Feinberg School of Medicine,
Northwestern University, Chicago, Illinois

ERIC S. LEE, MD
Clinical Research Investigator, Department
of Dermatology, Psoriasis and Skin Treatment
Center, University of California San Francisco
Medical Center, San Francisco, California;
University of Nebraska Medical Center,
College of Medicine, Omaha, Nebraska

MICHELLE M. LEVENDER, MD
Research Fellow, Department of Dermatology,
Center for Dermatology Research, Wake
Forest School of Medicine, Winston-Salem,
North Carolina; Department of Dermatology,
Columbia University Medical Center,
New York, New York

TIFFANY J. LIEU, BA, BS
Medical Student, University of Texas
Southwestern Medical Center, Dallas, Texas

ALAN MENTER, MD
Chief of Dermatology, Department of
Dermatology, Baylor University Medical
Center; Director, Baylor Psoriasis Research
Center; Clinical Professor,
University of Texas Southwestern Medical
Center, Dallas, Texas

**DÉDÉE F. MURRELL, MA, BMBCh,
FAAD, MD, FACD**
Professor and Head, Department of
Dermatology, St George Hospital, University
of New South Wales, Kogarah, Sydney,
New South Wales, Australia

TIEN V. NGUYEN, BA
Clinical Research Investigator, Department
of Dermatology, Psoriasis and Skin Treatment
Center, University of California San Francisco
Medical Center, San Francisco, California;
Medical Student, University of Texas Health
Science Center at San Antonio, School of
Medicine, San Antonio, Texas

AMIT G. PANDYA, MD
Professor, Department of Dermatology,
University of Texas Southwestern Medical
Center, Dallas, Texas

VINCENT PIGUET, MD, PhD
Professor, Department of Dermatology and
Wound Healing, Cardiff University School
of Medicine, Heath Park, Cardiff, Wales,
United Kingdom

C.A.C. PRINSEN, MSc
Department of Dermatology, Aquamarine
Foundation, Academic Medical Center,
University of Amsterdam, Amsterdam,
The Netherlands

ANNA ROGERS, BS
Medical Student, Department of Dermatology,
Emory University School of Medicine,
Atlanta, Georgia

MERRICK I. ROSS, MD
Department of Surgical Oncology, The
University of Texas MD Anderson Cancer
Center, Houston, Texas

DESHAN F. SEBARATNAM, MBBS (Hons)
Resident Medical Officer, Department of
Dermatology, St George Hospital; Research
Student, Faculty of Medicine, University of
New South Wales, Sydney, New South Wales,
Australia

ANNE M. SEIDLER, MD, MBA
Department of Dermatology, Emory University
School of Medicine, Atlanta, Georgia

EMMA V. SMITH, MRCP
Department of Dermatology, Welsh Institute
of Dermatology, University Hospital of Wales,
Heath Park, Cardiff, Wales, United Kingdom

M.A.G. SPRANGERS, MA, PhD
Department of Medical Psychology,
Academic Medical Center, University
of Amsterdam, Amsterdam,
The Netherlands

Ph.I. SPULS, MD, PhD
Department of Dermatology, Academic
Medical Center, University of Amsterdam,
Amsterdam, The Netherlands

O.D. van CRANENBURGH, MSc
Department of Dermatology, Aquamarine
Foundation, Academic Medical Center,
University of Amsterdam, Amsterdam,
The Netherlands

EMIR VELEDAR, PhD
Department of Dermatology, Emory University
School of Medicine, Atlanta, Georgia

JILLIAN W. WONG, BA
Clinical Research Investigator, Department
of Dermatology, Psoriasis and Skin Treatment
Center, University of California San Francisco
Medical Center, San Francisco, California;
Medical Student, University of Utah School
of Medicine, Salt Lake City, Utah

Contents

Improvement of health-related quality of life (HRQoL) is a major goal of dermatology. Identifying how the skin condition affects lives, quantifying this burden, and using this information to improve patients' lives on an individual basis are important targets in clinical dermatology. Using this information in clinical trials and on a health policy level is the objective of QoL research. This article introduces a compendium of articles that address HRQoL in dermatology across a spectrum of diseases and ways that HRQoL can be incorporated in the clinical and research settings.

The concept of quality of life (QOL) is becoming increasingly important in medicine, particularly in dermatology where many cutaneous diseases have the potential to affect the quality rather than the length of life. There is increasing interest in devising methodology to accurately measure the impact of disease on QOL for use in clinical practice, research studies, and economic analyses. The question of which dermatologic QOL instruments to choose inevitably arises. The aim of this article is to familiarize readers with health status measures and to review their use in dermatology.

In this overview of preference-based measures, utilities and willingness to pay (WTP) are discussed as measures relevant to dermatology for capturing the burden of skin diseases. An overview is provided of the concepts of utilities and WTP and their importance in decision making. Specific examples of elicitation methods for capturing utility and WTP measures are provided. Prior studies exploring utilities and WTP in dermatology are reviewed. Each of these measures has limitations and likely varying relevance to specific dermatologic diseases and to specific individuals.

Skindex-29 and Skindex-16 are validated measures of the effects of skin diseases on patients' quality of life. This article reviews the development of both versions of Skindex, discusses their measurement properties and interpretability, and gives examples of how they have been used and adapted for dermatologic research internationally. Studies of quality of life in patients with nonmelanoma skin cancer are described to illustrate the use of Skindex to understand quality of life and to compare effectiveness of different treatments for this highly prevalent condition.

The Dermatology Life Quality Index (DLQI) is an easy and practical way of quantifying the impact of skin disease. The role of DLQI in treatment guidelines and its emergence as an eligibility and response criterion in health technology appraisal are discussed. This review analyzes the current available literature on the clinical use of the DLQI, with particular reference to its relationship with disease severity and as a criterion in the assessment of health technology. The need for future studies of chronic hand eczema to incorporate DLQI to document quality-of-life outcomes with new treatments is also discussed.

The increasing public health burden of melanoma warrants evaluation of quality-of-life outcomes and the instruments most commonly used to measure quality of life in patients with melanoma. A review of the published literature focusing on quality-of-life outcomes in melanoma patients was performed to appraise the instruments used for assessment and the significant findings. In general, generic instruments continue to be most commonly used in the evaluation of quality of life despite the lack of responsiveness to changes in quality of life in subsets of patients. Cancer-specific and melanoma-specific instruments may be more suited for longitudinal clinical assessments.

Vitiligo, an acquired disease of depigmentation, affects millions worldwide. The psychosocial and health-related quality of life (HRQL) impact of the disease varies based on several parameters, including country of origin, skin type, gender, age, marital status, and involved body site. Many instruments, both dermatology specific and dermatology nonspecific, have been used to measure HRQL. Assessing HRQL in vitiligo is an important part of disease management.

The Melasma Quality of Life scale (MELASQOL) is a useful tool in assessing quality of life in patients with melasma. Initially developed in English, it has recently been translated into Spanish, Brazilian Portuguese, French, and Turkish. Development of a validated, translated, disease-specific quality of life questionnaire is a complex process which is further discussed in this article. When developing the MELASQOL in other languages, careful attention must be paid to cross-cultural adaptation and proper methods of translation and validation to have an accurate instrument. This article addresses these methods, which could be useful to those desiring to develop the MELASQOL in other languages.

The negative impact of psoriasis on a patient's quality of life (QoL) is well documented in the literature. Patients often suffer poor self-esteem, difficulties in social interactions, and significant psychological distress. It is, therefore, critically important that a clinician evaluate the extent to which the disease impacts a patient's QoL. This chapter reviews several validated and reliable generic, dermatology-specific, and disease-specific QoL instruments useful in measuring the impact of psoriasis on patient's QoL. These QoL instruments can be especially helpful in identifying those patients who would most benefit from systemic or biologic therapy.

Acne vulgaris affects most adolescents and two-thirds of adults and is associated with substantial psychosocial burden. Health-related quality of life (HRQOL) for patients with acne is an important factor of patient care, and several dermatologic and acne-specific measures have been created to assist in acne research, management, and care. This review describes several skin disease and acne-specific HRQOL measures and their applications in clinical care or research. The ideal HRQOL measure for the management of patients with acne is a concise questionnaire that places minimal burden on respondents and allows physicians to track improvement in HRQOL with successful treatment.

Both congenital and acquired bullous dermatoses have the potential to impose a significant burden of disease, and the impact exerted on the quality of life (QOL) of patients is often multifaceted. The qualitative and quantitative studies reviewing QOL in patients with bullous dermatoses have all reported a significant decrease in QOL scores compared with the greater population using a range of patient-based measures. Formal evaluation of QOL in the setting of bullous dermatoses facilitates the assessment of disease severity and mapping of disease trajectory and can capture outcomes of therapeutic intervention relevant to the patient.

Health-related quality of life (QoL) is a patient-reported outcome that describes the impact of the disease in question to all aspects of persons' life, including psychosocial, emotional, physical, and functional impact. As such, health-related QoL is particularly relevant in conditions that have no physical signs and need to rely on patient reports to know whether they are improving or not. Work is beginning in pruritus to develop instruments that can measure pruritus-related QoL. This article reviews the instruments that have been developed and used in pruritus and also reviews the literature regarding the impact of pruritus on QoL.

Health-related quality of life (HRQoL) is gradually becoming a standard outcome in clinical research and health care management. Nevertheless, application in dermatologic practice is not customary and many practical and attitudinal barriers need to be overcome. To contribute to the discussion on and the implementation of HRQoL assessment in routine dermatologic practice, this article describes (1) why HRQoL assessment is relevant for dermatologic practice, (2) which patients would benefit most from routine HRQoL assessment, and (3) how HRQoL assessment can be applied in clinical practice.

Clinical meaning can be assigned to scores of health status measures by using a variety of approaches. The anchor-based approach involves determining the difference on a quality of life (QOL) scale that corresponds to a self-reported small but important change on a global scale given concomitantly, which serves as an independent anchor. This article focuses on the anchor-based banding approach and reviews methods to assign clinical meaning to QOL measures, specifically the Dermatology Life Quality Index (DLQI) and Skindex. This article also includes pilot data that compares the DLQI and Skindex using these previously validated banding systems.

Within the last few decades, outcomes research, and in particular quality of life (QoL) outcomes research, has become integrated into clinical and research practices. QoL outcomes are important to dermatology, because many diseases carry significant psychosocial burdens and morbidity from appearance and symptoms with few cases of mortality. In this article, the authors discuss the future directions in QoL. Important areas are the determination, clinical significance and interpretation of measured QoL values. Additionally, the development of proxies for preference-based QoL measures and modules for health status QoL measures are discussed.

Dermatologic Clinics

THE CLINICS ARE NOW AVAILABLE ONLINE!

Access your subscription at:
www.theclinics.com

Preface

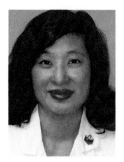

Suephy C. Chen, MD, MS
Guest Editor

Health-related quality of life (HRQoL) is increasingly being recognized as an important parameter to consider in research as well as in patient care. In fact, the Healthy People 2020 initiative, developed by lead federal agencies, such as the Centers for Disease Control and Prevention, Agency for Healthcare Research and Quality, National Institutes of Health, and Food and Drug Administration, to name a few, has named "health-related quality of life and well-being" as a new topic area for this decade as a high-priority national health objective.

HRQoL is particularly important in dermatology because a major goal of dermatology is to improve quality of life as it relates to the skin. In this issue of *Dermatology Clinics*, an attempt is made to organize a compendium of articles from experts in the field that address the HRQoL impact of different dermatologic conditions ranging from the relatively common (acne) to the more rare (blistering disorders) and also ranging from the chronic diseases (psoriasis) to the cancers (nonmelanoma and melanoma). Issues and applications for the practicing clinician as well as for researchers are carefully delineated.

I am grateful to all the authors for their countless hours and effort to this edition. I also want to thank Bruce Theirs for the opportunity to guest edit this issue and Stephanie Donley for her professional editorial assistance. Last, I want to recognize my family for their support of this scholarly endeavor.

Suephy C. Chen, MD, MS
Division of Dermatology
Atlanta Veterans Affairs Medical Center
Decatur, GA 30322, USA

Department of Dermatology
Emory University
101 Woodruff Circle
Atlanta, GA 30322, USA

E-mail address:
Schen2@emory.edu

Dermatol Clin 30 (2012) xiii
doi:10.1016/j.det.2011.11.014
0733-8635/12/$ – see front matter

derm.theclinics.com

Health-Related Quality of Life in Dermatology: Introduction and Overview

Suephy C. Chen, MD, MS[a,b,*]

KEYWORDS

- Health-related quality of life • Health status instruments
- Dermatology • Guidelines

The World Health Organization defines quality of life (QoL) as "the individuals' perception of their position in life, in the context of the cultural and value system in which they live and in relation to their goals, expectations, standards and concerns."[1] QoL is a multidimensional construct used to evaluate the general well-being of an individual and encompasses physical, functional, emotional, social, and family well-being.[2] Although QoL can be influenced by nonmedical factors, such as environmental, financial status, political, and other phenomenon, health-related QoL (HRQoL) is a more limited concept that captures the effects of a health condition on a persons' quality of life, as perceived by that person.

HRQoL is particularly important in dermatology because a major goal of dermatology is to improve QoL as it relates to the skin. Although there are a few dermatologic conditions that can affect survival, such as melanoma, cutaneous T-cell lymphomas, and Merkel cell carcinomas, most dermatologic conditions do not shorten life expectancy. Rather, most dermatologic conditions affect patients' lives in a physical, emotional, or functional manner. Identifying how a skin condition affects lives, quantifying this burden, and using this information to improve patients' lives on an individual basis are important targets in clinical dermatology.

Using this information in clinical trials and on a health policy level is the goal of QoL research. As such, HRQoL can be viewed as another "vital sign" that should be consistently measured in dermatology.[3]

RECOMMENDATIONS FROM THE INTERNATIONAL DERMATOEPIDEMIOLOGY ASSOCIATION MEETING

This introduction would not be complete without citing findings and recommendations from the last International DermatoEpidemiology Association (IDEA) meeting held jointly with the Americas DermatoEpidemiology Network (ADEN) in Nottingham, Great Britain, in 2008. This meeting, which occurs every 3 to 4 years, invites dermatologists interested in epidemiology, outcomes research, and health services research to convene to share research ideas and interests. This particular meeting was also charged with making broad recommendations to improve research and reporting in three aspects of the burden of skin disease: (1) epidemiology, (2) QoL, and (3) economics. This article focuses on the QoL discussion.

Health Status Versus HRQoL

The first major concern of the IDEA group was a lack of consensus and thus transparency in

Financial disclosures and Conflicts of Interest: None.

[a] Division of Dermatology, Atlanta Veterans Affairs Medical Center, Decatur, GA 30322, USA
[b] Department of Dermatology, Emory University, 101 Woodruff Circle, Atlanta, GA 30322, USA
* Department of Dermatology, Emory University, 101 Woodruff Circle, Atlanta, GA 30322.
E-mail address: schen2@emory.edu

Dermatol Clin 30 (2012) 205–208
doi:10.1016/j.det.2011.12.001
0733-8635/12/$ – see front matter © 2012 Published by Elsevier Inc.

research of the construct being measured: HRQoL versus health status. Although many investigators use health status and HRQoL interchangeably, others distinguish measures of health status from true QoL instruments. HRQoL refers to domains of health that are important to patients' QoL and takes into account the patient's own expectations or internal standards. Health status questionnaires are standardized for "typical patients" and as such, scores provide measures of the effects of disease or treatment, but do not measure the impact of the disease itself or the probability of benefit of treatment to the patient.[4,5] The term "HRQoL" is also considered problematic by some in that although health impacts QoL, health cannot be equated with QoL. There are those in bad health and good QoL, and vice versa. Additionally, researchers claim that HRQoL implies that QoL can be separated into health and non-health, although there is little evidence that patients can make this distinction when reflecting on their own QoL.[6]

Supporting this concern is a review of 75 articles that reported to evaluate HRQoL by Gill and Feinstein.[7] The authors found that only 15% of these papers provided conceptual definitions of HRQoL or health status. HRQoL was often used as a generic label for an assortment of physical functioning and psychosocial variables. Smith and colleagues[6] performed a structural equation analysis of several published papers. Their goal was to determine whether health status (defined by them as "perceived health") differs from HRQoL. They found that perceived health most strongly related to physical functioning, energy and fatigue, and pain, whereas HRQoL related more to mental health. They concluded that only two domains, mental health and physical functioning, are key determinants of HRQoL judgment. Other domains, such as social support or cognitive functioning, are relevant to HRQoL only to the extent that they affect mental or physical functioning. Implications for HRQoL research from their research are that questionnaires designed to measure health status may be inappropriate for assessing HRQoL. Those measures that do not tap psychologic functioning may be inadequate for monitoring HRQoL.

Streamlining of HRQoL and Health Status Instruments

Another concern from the IDEA group is the multitude of instruments available for particular diseases. The group agreed that some method should be used to evaluate these instruments carefully and that only a few should be used in trials such that the results can be compared and contrasted across studies. One idea was to use an organization, such as the Outcome Measures in Rheumatoid Arthritis Clinical Trials (OMERACT). The OMERACT initiative has turned into an international informal network, with a five-member Organizing Committee consisting of members from three continents, and a 15-member Scientific Advisory Committee composed of international opinion leaders from nine countries, all interested in outcome measurement across the spectrum of rheumatology intervention studies. The acronym has been broadened to now stand for "Outcome Measures in Rheumatology."[8] Others pointed to a recent compilation and evaluation of health status and HRQoL measures, commissioned by the National Institutes of Arthritis, Musculoskeletal and Skin.[9] However, despite the thorough evaluation, there was no recommendation made as to the few measures to use. Moreover, the effort was only one-time and no group, such as the OMERACT, exists to continually evaluate new instruments. The group concluded by recommending a World Wide Web–based initiative, such as OMERACT, to oversee the effort of critiquing and recommending health status and HRQoL measures to be adopted in research.

Minimum Criteria for Dermatologic HRQoL and Health Status Instruments

The next major point of discussion was to articulate a shortlist of minimum criteria to develop and report HRQoL and health status instruments in dermatology. The consensus of ideas includes three major points, listed next. Ideally, a guidance statement, such as the CONSORT for randomized controlled trials or the STROBE for observational studies in epidemiology, would be ideal. However, these statements involve development with editors of major medical journals, none of whom were present at the IDEA meeting.

1. Declaration of domains or constructs that the instrument is to measure so that the distinction of health status versus HRQoL measures can be discerned. At the minimum, a statement of whether health status is being measured or whether a mental functioning component is also included, thus measuring HRQoL.
2. Psychometric testing of instruments to demonstrate reliability, reproducibility, validity, and responsiveness.
3. Guidance on clinically relevant difference in scores. The scores on HRQoL or health status instruments would be more useful if there were clinical meaning to either the scores themselves or to a minimum difference in the scores.

Audience for HRQoL Information

The last point that the IDEA group discussed was the target audience for the information gathered from health status and HRQoL measures. Possible users of this information include researchers, pharmaceutical companies, insurance companies, politicians, and patients. Several of the European participants shared their experiences in that their healthcare system has mandated measuring QoL, and encouraged the group to use the existing health status and HRQoL instruments in dermatology and translate such patient-reported outcome measures into quality of care. From a patient care standpoint, several participants point out that dermatologists are not good at detecting depression. HRQoL instruments can help detect signs of depression and start communication between the physician and patient. Because the items that relate to psychosocial issues are imbedded in the instrument, administration of the questionnaire to the patient facilitates initiation of discussion of such awkward issues during the clinic visit.

OVERVIEW OF COMPENDIUM

This compendium of articles addresses the issues that were raised by the IDEA meeting. These articles hinge on the conceptual framework that dermatology HRQoL can be viewed as two distinct but somewhat overlapping constructs: health status QoL measures and preference-based QoL measures. The papers were not scrutinized for differences between health status and QoL. However, a conceptual framework (**Fig. 1**) is proposed to distinguish between those HRQoL measures that explicitly describe the domains of how a skin condition affects one's HRQoL (termed here as "health status QoL") versus measures that incorporate patients' preference for a given state of a skin condition (termed here as "preference-based QoL").

Within the proposed conceptual framework, the compendium of papers starts with several articles that overview health status QoL measures, including the two most commonly used, the Dermatology Life Quality Index (DLQI) and the Skindex, and preference-based HRQoL measures in dermatology. The compendium also seeks to provide an overview of skin disease–specific issues for a variety of dermatologic conditions ranging from the relatively common (acne) to the more rare (blistering disorders) and also ranging from chronic diseases (psoriasis) to cancers (nonmelanoma and melanoma). Unfortunately, HRQoL measures for children and families are currently limited, and thus are not reviewed in this compendium. Future work needs to focus on these populations. Nevertheless, the articles in this compendium address unique issues as they relate to HRQoL, information that will help clinicians and guide future researchers.

For the Practicing Clinician

Several articles review the impact of a particular skin disease relative to other skin diseases and nondermatologic diseases. This is made possible by using either skin-specific HRQoL measures (to compare against other skin conditions) or general health instruments (to compare across all diseases). Clinicians can benefit by appreciating the impact of these skin disorders on their patients because a multitude of studies have demonstrated that clinicians are poor proxies in estimating the HRQoL impact of skin conditions on their patients. The vitiligo article by Kundu and Bhandarkar points out how the impact of vitiligo can differ in different cultures. This information may be helpful to those who treat vitiligo. Also useful to practitioners are the papers by Heller and Koo and Basra and colleagues outlining how health status QoL instruments have been used during the consideration of recommending high-cost treatments. The paper by Rogers and colleagues reviews how to interpret scores from the DLQI and Skindex, providing clinical meaning, such as "little impact versus great impact" for a band of scores. Knowing the clinical meaning helps clinicians when they review journal articles that use these instruments. For instance, they will be able to appreciate that a difference in two reported scores may be statistically significant, but did not change the impact in a clinically meaningful way because the preintervention and postintervention scores are in the same band of scores (eg, "great impact" to "great impact"). Finally, the article by deKorte

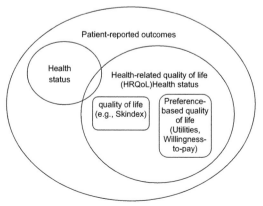

Fig. 1. Conceptual framework for patient-reported outcomes.

and colleagues builds on the suggestion that HRQoL be considered a vital sign in dermatology. They describe how HRQoL assessment can be applied in clinical practice. Similarly, Barnes and Feldman review a suggestion as to how acne-specific HRQoL measures can be incorporated into the clinical setting.

For Researchers

For investigators pursuing research in preference-based HRQoL, Seidler and coworkers' paper gives a comprehensive overview of the pitfalls of using proxies to estimate utilities. Basra and coworkers' paper gives an example of how the DLQI, a health status instrument, has been mapped into an estimate of utilities, but cautions that the approach has yet to be validated. For researchers interested in health status QoL measures, the melasma paper by Lieu and Pandya highlights the issues of translating their MELASQoL questionnaire into other languages, such as the need to address awkward phrasing and syntax and to address more fundamental issues, such as lack of an equivalent idea or phenomenon in the second language. This paper gives a dermatologic example of how guidelines to translate HRQoL questionnaires can be applied to dermatology.[10–12] Cormier's melanoma paper gives an example of how future health status QoL measures may be developed, by adding a disease-specific module onto an existing validated instrument. Other approaches to the development of future health status QoL measures are discussed in DeLong and Chen's "Future Directions" paper. This last paper also encourages researchers to investigate the minimally important difference in existing health status QoL measures, the smallest change in QoL scores that the patients perceive is important.

SUMMARY

This compendium of articles represents the latest update of HRQoL and health status work in dermatology and provides information of interest and use for clinicians and researchers.

ACKNOWLEDGMENTS

Participants of the 2008 International Dermato-Epidemiology Association Meeting include Hywel Williams, Luigi Naldi, Alan Tenant, Martin Weinstock, Mary-Margaret Chren, Christian Apfelbacher, Phyllis Spuls, Bob Dellavalle, Rob Stern, Julia Schofield, Andrew Finlay, Laura von Kobyletzki, Frances Sampogna, and Jen Jacques Grob.

REFERENCES

1. WHOQoL measuring quality of life from division of mental health and prevention of substance abuse. Geneva (Switzerland): World Health Organization; 1997.
2. Schipper H, Clinch J, Olweny C. Quality of life studies: definitions and conceptual issues. In: Spilker B, editor. Quality of life and pharmacoeconomics in clinical trials. 2nd edition. Philadelphia: Lippincott-Raven; 1996. p. 11–23.
3. Chren M. Measurement of vital signs for skin diseases. J Invest Dermatol 2005;125(4):viii–viix.
4. Doward L, McKenna S. Defining patient-reported outcomes. Value Health 2004;7:S4–8.
5. Jones P. Health status: what does it mean for payers and patients? Proc Am Thorac Soc 2006;3:222–6.
6. Smith K, Avis N, Assmann S. Distinguishing between quality of life and health status in quality of life research: a meta-analysis. Qual Life Res 1999;8(5):447–59.
7. Gill T, Feinstein A. A critical appraisal of the quality of quality-of-life measurements. JAMA 1994;272:619–26.
8. Tugwell P, Boers M, Brooks P, et al. OMERACT: an international initiative to improve outcome measurement in rheumatology. Trials 2007;8:38.
9. NIAMS. Workshop on the burden of skin diseases summary. 2002. Available at: http://www.niams.nih.gov/News_and_Events/Meetings_and_Events/Reports/2002/burden_skin_disease.asp. Accessed November 4, 2011.
10. Guillemin F, Bombardier C, Beaton D. Cross-cultural adaptation of health-related quality of life measures: literature review and proposed guidelines. J Clin Epidemiol 1993;46(12):1417–32.
11. Cestari T, Hexsel D, Viegas M, et al. Validation of a melasma quality of life questionnaire for Brazilian Portuguese language: the MelasQoL-BP study and improvement of QoL of melasma patients after triple combination therapy. Br J Dermatol 2006; 156(Suppl 1):13–20.
12. WHO. Process of translation and adaptation of instruments. Geneva (Switzerland): Available at: http://www.who.int/substance_abuse/research_tools/translation/en/. Accessed 2010.

Overview of Health Status Quality-of-Life Measures

Seema P. Kini, MD, MS[a], Laura K. DeLong, MD, MPH[a,b,*]

KEYWORDS

• Health status • Quality of life • Dermatology

The concept of quality of life (QOL) is becoming increasingly important in medicine, particularly in dermatology where many cutaneous diseases have the potential to affect the quality rather than the length of life. As such, there has been increasing interest in devising methodology to accurately measure the impact of disease on QOL for use in clinical practice, research studies, and economic analyses. The aim of this article is to familiarize readers with health status QOL instruments and to review their use in dermatology.

There are several instruments used to capture the impact of disease on QOL, which can be categorized into 2 principal categories: preference-based measures and health status QOL assessments. Preference-based measures are derived from decision-making theory and determine patient preferences for a specific health state by inviting patients to hypothetically give up something of value, such as money, years of life, and so forth. A detailed discussion of preference-based measures can be found in the article by Seidler and colleagues elsewhere in this issue. In contrast, health status QOL measures capture the impact of disease on various dimensions of QOL, such as the cognitive, social, and emotional aspects, as well as physical discomfort and limitations. Of note, the authors acknowledge that some investigators distinguish between "health status" and "health-related quality of life" as discussed in the introduction to this issue. Here, the authors use the term "health status QoL" to distinguish from preference-based measures.

For the purposes of this discussion, the authors are loosely combining both instruments that focus more on disability (health status) with those that integrate the psychosocial aspects (health-related QoL). The dimensions that compose health status are well established and make up the conceptual framework on which many health status QOL measures are based. Health status QOL measures quantitatively represent the impact of disease on health status through a single summary score or a profile of interrelated subscale scores. A college-aged female patient with psoriasis might consider her skin condition more burdensome than an 85-year-old man with the same skin condition who is less concerned with his appearance. Health status QOL instruments allow distinguishing between individuals who may bear the same skin pathology but experience different burden of disease. Health status measures can generally be classified into 3 main categories: generic, dermatology-specific, and condition-specific instruments, which are discussed in detail.

In 2002, the United States Congress requested further investigation by the National Institute of Arthritis and Musculoskeletal and Skin Disease (NIAMS) into the burden of skin disease. In response, the NIAMS sponsored the Workshop on the Burden of Skin Disease in 2002 to discuss elements that compose the burden of skin diseases and their impact on public health and daily living. One of the project recommendations from this working group was a need for additional adult

The authors have nothing to disclose.

[a] Department of Dermatology, Emory University School of Medicine, Emory Clinic, Building A, 1365 Clifton Road Northeast, Suite 1100, Atlanta, GA 30322, USA
[b] Division of Dermatology, Atlanta Veterans Affairs Medical Center, Decatur, GA 30322, USA
* Corresponding author. Department of Dermatology, Emory University School of Medicine, Emory Clinic, Building A, 1365 Clifton Road Northeast Suite 1100, Atlanta, GA 30322.
E-mail address: lkdelon@emory.edu

Dermatol Clin 30 (2012) 209–221
doi:10.1016/j.det.2011.11.007
0733-8635/12/$ – see front matter Published by Elsevier Inc.

skin–specific QOL instruments for the more prevalent skin diseases that capture not only the symptomatic but also the functional, psychological,
social, and emotional impact of skin disease. Additionally, the development of skin-specific QOL
measures for children and family impact was recommended to characterize QOL impact more
comprehensively.[1]

In 2007, a NIAMS-funded working group[1] published a summary of their work in response to the
Workshop's recommendation. They systematically
and comprehensively searched for all available
health status QOL instruments that had been either
applied to or developed for skin diseases. They
found a total of 40 health status QOL instruments:
6 generic, 11 adult skin specific, and 15 adult
condition specific. This article does not seek to
be comprehensive like the 2007 effort. Rather,
it highlights the most commonly used generic,
skin-specific, and condition-specific health status
measures for dermatology and summarizes the
appropriate usage of these instruments.

CONSIDERATIONS IN SELECTING A HEALTH STATUS QOL INSTRUMENT

Although there is no simple formula for selecting
a health status QOL measure, there are several
considerations in deciding which health status
QOL instrument is most appropriate for use. The
setting, time course, and psychometric properties
of the instrument are all factors in guiding questionnaire selection.

Although the use of QOL measures in routine
clinical practice has been sparse, in recent years
there has been increased interest in the use of
QOL assessments in clinical settings to prioritize
problems, evaluate physical or psychosocial problems that might otherwise be overlooked, monitor
the therapeutic process and assess treatment
outcomes, and improve clinical care.[2] In the clinical setting, measures that are concise, have
a straightforward scoring system, and are dermatology specific or condition specific may be most
useful to clinicians.

The use of health status QOL instruments in clinical research is dependent on the specific aim of
the study itself. If the purpose is to evaluate treatment outcomes of a therapy, condition-specific
measures may be most sensitive in capturing the
small changes in therapeutic response. If the
purpose is to compare different skin diseases,
the use of a dermatology-specific instrument alone
or in conjunction with a condition-specific instrument may be more appropriate. In health-
economic analyses, the use of generic health
status QOL measurements, alone or in conjunction

with a dermatology or condition-specific measure,
is necessary to compare burden of dermatologic
disease with non-dermatologic pathology.

Although time constraints may not be as much of
a concern in clinical research or economic analyses, care should be taken to consider the total
time required to answer a questionnaire, particularly when multiple instruments are administered.
The accuracy of completion of questionnaires likely
wanes as more questionnaires are administered.

The time course over which health status is
assessed is also an important consideration.
Some health status QOL instruments assess only
the day of completion itself. Although this allows
for an accurate assessment of a patient's symptoms in real time, the disadvantage of only assessing symptoms "today" or "currently" is that this
only provides a brief snapshot of burden of
disease. This may be appropriate for chronic
diseases where the symptoms occur daily with
little fluctuation but may be less relevant for
diseases that are relapsing and remitting in nature.
Questionnaires that provide a longer time course,
such as 1 week or 4 weeks, may be more reasonable alternatives. If an instrument is re-
administered for meaningful comparison, the
frequency of administration should not be less
than the time course used.

In addition, the psychometric properties of the
measurement tools themselves must be considered. The primary properties used to evaluate
health status instruments are reliability, validity,
and responsiveness.

Reliability

Reliability is the degree to which an instrument is
free from random error. That is, the more reliable
an instrument, the more it produces the same
results when used repeatedly under the same
conditions. Two types of reliability are considered
important with regard to health status QOL
measures: test-retest reliability and internal consistency reliability. Test-retest reliability is the
degree to which an instrument yields stable scores
over time among respondents who are assumed
not to have changed with regard to the domains
assessed. The correlation is usually expressed
by an intraclass correlation coefficient (ICC). An
ICC greater than 0.70 is desirable for group
comparisons and 0.90 to 0.95 is desirable for
individual measurements over time.

Internal consistency reliably reflects the extent
to which all items of a questionnaire address the
same theoretic construct. A questionnaire is
considered internally consistent when there is
a high intercorrelation among the item scores.

The intercorrelation is usually expressed by the Cronbach α coefficient. Commonly acceptable standards for reliability coefficients, similar to ICC, are 0.70 for group comparisons and 0.90 to 0.95 for individual comparisons.[3]

Validity

Validity is the degree to which a questionnaire measures what it intends to measure. Validity is particularly important with respect to the language, cultural, and clinical settings in which an instrument was developed—an instrument validated in one language or in a specific population may not be valid in other groups. Revalidation may be necessary in a new environment. Although there are many types of validity, those most commonly used for testing the psychometrics of dermatology health status QOL measures are content validity and construct validity.

Content validity is defined as the extent to which the content of an instrument is appropriate for its intended use. The items should adequately represent the entire construct measured and questions should be clear and free of redundant items. For example, when generic measures are used in dermatology, they generally have lower content validity in comparison with dermatology-specific measures since they contain items not applicable to dermatology patients.

Construct validity is the degree to which a questionnaire agrees with a priori theorized constructs. The RosaQoL, a rosacea-specific QOL instrument, was theorized to measure three constructs: symptom, emotional, and functional impairment of rosacea. Using principal components analysis, the three main factors correlated to the three main theorized constructs with statistical significance—indicating that the RosaQoL actually measures the three domains as was intended.

Responsiveness

Responsiveness to change is the extent to which a questionnaire can be used to detect changes over time. Responsiveness is supported when a measure can detect differences in outcomes even if those differences are small. Common methods of assessing responsiveness include comparing scale scores before and after an intervention expected to affect the construct and comparing changes in scale scores with changes in other related measures assumed to move in the same direction as the target measure.[3] Condition and dermatology-specific measures are more sensitive to small changes in disease status and are generally regarded as more responsive than generic measures.

Selecting the appropriate instrument often involves trade-offs between short, simple measures and lengthier more comprehensive measures in terms of reliability, validity, and responsiveness.

GENERIC HEALTH STATUS QOL MEASURES

Generic measures (**Table 1**) are designed to comprehensively capture the many aspects of health as it relates to QOL in different diseases, patients, and populations of health status. As such, generic instruments have the advantage that they can be applied across varying types and severity of disease, medical treatments or therapeutic interventions, and demographic and cultural subgroups.

Although generic measures may have robust psychometric properties, they may suffer from low content validity because they contain items of little or no relevance to dermatology patients.[4] As such, they may not detect small changes in QOL and thus are not helpful in following dermatologic impact across time in the clinical or research setting. Because of these issues, generic health instruments should be used in a limited capacity. One scenario where they may be helpful is if a clinician or researcher wants to compare a dermatologic condition with a nondermatologic condition in terms of QOL impact. The other scenario is to use a generic QOL instrument in conjunction with dermatology-specific or condition-specific instruments when the skin condition in question has substantial health-related QOL impact beyond the disease specific impact.[5] For example, Sampogna and colleagues[6] compared results from the Medical Outcomes Study 36-Item Short Form Health Survey (SF-36) with dermatology-specific instruments (discussed later), the Skindex-29 and Dermatology Life Quality Index (DLQI), in psoriasis patients and concluded that generic QOL instruments (eg, the SF-36) served as a useful adjunct to dermatology-specific questionnaires and allowed for a more comprehensive assessment of burden in psoriasis patients than would otherwise have been gained from using dermatology-specific instruments alone. This article reviews 4 of the more common generic QOL instruments that have been applied to dermatology. The decision to select of these 4 instruments should be based on the construct and domains that the instrument covers and if the instrument has been applied to the dermatologic disease in question. The latter criteria allow clinician/researchers to compare their data with those of a previous population with the same skin condition.

Table 1
Generic health instruments and their properties

Generic Health Instrument	Number of Questions	Time (min) for Administration	Health Domains	Advantages/ Disadvantages
MOS 36-Item Short Form Health Survey (SF-36)	36	5 to 10	Physical functioning Role limitations due to physical problem Bodily pain General health Vitality Social functioning Role limitations due to emotions Mental health Health transition	Considered the most studied and well-validated instrument available and the reference instrument by most researchers. Applicable across a broad range of clinical conditions. Structure and restest reliability are controversial.
Sickness Impact Profile (SIP)	136	20 to 30	Physical Dimension Ambulation Mobility Body care and movement Psychosocial Dimension Communication Alertness behavior Emotional behavior Social interaction Independent Categories Sleep and rest Eating Work Home management Recreation and pastimes	Long time for completion, focused on disability
Nottingham Health Profile (NHP)	38	10 to 15	Energy level Emotional reactions Physical mobility Pain Social isolation Sleep	Easy to administer
WHOQOL-100	100	20 to 30	Physical Psychological Level of independence Social relationships Environment Spirituality	Truly cross-culturally equivalent

The Sickness Impact Profile (SIP) is a 136-item measure developed in the United States to provide a broad measure of disease impact on physical and emotional functioning. The SIP assesses disability due to disease across 12 domains: physical (ambulation, mobility, and body care/movement) and psychosocial dimensions (social interaction, communication, alertness behavior, emotional behavior, sleep, eating, home management, recreation, and work).[7] The SIP percentage score can be calculated for the total instrument (an index score) or for each domain, where 0 indicates better health and 100 worse health status. Two summary scores, a physical function and psychosocial function, may also be calculated. The instrument may be self-administered or interview-administered. An abbreviated version of the SIP with 68 items, the SIP68, has been developed.[8] The SIP has been used in psoriasis,[9,10] atopic dermatitis,[11] acne,[12] and basal cell carcinoma.[13]

The Nottingham Health Profile (NHP) was developed in the United Kingdom in the 1970s. Part I of the NHP contains 38 items that cover 6 domains of experience (physical ability, energy level, emotional reaction, sleep, social isolation, and pain) with individual scores for each domain. Part II of the NHP contains statements about areas of daily life most often affected by health. Results are analyzed by summing the number of positive responses in a dimension or weighting items to calculate a dimension score (range 0–100).[14] The instrument may be administered by self, interviewer, or via telephone. The NHP has been used in patients with psoriasis,[15] palmar hyperhydrosis,[16] chronic urticaria,[17,18] chronic leg ulcers,[19] and herpes zoster.[20]

The SF-36 is designed for use in clinical practice and research, health policy evaluations, and general population surveys. The questionnaire contains 36 items measuring 8 dimensions: physical functioning, emotional role functioning, physical role functioning, social role functioning, mental health, vitality, bodily pain, and general health perception. The 8 dimensions of the SF-36 can be combined into 2 summary scores, the physical component score and the mental component score. Scoring is on a 100-point scale with a change of 5 points considered clinically significant.[21] The SF-36 has been used in psoriasis,[22–25] acne,[26,27] and atopic dermatitis,[22,28,29] chronic urticaria[30,31] and has been demonstrated to enhance the information derived from dermatology-specific questionnaires. Abbreviated versions of the SF-36, including the 20-Item Short Form Health Survey (SF-20) and 12-Item Short Form Health Survey (SF-12), were developed from the SF-36 for use in large surveys and longitudinal studies. Seven items of the SF-12 correspond to the physical component score whereas 5 comprise the mental component score.[32] The SF-12 has been used in dermatology, albeit less than the SF-36, in studies of hyperhidrosis,[33,34] atopic dermatitis,[35,36] onychomycosis,[37] alopecia,[38–40] nonmelanoma skin cancer[41,42] oral mucosal conditions,[43] and melisma.[44]

The WHOQOL-100 is a 100-item questionnaire developed in 1994 by the World Health Organization that evaluates QOL in 6 domains: physical, psychological, level of independence, social relationships, environment, and spirituality.[45,46] The WHOQOL-100 was developed with the aim of being able to identify aspects of QOL that are cross-culturally important[47] and has been used in studies around the world. Compared with the SF-36, the WHOQOL-100 has demonstrated good concurrent validity, greater comprehensiveness, and very good responsiveness to clinical change in a cohort of chronic pain patients[48] and has proved a valuable instrument for measuring QOL in depressed patients.[49,50]

The WHOQOL-BREF is a more concise 26-item questionnaire with 2 items dedicated to assessing overall health and the remaining items adapted from the physical, psychological, social relations, and environment domains of the WHOQOL-100.[51] The WHOQOL-100 has been used in psoriasis[52,53] and the WHOQOL-BREF in atopic dermatitis,[54,55] acne,[56,57] chronic urticaria,[54,58] melasma,[59] and vitiligo.[60]

DERMATOLOGY-SPECIFIC INSTRUMENTS

Because of the limited ability of generic health status QOL instruments to capture important aspects of QOL, dermatology-specific QOL measures with higher content validity, such as the DLQI, Skindex, and Dermatology-Specific Quality of Life (DSQL), have been developed. Although these measures are more sensitive to QOL aspects of dermatologic disease, they only allow for comparison of health status among cutaneous diseases. This article reviews 4 dermatology-specific QOL measures and suggests optimal scenarios in which to use them.

The DLQI was the first dermatology-specific QOL instrument created[61] and to date is the most commonly used in clinical practice and in randomized controlled trials in dermatology.[62,63] The DLQI consists of 10 questions that assess how symptoms and feelings, daily activities, leisure, work, school, personal relationships, and treatment were affected by skin disease over the previous week. Questions are scored on a 0 to 3 Likert based scale and the sum of the scores provides a value between 0 (no involvement) and 30 (maximum impact on QOL of patient). The DLQI was initially developed in 120 patients with different skin conditions and consequently is applicable to most dermatology patients.[61] A systematic review by Basra and colleagues[62] found that by the end of 2007, a total of 272 full articles and 291 abstracts had been published using the DLQI. Additionally, the psychometric properties of the instrument, such as validity, reliability, responsiveness to change, factor structure, and minimal important difference, have been described in 115 studies. The DLQI has demonstrated excellent discriminant and construct validity as well as high reliability and internal consistency.[61,64] An additional advantage of the DLQI is that it is sensitive and responsive to clinical change and, therefore, able to capture the evolving effect of various therapies on QOL. The DLQI has been translated into more than 55 languages, and studies of the instrument in different countries (including developing countries) have found the instrument valid, reliable, and responsive to change.[65–67]

With such an impressive background, the DLQI can be recommended broadly for clinical and research scenarios to track changes in skin-specific QOL. One limitation to the DLQI, however, is the paucity of emotion-based questions compared with symptoms and functional impact and thus it can be argued to measure health status rather than true health-related QOL. If future users are seeking to focus on the emotional impact of skin disease, other instruments may be more enlightening.

The Skindex-29 was designed to measure the effects of skin disease on health-related QOL across different populations and to aid in assessing change in this parameter in individual patients. Originally, the Skindex consisted of 61 items, but a refinement study resulted in a 30-item instrument with improved discriminative and evaluative capacity.[68,69] Twenty-nine of the 30 items are reported as 3 subscale scores representing the frequency of 3 dimensions of QOL (functioning, emotions, and physical symptoms). A composite score is calculated from the average of the 3 subscale scores and transformed to a percentage, with higher scores indicating greater effect of skin disease on QOL. Reliability and validity of the Skindex-29 have been tested in patients with various diseases and found to be high. Internal consistency, reliability, and test-retest reliability are excellent (0.87–0.96). Responsiveness has also been demonstrated. More concise versions of the Skindex-29 exist: the Skindex-16 and Skindex-17. The Skindex-16 was revised to omit items in the Skindex-29 to which a majority of patients chose the same response and include measurement of bother rather than frequency of patient experiences.[70]

Similar to the DLQI, the Skindex has been extensively tested and can be used comfortably in clinical and research scenarios that need to measure changes in skin-specific QOL impact. Additionally, the Skindex has a broad emotional component and can be used if the need is to further characterize the emotional impact of the skin disease. While the Skindex-16 is more concise than the Skindex 29, the latter is preferred when used in conjunction with other frequency based measures, such as the SF-12.

The DSQL is a 52-item QOL instrument developed from the SF-36 in patients with contact dermatitis and acne vulgaris.[71] Studies to assess item behavior have been limited to these two conditions[72,73] and this tool has not been used or tested in other dermatologic conditions. This instrument may be helpful when used with the SF-36 or SF-12 because it should parallel the generic instrument. Further psychometric testing, however, is warranted.

CONDITION-SPECIFIC MEASURES

Compared with generic measures, condition-specific measures tend to have higher content validity and are more responsive because they are designed to assess specific groups or patient populations and are, therefore, more sensitive to small changes considered clinically important to the disease in question (**Table 2**). The main disadvantage of condition-specific measures is that data cannot be compared across diseases. In dermatology, condition-specific measures have been developed in a wide variety of cutaneous conditions. This article concentrate on measures developed for psoriasis, acne, atopic dermatitis, rosacea, onychomycosis, diabetic foot ulcers, urticaria, and nonmelanoma skin cancer.

Psoriasis

Psoriasis is a common, chronic, relapsing disease with cutaneous and systemic manifestations affecting approximately 4.5 million adults in the United States.[74] Although historically regarded as simply a cosmetic problem, psoriasis can have considerable impact on the physical, emotional, and psychosocial well-being of affected patients. Traditional endpoints to measure disease involvement as burden of disease (eg, percentage of body surface area involved), although useful, do not often correlate with burden of disease experienced by patients. A study of 601 psoriasis patients revealed that approximately 60% of patients reported their disease to be a large problem and approximately 80% of patients who were very dissatisfied with their treatment had less than 10% body surface area affected.[74] Similarly, a study of QOL in psoriasis by Fortune and colleagues[75] found that QOL impact did not correlate overall with clinical severity and duration of disease.

The Psoriasis Disability Index (PDI) is a 15-item self-administered questionnaire that assesses impact of psoriasis on 5 main domains: daily activities, work/school, personal relationships, leisure, and treatment during the previous 4 weeks. The PDI is scored on a visual analog scale ranging from 1 to 7, with a maximum score of 105, or

Table 2
Characteristics of selected condition-specific measures in dermatology

Abbreviation	Instrument	Source Reference	Number of Questions	Question Time Course (Days)
PDI	Psoriasis Disability Index	Finlay and Coles[77]	15	28
PLSI	Psoriasis Life Stress Inventory	Gupta and Gupta[80]	15	30
SPI	Salford Psoriasis Index	Kirby et al[82]	3 figures	Current
ADI	Acne Disability Index	Motley and Finlay[84]	10	Current
CADI	Cardiff Acne Disability Index	Motley and Finlay[85]	5	30
AQOL	Acne Quality of Life	Gupta et al[86]	9	Current
Acne-QOL	Acne-Specific Quality of Life	Girman et al[87]	24	7
QoLIAD	Quality of Life Index for Atopic Dermatitis	Whalley et al[89]	25	Current
RosaQoL	RosaQoL	Nicholson et al[90]	21	Current
Onychomycosis	Onychomycosis	Lubeck et al[91,92]	55	28
DFS	Diabetic Foot Ulcer Scale	Bann et al[94]	64	Current
CU-Q2oL	Chronic Urticaria Quality of Life Questionnaire	Baiardini et al[95]	23	Current
SCI	Facial Skin Cancer Index	Rhee et al[96]	15	Current

graded on a 4-point tick-box system, with greater scores representing greater burden of disease.[76,77] The PDI has been shown to have good concurrent validity with the SIP[9] (although no other validation studies have been performed on the instrument) and has met good criteria for responsiveness.[78] One of the main concerns with the PDI is a possible floor effect in that the instrument demonstrates greater sensitivity in patients with moderate to severe disability compared with mildly affected patients.[79] Nevertheless, the PDI is the most widely used psoriasis-specific health status QOL instrument in more than 31 published articles.

Given its extensive testing and popularity, the PDI is appropriate for moderate-to-severe psoriasis in the clinical and research setting where changes in psoriasis-specific QOL impact are important. The measurement time frame is 4 weeks, so any intervention that is intended to work in a smaller time frame may not be well-suited for the PDI. Also, the PDI is a disability index and, thus, similar to the DLQI, does not elaborate on the emotional aspects of psoriasis.

The Psoriasis Life Stress Inventory (PLSI) is a 15-item instrument based on a study of 50 psoriatic patients designed to measure psoriasis-related stress associated with cosmetic disfigurement, social stigma, symptoms of disease, and treatment effects. Each of the 15 items is rated on a scale ranging from 0 (not at all) to 3 (a great deal) for a maximum score of 45, with higher scores indicating greater burden of disease.[80] A factor analysis by Fortune and colleagues[75] found that items cluster into 2 factors: (1) stress resulting from anticipation of other people's possible reactions leading to avoidance of worrying situations (eg, not going to public places when you would have liked to) and (2) stress resulting from patients' beliefs or actual experiences of being evaluated by others solely on the basis of their skin condition (eg, people making a conscious effort not to touch you). Compared with the PDI, the PLSI provides a better measurement of health-related QOL in patients with mild to moderate psoriasis because of its greater emphasis on psychosocial stressors. Although the PDI has been validated against the SF-36, sensitivity of the PLSI to changes in health-related QOL has not been assessed.[81]

The Salford Psoriasis Index (SPI) assesses 3 aspects of psoriasis: the current clinical extent of disease based on the Psoriasis Area and Severity Index, a score indicating psychosocial disability, and past severity based on treatment history. Each of the 3 dimensions of the SPI is scored separately and expressed as a distinct independent value: the Psoriasis Area and Severity Index score is expressed on a 0 to 10 scale, psychosocial disability is also measured on a visual analog scale from 0 to 10, and historical severity is graded by assigning points to patients who had previous systemic treatment, who were hospitalized, and who experienced erythroderma as a result of their disease.[82] The SPI brings an interesting dimension to chronic disease evaluation. The personal history and experiences of individual patients are sure to influence their QOL. Clinicians/researchers who are interested in exploring this aspect of QOL should consider using the SPI. For those interested in measuring changes across time, however, the other psoriasis instruments might provide a more efficient assessment.

Acne

In acne vulgaris, as in psoriasis, there are several condition-specific instruments dedicated to assessing acne-specific QOL impact. A study by Lasek and Chren[83] found that patients with acne vulgaris reported emotional effects similar in magnitude to those reported by patients of psoriasis. Health status QOL instruments serve an important role in acne because the disease often first manifests during adolescence—a time of relative insecurity, self-consciousness, and psychosocial instability. Acne-specific instruments are important not just for youth—in the previously referenced study, older adults with acne vulgaris reported significantly greater effects on their QOL than did younger patients, even when controlling for clinical severity of acne as judged by the dermatologist.[83]

The Acne Disability Index (ADI) is a 10-item questionnaire assessing the impact of acne on QOL during the prior 4 weeks. In the pilot study, the ADI correlated with the severity of facial acne, chest acne, and back acne.[84]

The Cardiff Acne Disability Index (CADI) is a 5-item questionnaire derived from the ADI and designed for use in teenagers and young adults with acne. Each item is expressed on a Likert-type scale ranging from 0 to 3; the total score ranges from 0 to 15 and may be expressed as a percentage.[85] Because the CADI is so concise, it is particularly useful in busy clinical practices.

The Acne Quality of Life (AQOL) is a 9-item scale created by Gupta and colleagues[86] in 1998 to be sensitive to changes in patient-rated indices of acne severity and the psychological morbidity associated with acne. The scale has demonstrated to have a high degree of internal consistency particularly among mildly to moderately affected patients.

The Acne-Specific Quality of Life (Acne-QOL) is a 24-item questionnaire developed in 165 acne patients by Girman and colleagues[87] in 1996. Questions are scaled on a 7-point scale and take 10 minutes to complete. The instrument has been found reliable, valid, and able to distinguish differences across severity groups after 16 weeks of acne therapy.

Dréno[88] evaluated health status QOL instruments in acne and found that of the dermatology-specific scales, only the Skindex, DSQL, and DLQI have been adequately evaluated and validated in acne patients (the Skindex has been validated in Japanese patients). With regard to the acne-specific scales, the CADI has been found to correlate well with the response to treatment in published studies. Because the CADI and AQOL are concise, they are most appropriate for clinical practice, whereas the longer Acne-QoL is more suitable for clinical trials.

There have been efforts to develop other condition-specific instruments in less common diseases. A few that are not discussed in other articles in this issue include atopic dermatitis, rosacea onychomycosis, diabetic foot ulcers, urticaria, and nonmelanoma skin cancer.

Atopic Dermatitis

The Quality of Life Index for Atopic Dermatitis (QoLIAD) is a 25-item instrument with dichotomous responses developed in patients in the United States and Europe.[89] The instrument is available in UK English, US English, Dutch, French, German, and Spanish. All language versions with the exception of the Dutch measure have test-retest reliability coefficients in excess of 0.85. The test-retest reliability in the Netherlands was 0.80. The QoLIAD has adequate internal consistency and initial indications of construct validity are good.

Rosacea

The RosaQoL is a 21-item survey containing rosacea-specific items grouped into 3 subscales: symptom, emotion, and function. Questions are scaled from 1 (never) to 5 (all the time). The total score is averaged so the ranges for both the total score and the subscores are from 1 to 5, with a higher score translating to a worse QOL.[90] The instrument was developed in the United States and includes 10 items from the Skindex-29 and 11 rosacea-specific items. The RosaQoL has demonstrated high reliability (Cronbach α 0.82–0.97, ICC 0.70–0.95), and preliminary responsiveness in patients with improving rosacea.

Onychomycosis

Lubeck and colleagues created a 55-item onychomycosis-specific questionnaire. The subscales of the instrument showed high internal consistency reliability (range 0.63–0.95). Construct validity reflected the close association of physical functioning scores with onychomycosis impairment. Test-retest reliability was good to excellent for all scales (ICC 0.52–0.89). Responsiveness to clinical changes was noted for all disease-specific scale scores for improved patients.[91,92]

Diabetic Foot Ulcers

The Diabetic Foot Ulcer Scale (DFS) was developed to measure the impact of diabetic foot ulcers on QOL issues most important to patients. The scale contains a total of 64 items and demonstrates good scaling properties and has good reliability and validity. Moreover, the DFS shows good construct validity compared with the SF-36 and is able to discriminate between patients with healed ulcers and patients with current ulcers for the leisure, emotions, and financial domains.[93] More recently a shortened version of the DFS, the DFS-SF, was created and is composed of 6 subscales with considerable internal consistency, test-retest reliability, and marked construct validity. The shortened version of the questionnaire may detect changes in clinical condition more consistently than the DFS.[94]

Urticaria

The Chronic Urticaria Quality of Life Questionnaire (CU-Q2oL) is a 23-item questionnaire expressed on a Likert scale from 0 to 5 developed in 80 patients with chronic urticaria. The questionnaire requires approximately 5 minutes to complete and has showed good levels of internal consistency for pruritus (0.79), swelling (0.65), impact on life activities (0.83), sleep problems (0.77), looks (0.83), and limits (0.74). In stable conditions, the CU-Q2oL showed good reliability, ranging from 0.64 to 0.92, and excellent responsiveness to clinical changes.[95]

Nonmelanoma Skin Cancer

The Facial Skin Cancer Index (SCI) is a 15-item, validated, disease-specific QOL instrument created to capture the relevant QOL issues for nonmelanoma skin cancer patients with regard to 3 distinct domains: emotion, social, and appearance. Higher scores reflect improved QOL (less burden of disease). The 3 subscales have demonstrated excellent internal validity and convergent validity with other validated scales (eg, DLQI and SF-12). SCI is a highly sensitive and clinically responsive measure of QOL changes for nonmelanoma skin cancer patients.[96]

USES FOR HEALTH STATUS QOL MEASURES IN DERMATOLOGY

This article provides a review of general, dermatology-specific, and disease-specific health status QOL instruments and discusses important considerations in deciding which health status QOL instrument is most appropriate for use.

Health status QOL measures in dermatology are of value because they give both clinicians and researchers an objective way to see how skin disease has an impact on a patient's QOL. Recent studies, however, suggest that little QOL-related discussion takes place in the average dermatology outpatient consultation.[97] Moreover, although most dermatologists believe that they have good insight into how their patients are affected by their skin condition, their views are often not as accurate as they believe. Often when physician assessment of QOL impairment is low, patients estimate disease burden at a higher level, and where physician assessment is high, patients note lower QOL impact from their disease.[98,99] Nevertheless, there is evidence to suggest that in settings where health status QOL instruments are used, patient-physician communication is significantly increased, particularly in the discussion of health-related QOL issues that were less observable (ie, social functioning) or are more diffuse and chronic in nature (ie, fatigue)—often left unaddressed by health care providers.[2]

Furthermore, if a clinician knows which disease aspect has the most significant impact on a patient's health-related QOL (symptom vs emotional vs functional impact), then treatments can be tailored to match, providing optimum relief to the patient. For example, some systemic therapies have significant side effects and should only be used in patients who have severe disease or whose QOL is severely affected. Additionally, these measures can help clinicians and researchers know if treatments are working over time through repeated measures.

Although health status QOL measurements are increasingly used in clinical trials in dermatology, the use of patient reported outcomes as a primary and even secondary endpoint in dermatology research has been traditionally sparse.[63,100] Much of this stems from a perceived lack of credibility on the part of health status QOL instruments: even when these measures have been tested to be reliable, reproducible, and valid, they may still be viewed as a largely subjective assessment of health status. This perspective is compounded by doubts regarding the cultural cross-equivalence of many of these instruments. Multinational trials often require dermatology and disease-specific instruments that, although responsive, may not be validated in different cultural and linguistic settings. Lastly, even if health status QOL instruments are accepted as a valid measure of burden of disease, it is difficult to know how these scores translate clinically.[101] Despite these concerns, the use of health status QOL instruments in clinical research remains paramount because many aspects of health status, particularly in chronic skin diseases, are difficult for physicians to accurately assess. In addition, health status assessments may relay important information about compliance and efficacy of treatments that otherwise would not be observed from physician assessments alone.

Given growing health care costs and demand, the question of the cost-effectiveness of treatments and practices is of increasing importance. Health status QOL measures have a role in clinical outcomes, clinical trials, and health services research.

SUMMARY

This article provides a broad overview of general, dermatology-specific, and disease-specific health status QOL instruments; considerations for selecting an instrument; and their use in dermatology. Although the use of health status QOL measures is well established in dermatology, continued efforts are needed to devise measures that are standardized and cross-culturally equivalent. In addition, providing clinical relevance of scores and developing consistent frameworks for the application and reporting of patient reported outcomes will be important factors in determining how frequently health status QOL measures are used in clinical and research settings. Ultimately, standardization in the assessment and reporting of health status QOL will allow for a more rigorous understanding of the burden of cutaneous diseases.

REFERENCES

1. NIAMS. Workshop on the Burden of Skin Diseases Summary 2002. Available at: http://www.niams.nih.gov/News_and_Events/Meetings_and_Events/Reports/2002/burden_skin_disease.asp. Accessed October 23, 2011.
2. Detmar SB, Muller MJ, Schornagel JH, et al. Health-related quality-of-life assessments and patient-physician communication. JAMA 2002; 288(23):3027–34.
3. Scientific Advisory Committee of the Medical Outcomes Trust. Assessing health status and quality-of-life instruments: attributes and review criteria. Qual Life Res 2002;11(3):193–205.
4. Chen SC. Dermatology quality of life instruments: sorting out the quagmire. J Invest Dermatol 2007; 127:2695–6.
5. Both H, Essink-Bot ML, Busschbach J, et al. Critical review of generic and dermatology-specific health-related quality of life instruments. J Invest Dermatol 2007;127(12):2726–39.
6. Sampogna F, Tabolli S, Soderfelt B, et al. Measuring quality of life of patients with different clinical types of psoriasis using the SF-36. Br J Dermatol 2006;154(5):844–9.
7. Bergner M, Bobbitt RA, Pollard WE, et al. The sickness impact profile: validation of a health status measure. Med Care 1976;14(1):57–67.
8. de Bruin AF, Buys M, de Witte LP, et al. The sickness impact profile: SIP68, a short generic version. First evaluation of the reliability and reproducibility. J Clin Epidemiol 1994;47(8):863–71.
9. Finlay AY, Khan GK, Luscombe DK, et al. Validation of sickness impact profile and psoriasis disability index in psoriasis. Br J Dermatol 2006;123(6):751–6.
10. Salek MS, Finlay AY. Cyclosporin improves quality of life in psoriasis—does this matter? Br J Dermatol 1993;189:234–7.
11. Salek MS, Finlay AY. Cyclosporin greatly improves quality of life of adults with severe atopic dermatitis. Br J Dermatol 1993;129:422–30.
12. Salek MS, Khan GK, Finlay AY. Questionnaire techniques in assessing acne handicap: reliability and validity study. Qual Life Res 1996;5:131–8.
13. Blackford S, Roberts DL, Salek MS, et al. Basal cell carcinomas and their treatment cause little handicap—the reason for delayed presentation? Qual Life Res 1996;5:191–4.
14. McEwen J, McKenna SP. Nottingham health profile. Quality of life pharmacoeconomics in clinical trials. 2nd edition. Philadelphia: Lippincott Williams & Wilkins; 1996. p. 281–6.
15. Billing E, McKenna S, Staun M, et al. Adaptation of the Psoriatic Arthritis Quality of Life (PsAQoL) instrument for Sweden. Scand J Rheumatol 2010; 39(3):223–8.
16. Ambrogi V, Campione E, Mineo D, et al. Bilateral thoracoscopic T2 to T3 sympathectomy versus botulinum injection in palmar hyperhidrosis. Ann Thorac Surg 2009;88(1):238–45.
17. O'Donnell B, Lawlor F, Simpson J, et al. The impact of chronic urticaria on the quality of life. Br J Dermatol 1997;136(2):197–201.
18. Berrino AM, Voltolini S, Fiaschi D, et al. Chronic urticaria: importance of a medico-psychological approach. Eur Ann Allergy Clin Immunol 2006;38: 149–52.
19. Moffatt CJ, Franks PJ, Doherty DC, et al. Psychological factors in leg ulceration: a case–control study. Br J Dermatol 2009;161(4):750–6.
20. Mauskopf J, Austin R, Dix L, et al. The Nottingham Health Profile as a measure of quality of life in zoster patients: convergent and discriminant validity. Qual Life Res 1994;3(6):431–5.
21. Ware J, Sherbourne C. The MOS 36-item short-form health survey (SF-36). Conceptual framework and item selection. Med Care 1992;30(6):473–83.

22. Lundberg L, Johannesson M, Silverdahl M, et al. Health-related quality of life in patients with psoriasis and atopic dermatitis measured with SF-36, DLQI, and a subjective measure of disease activity. Acta Derm Venereol 2000;80:430–4.

23. Nichol MB, Margolies J, Lippa E, et al. The application of multiple quality-of-life instruments in individuals with mild-to-moderate psoriasis. Pharmacoeconomics 1996;10(6):644–53.

24. Rapp S, Feldman SR, Exum M, et al. Psoriasis causes as much disability as other major medical diseases. J Am Acad Dermatol 1999;41(3):401–7.

25. Heydendael M, de Borgie C, Spuls P, et al. The burden of psoriasis is not determined by disease severity only. J Investig Dermatol Symp Proc 2004; 9(2):131–5.

26. Mallon E, Klassen A, Stewart-Brown SL, et al. The quality of life in acne: a comparison with general medical conditions using generic questionnaires. Br J Dermatol 1999;140(4):672–6.

27. Newton J, Mallon E, Klassen A, et al. The effectiveness of acne treatment: an assessment by patients of the outcome of therapy. Br J Dermatol 2006; 137(4):563–7.

28. Kiebert G, Sorensen S, Revicki D, et al. Atopic dermatitis is associated with a decrement in health-related quality of life. Int J Dermatol 2002; 41(3):151–8.

29. Fivenson D, Arnold R, Kaniecki D, et al. The effect of atopic dermatitis on total burden of illness and quality of life on adults and children in a large managed care organization. J Manag Care Pharm 2002;8(5):333–42.

30. Baiardini I, Giardini A, Pasquali M, et al. Quality of life and patients' satisfaction in chronic urticaria and respiratory allergy. Allergy 2003;58(7): 621–3.

31. Özkan M, Oflaz SB, Kocaman N, et al. Psychiatric morbidity and quality of life in patients with chronic idiopathic urticaria. Ann Allergy Asthma Immunol 2007;99(1):29–33.

32. Ware J, Kosinski M, Keller S. A 12-item short form health survey: construction of scales and preliminary tests of reliability and validity. Med Care 1996;34(3):220–33.

33. Hamm H, Naumann MK, Kowalski JW, et al. Primary focal hyperhidrosis: disease characteristics and functional impairment. Dermatology 2006;212:343–53.

34. Naumann MK, Hamm H, Lowe NJ. Effect of botulinum toxin type A on quality of life meaures in patients with excessive axillary sweating: a randomized controlled trial. Br J Dermatol 2002;147(6): 1218–26.

35. Misery L, Finlay AY, Martin N, et al. Atopic dermatitis: impact on the quality of life of patients and their partners. Dermatology 2007;215:123–9.

36. Warschburger P, Buchholz H, Petermann F. Psychological adjustment in parents of young children with atopic dermatitis: which factors predict parental quality of life? Br J Dermatol 2004;150(2):304–11.

37. Drake L, Patrick D, Fleckman P, et al. The impact of onychomycosis on quality of life: development of an onychomycosis-specific questionnaire to measure patient quality of life. J Am Acad Dermatol 1999;41(2):189–96.

38. Cirman CJ, Rhodes T, Lilly FR, et al. Effects of self-perceived hair loss in a community sample of men. Dermatology 1998;197(3):223–9.

39. DeMuro-Mercon C, Rhodes T, Girman C, et al. Male-pattern hair loss in norwegian men: a community based study. Dermatology 2000;200(3): 219–22.

40. Budd D, Himmelberger D, Rhodes T, et al. The effects of hair loss in European men: a survey in four countries. Eur J Dermatol 2000;10(2):122–7.

41. Rhee J, Matthews A, Neuburg M, et al. Validation of a quality-of-life instrument for patients with non-melanoma skin cancer. Arch Facial Plast Surg 2011;8(5):314–8.

42. Chen T, Bertenthal T, Sahay A, et al. Predictors of skin-related quality of life after treatment of cutaneous basal-cell carcinoma and squamous cell carcinoma. Arch Dermatol 2007;143(11): 1386–92.

43. Tabolli S, Bergamo F, Alessandroni L, et al. Quality of life and psychological problems of patients with oral mucosal disease in dermatological practice. Dermatology 2009;218(4):314–20.

44. Misery L, Schmitt A, Boussetta S, et al. Melasma: measure of the impact on quality of life using the french version of melasqol after cross-cultural adaptation. Acta Derm Venereol 2010;90:331–2.

45. WHOQOL Group. Development of the WHOQOL: rationale and current status. Int J Ment Health 1994;23:24–56.

46. WHOQOL Group. The World Health Organization Quality of Life Assessment (WHOQOL): development and general psychometric properties. Soc Sci Med 1998;46:1569–85.

47. The WHOQOL Group, Power M, Bullinger M, et al. The World Health Organization WHOQOL-100: tests of the universality of quality of life in 15 different cultural groups worldwide. Health Psychol 1999;18(5):495–505.

48. Skevington S, Carse M, Wiliams A. Validation of the WHOQOL-100: pain management improves the quality of life for chronic pain patients. Clin J Pain 2001;17:264–75.

49. Bonicatto S, Dew M, Zaratiegui R, et al. Adult outpatients with depression: worse quality of life than in order chronic medical diseases in Argentina. Soc Sci Med 2001;52(6):911–9.

50. Skevington S, Wright A. Changes in the quality of life of patients receiving antidepressant medication in primary care: validation of the WHOQOL-100. Br J Psychiatry 2001;178(3):261–7.

51. WHOQOL Group. Development of the World Health Organization WHOQOL-BREF quality of life assessment. Psychol Med 1998;28:551–8.

52. Skevington SM, Bradshaw J, Hepplewhite A, et al. How does psoriasis affect quality of life? Assessing an Ingram-regimen outpatient programme and validating the WHOQOL-100. Br J Dermatol 2006; 154(4):680–91.

53. Ryu JH, Kim KH, Kim KJ, et al. Quality of life in patients with psoriasis. Korean J Dermatol 2004; 42(3):264–71.

54. Engin B, Uguz F, Yilmaz E, et al. The levels of depression, anxiety and quality of life in patients with chronic idiopathic urticaria. J Eur Acad Dermatol Venereol 2008;22(1):36–40.

55. Kawashima M. Quality of life in patients with atopic dermatitis: impact of tacrolimus ointment. Int J Dermatol 2006;45(6):731–6.

56. Matsuoka Y, Yoneda K, Sadahira C, et al. Effects of skin care and makeup under instructions from dermatologists on the quality of life of female patients with acne vulgaris. J Dermatol 2006; 33(11):745–52.

57. Ng CH, Tam MM, Celi E, et al. Prospective study of depressive symptoms and quality of life in acne vulgaris patients treated with isotretinoin compared to antibiotic and topical therapy. Australas J Dermatol 2002;43(4):262–8.

58. Uguz F, Engin B, Yilman E. Quality of life in patients with chronic idiopathic urticaria: the impact of axis I and axis II psychiatric disorders. Gen Hosp Psychiatry 2008;30:453–7.

59. Dogramaci AC, Havlucu DY, Inandi T, et al. Validation of a melasma quality of life questionnaire for the Turkish language: the MelasQoL-TR study. J Dermatolog Treat 2009;20(2):95–9.

60. Agarwal S, Ramam M, Sharma VK, et al. A randomized placebo-controlled double-blind study of levamisole in the treatment of limited and slowly spreading vitiligo. Br J Dermatol 2005; 153(1):163–6.

61. Finlay AY, Khan GK. Dermatology Life Quality Index (DLQI): a simple practical measure for routine clinical use. Clin Exp Dermatol 1994;19:210–6.

62. Basra MK, Fenech R, Gatt RM, et al. The Dermatology Life Quality Index 1994–2007: a comprehensive review of validation data and clinical results. Br J Dermatol 2008;159(5):997–1035.

63. Le Cleach L, Chassany O, Levy A, et al. Poor reporting of quality of life outcomes in dermatology randomized controlled clinical trials. Dermatology 2008;216(1):46–55.

64. Shikiar R, Bresnahan B, Stone S, et al. Validity and reliability of patient reported outcomes used in psoriasis: results from two randomized clinical trials. Health Qual Life Outcomes 2003;1(53):1–9.

65. Henok L, Davey G. Validation of the Dermatology Life Quality Index among patients with podoconiosis in southern Ethiopia. Br J Dermatol 2008;159(4): 903–6.

66. Takahashi N, Suzukamo Y, Nakamura M, et al. Japanese version of the Dermatology Life Quality Index: validity and reliability in patients with acne. Health Qual Life Outcomes 2006;4(46):1–7.

67. Madarasingha N, de Silva P, Satgurunathan K. Validation study of Sinhala version of the dermatology life quality index (DLQI). Ceylon Med J 2011;56(1): 18–22.

68. Chren MM, Lasek R, Flocke S, et al. Improved discriminative and evaluative capability of a refined version of Skindex, a quality-of-life instrument for patients with skin diseases. Arch Dermatol 1997; 133:1433–40.

69. Chren MM, Lasek R, Quinn L, et al. Skindex: a quality-of-life measure for patients with skin disease: reliability, validity, and responsiveness. J Invest Dermatol 1996;107(5):707–13.

70. Chren MM, Lasek R, Sahay A, et al. Measurement properties of Skindex-16: a brief quality of life measure for patients with skin diseases. J Cutan Med Surg 2001;5(2):105–10.

71. Anderson R, Rajagopalan R. Development and validation of a quality of life instrument for cutaneous disease. J Am Acad Dermatol 1997;37(1): 41–50.

72. Anderson R, Rajagopalan R. Responsiveness of the Dermatology-specific Quality of Life (DSQL) instrument to treatment for acne vulgaris in a placebo-controlled clinical trial. Qual Life Res 1998;7(8):723–34.

73. Rajagopalan R, Anderson R. Impact of patch testing on dermatology-specific quality of life in patients with allergic contact dermatitis. Am J Contact Dermatitis 1997;8(4):215–21.

74. Stern RS, Nijsten T, Feldman SR, et al. Psoriasis is common, carries substantial burden even when not extensive and is associated with widespread treatment dissatisfaction. J Investig Dermatol Symp Proc 2004;9:136–9.

75. Fortune DG, Main CJ, O'Sullivan TM, et al. Quality of life in patients with psoriasis: the contribution of clinical variables and psoriasis-specific stress. Br J Dermatol 1997;137(5):755–60.

76. Finlay AY, Kelly SE. Psoriasis-an index of disability. Clin Exp Dermatol 1987;12(1):8–11.

77. Finlay AY, Coles EC. The effect of severe psoriasis on the quality of life of 369 patients. Br J Dermatol 1995;132(2):236–44.

78. Bronsard V, Paul C, Prey S, et al. What are the best outcome measures for assessing quality of life in plaque type psoriasis? A systematic review of the literature. J Eur Acad Dermatol Venereol 2010;24:17–22.

79. Nijsten T, Whalley D, Gelfand J, et al. The psychometric properties of the psoriasis disability index in United States patients. J Invest Dermatol 2005;125(4):665–72.

80. Gupta MA, Gupta A. The Psoriasis Life Stress Inventory: a preliminary index of psoriasis-related stress. Acta Derm Venereol 1995;75(3):240–3.

81. Mease PJ, Menter MA. Quality-of-life issues in psoriasis and psoriatic arthritis: outcome measures and therapies from a dermatological perspective. J Am Acad Dermatol 2006;54(4):685–704.

82. Kirby B, Fortune DG, Bhushan M, et al. The Salford Psoriasis Index: an holistic measure of psoriasis severity. Br J Dermatol 2000;142(4):728–32.

83. Lasek RJ, Chren MM. Acne vulgaris and the quality of life of adult dermatology patients. Arch Dermatol 1998;134(4):454–8.

84. Motley RJ, Finlay AY. How much disability is caused by acne? Clin Exp Dermatol 1989;14(3):194–8.

85. Motley RJ, Finlay AY. Practical use of a disability index in the routine management of acne. Clin Exp Dermatol 1992;17(1):1–3.

86. Gupta M, Johnson A, Gupta A. The development of an acne quality of life scale: reliability, validity, and relation to subjective acne severity in mild to mdoerate acne vulgaris. Acta Derm Venereol 1998;78:451–6.

87. Girman CJ, Hartmaier S, Thiboutot D, et al. Evaluating health-related quality of life in patients with facial acne: development of a self-administered questionnaire for clinical trials. Qual Life Res 1996;5(5):481–90.

88. Dréno B. Assessing quality of life in patients with acne vulgaris: implications for treatment. Am J Clin Dermatol 2006;7(2):99–106.

89. Whalley D, McKenna SP, Dewar AL, et al. A new instrument for assessing quality of life in atopic dermatitis: international development of the Quality of Life Index for Atopic Dermatitis (QoLIAD). Br J Dermatol 2004;150(2):274–83.

90. Nicholson K, Abramova L, Chren MM, et al. A pilot quality-of-life instrument for acne rosacea. J Am Acad Dermatol 2007;57(2):213–21.

91. Lubeck DP, Patrick DL, McNulty P, et al. Quality of life of persons with onychomycosis. Qual Life Res 1993;2(5):341–8.

92. Lubeck DP, Gause D, Schein JR, et al. A health-related quality of life measure for use in patients with onychomycosis: a validation study. Qual Life Res 1999;8(1/2):121–9.

93. Abetz L, Sutton M, Brady L, et al. The Diabetic Foot Ulcer Scale (DFS): a quality of life instrument for use in clinical trials. Practical Diabetes Int 2002;19(6):167–75.

94. Bann CM, Fehnel SE, Gagnon DD. Development and validation of the Diabetic Foot Ulcer Scale-short form (DFS-SF). Pharmacoeconomics 2003;21(17):1277–90.

95. Baiardini I, Pasquali M, Braido F, et al. A new tool to evaluate the impact of chronic urticaria on quality of life: chronic urticaria quality of life questionnaire (CU-Q2oL). Allergy 2005;60(8):1073–8.

96. Rhee JS, Matthews BA, Neuburg M, et al. The skin cancer index: clinical responsiveness and predictors of quality of life. Laryngoscope 2007;117(3):399–405.

97. David SE, Ahmed Z, Salek MS, et al. Does enough quality of life-related discussion occur during dermatology outpatient consultations? Br J Dermatol 2005;153(5):997–1000.

98. Jemec GB, Wulf HC. Patient–physician consensus on quality of life in dermatology. Clin Exp Dermatol 1996;21(3):177–9.

99. Hermansen SE, Helland CA, Finlay AY. Patients' and doctors' assessment of skin disease handicap. Clin Exp Dermatol 2002;27(3):249–50.

100. Townshend AP, Chen CM, Williams HC. How prominent are patient-reported outcomes in clinical trials of dermatological treatments? Br J Dermatol 2008;159(5):1152–9.

101. Grob JJ. Why are quality of life instruments not recognized as reference measures in therapeutic trials of chronic skin disorders? J Invest Dermatol 2007;127(10):2299–301.

Preference-Based Measures in Dermatology: An Overview of Utilities and Willingness to Pay

Anne M. Seidler, MD, MBA[a,*], Seema P. Kini, MD, MS[b],
Laura K. DeLong, MD, MPH[b,c], Emir Veledar, PhD[a],
Suephy C. Chen, MD, MS[c,d]

KEYWORDS

- Utility • Willingness to pay • Preference-based measure
- Time trade-off

UTILITIES: DEFINITIONS AND METHODS

Utilities are preference-based measures that aim to assess the desirability of certain health states. Such measures are important for decision analysis and cost-effectiveness analysis for which an assessment of the desirability of certain outcomes is crucial. Preference-based measures add the dimension of desirability to a simple assessment of a health status that is crucial for decision making.[1] Well-known methods of assessing utilities empirically include the standard gamble method and the time trade-off method. There are also population-based methods to estimate utilities. No matter the method, the utility is one number; a utility of 1 indicates the health state is equivalent to perfect health, and a utility of 0 indicates a preference for death over the current health state.[1]

Standard Gamble Method

The standard gamble method is used to assess the risk of death (without suffering) that individuals are willing to accept to be restored to perfect health or to rid them of a given disease. The respondent is asked to compare 2 outcomes: one is the best health state under consideration, and the other is the worst health state under consideration (which would be death without suffering). The outcomes are varied in a ping-pong fashion until the decision maker is indifferent between the gamble and the intermediate health state. For instance, if a subject is willing to take a 10% risk of death in exchange for a 90% chance of perfect health, then the utility of the intermediate state is 90% or 0.9.[1]

Time Trade-Off Method

The time trade-off method is an assessment of a person's willingness to live a shorter but healthier life without the current health condition. Patients are asked to select between 2 choices: living their normal life expectancy with their current skin disease or giving up a defined amount of time from their life in exchange for living disease free. Patients are asked about varying lengths of time they would be willing to give up, by varying from

[a] Department of Dermatology, Emory University School of Medicine, 5001 Woodruff Memorial Building, 1639 Pierce Drive, Atlanta, GA 30322, USA
[b] Department of Dermatology, Emory University School of Medicine, Emory Clinic, Building A, 1365 Clifton Road Northeast Suite 1100, Atlanta, GA 30322, USA
[c] Division of Dermatology, Atlanta Veterans Affairs Medical Center, Decatur, GA 30032, USA
[d] Department of Dermatology, Emory University, 101 Woodruff Circle, Atlanta, GA 30322, USA
* Corresponding author.
E-mail address: seidleranne@gmail.com

Dermatol Clin 30 (2012) 223–229
doi:10.1016/j.det.2011.12.002
0733-8635/12/$ – see front matter © 2012 Elsevier Inc. All rights reserved.

one extreme to the other in a ping-pong fashion.[2] The upper and lower bounds of time traded are then altered gradually, lessening the extremes. The task concludes when subjects indicate that they are indifferent between the 2 choices. The utility is calculated as the ratio of the time in best health to the life expectancy with skin disease. Lower scores indicate increased disease burden. Some believe this method is more comprehensible and simpler than the standard gamble method,[3] especially for health states in which very small risk (or small amounts of time) are to be considered. If the subject is willing to give up one-tenth of his or her life expectancy in return for perfect health, then the utility of the intermediate health state is 1 minus 0.10 or 0.90.[1]

Initially, the standard gamble technique was considered the best method of measuring utilities. This is because it is based directly on the fundamental components of utility theory. However, the time trade-off method is now accepted as the better option because it is more feasible, has a higher discriminating power, and has better face validity.[3]

Utility measurements have many challenges. Investigators need to make sure that the questions are explained clearly and patients are fully informed and comfortable and are in an environment conducive to answering such questions. Because the questions involve theoretical trading of time or taking hypothetical risks, patients may be unfamiliar and may feel that the process is awkward. The iterative process of eliciting these utilities also makes for a very time-consuming endeavor.

Population-based utility assessments

In contrast to the direct utility assessment methods described, utilities can also be assessed indirectly, through population-based measures, whereby health state classification systems are used to assign a utility value to a patient who meets criteria defined by a reference group. The reference group is created based on calculating mean responses from the general public rather than from subjects with the disease. These methods have been embraced because it is less time consuming than empirically assessing utilities by the standard gamble or time trade-off approaches. Population-based utility estimations have been used mostly in the nondermatology literature, but dermatology studies have started to use them.[4] The most popular population-based estimate used in dermatology is the European Quality of Life (EuroQoL) survey (EQ-5D).

The EQ-5D is a paper questionnaire in which subjects classify their health state according to a generic comprehensive health status classification system based on 5 dimensions, including mobility, self-care, usual activity (work, study, housework, family, and leisure), pain/discomfort, and anxiety/depression. Each of the dimensions has 3 levels: no, some, and extreme problems. For each respondent, a profile of health status is formed, and a corresponding health status valuation is matched to a corresponding utility derived from a reference population composed of members of the general public, not subjects with the disease in question. Weighted valuations for each health state have been elicited from respondents in the general population for 8 different countries, including the United States.

Despite the relative ease of using the EQ-5D and other similar population-based utility estimates, very few studies have been performed to validate these methods in the population with dermatologic concerns. The EQ-5D has been found to have limitations when compared with utilities elicited empirically from patients. A study by Lidgren and colleagues[5] assessed the impact of quality of life (QoL) of breast cancer by administering both the EQ-5D and a directly elicited time trade-off question to women with different stages of breast cancer. Across all stages, directly elicited time trade-off values were greater than EQ-5D values. Similarly, a study by Zethraeus and Johannesson[6] found that patient time trade-off values were similar to social UK EQ-5D index values for mild health states but that patient time trade-off values were higher for more severe health states.

These studies suggest that population-based measures may have the capacity to assess health states mild in severity but not more severe health states. Because of this limitation, generic QoL instruments such as the EQ-5D may not accurately capture disease or condition-specific impact. In the context of cost-effectiveness analyses, using the EQ-5D may overestimate QoL impact, translating to overestimation of the cost-effectiveness of a new drug.

A pilot study was performed involving a population with pruritus to examine the potential applicability of population-based utility measures in dermatology.[7] In this study, 58 subjects with chronic pruritus were recruited from the Emory Dermatology clinic. These subjects were interviewed via the time trade-off approach for empirically derived utilities and also given 3 paper-based questionnaires: a demographic survey, the EuroQoL, and a paper time trade-off survey. The paper-based survey consisted of 3 questions in which participants are asked to make hypothetical choices about improvement in their pruritic health state and duration of life. The 3 questions pose 3 different scenarios: (1) 100% relief from current itch, (2) 50% relief from current itch, and (3) never having itch. Rather than an iterative approach with the time trade-off method in the face-to-face interview, the subject is given 4 choices to each question: (1) give up 5 years of life; (2) give up 10 years of life; (3) give up more than 10 years, with a blank for the subject to fill in the number of years; and (4) none of the above, with a blank for the subject to complete. The last option allows for a choice less than 5 years.

The mean (standard deviation [SD]) age of the subjects was 56 (17) years; 38% were men and 64% were white. Of the subjects, 16 (28%) reported experiencing mild pruritus, with 28 (48%) and 13 (22%) experiencing moderate and severe pruritus, respectively. Paired t tests of the data revealed that mean (SD) EuroQoL utility scores 0.80 (0.13) were significantly lower (overestimating burden of disease) than face-to-face time trade-off derived scores (0.87 [0.27], P = .03). When utility scores were stratified by severity, a significant mean difference in valuation was observed for the moderate health state (0.14 [0.17], P<.01) between the 2 methods. Paper time trade-off utilities were overall greater than those derived by the face-to-face time trade-off method (mean [SD] difference −0.04 [0.17], P = .11).

These data indicate that population-based measures for eliciting utilities such as the EuroQoL may demonstrate a ceiling effect. The EQ-5D only includes the most basic measures of health status and does not account for emotional impact such as frustration, anger, helplessness, and stigmata—issues that significantly contribute to the overall QoL impact of cutaneous diseases.[8–10] Inclusion of these factors may assist in raising the ceiling effects observed. However, the paper version of the time trade-off did not fare better and seemed to underestimate QoL burden of chronic pruritus. These findings provide preliminary evidence that current proxy measures for utilities in chronic pruritus may not be accurate. Further studies should investigate the potential role of other population-based utility measures as proxy measures for eliciting utilities.

WILLINGNESS TO PAY: DEFINITIONS AND METHODS

Willingness to pay (WTP) is also considered a preference-based health status measure, but, rather than trading time or taking risks, QoL is quantified in monetary terms. Respondents consider how much they would be willing to pay either as a lump sum or as small payments over time to get rid of an undesirable health state. The expectation is

that a health state that is more bothersome to the patient will involve a greater burden of disease, and thus a patient will be able to be willing to make relatively more financial sacrifices to get rid of the disease. Information on annual income is also gathered so that WTP amounts can be expressed as percentages of income to help standardize these measures across income levels.

There have been some WTP studies that have varied from this method. Common variations include asking the payment amounts as predefined payment scale categories rather than in an open-ended format.

A variation from a prior study[11] is inserted here as an example to illustrate the ways in which this method may slightly differ but may still capture this preference-based measure: "You are offered a one-time treatment for your nail fungus. The treatment has an 85% cure rate, almost no side effects, and consists of taking a pill for 3 months. Think about all the things for which you spend money—food, rent/mortgage, bills, etc. How much would you be willing to pay out-of-pocket for this?"[11] In this study, patients selected their responses from predefined payment scale categories. Patients were also asked about their annual income, and they responded in predefined income range categories.

APPLICATIONS OF UTILITIES AND WTP

One of the most important roles of utility and WTP measures is their incorporation in cost-effectiveness analyses and cost-benefit analyses, respectively. Without these measures, therapeutics will be compared only via dollars and survival. In addition, these preference-based measures can be used on the individual level in the everyday care of patients. A discussion with patients assessing their willingness to trade time or WTP can provide a good idea of a patient's preferences, risk profile, and how much a given treatment course might be worth.[1]

Cost-Effectiveness Analysis

Utilities are used in cost-effectiveness analyses. The cost-effectiveness analysis is the ratio of additional cost of the health care intervention over the additional effectiveness it provides compared with the next best treatment alternative.

The effects may be measured in life-years, or they may be quality adjusted and include the QoL in each year as a weighting factor. The utility is the weighting factor used to calculate a quality-adjusted life year (QALY). For instance, if the life-year prolonged by a therapy is, say, 10 years and the utility indicating quality of those life-years is, say, 0.98, then the QALY is 9.8 years.

Obtaining utilities for incorporation in cost-effectiveness analyses is time consuming, and the varying methodologies yield different results. An alternative to obtaining utilities directly from patients is to use previously published utility values directly from the literature. Investigators in dermatology have attempted to take steps toward developing a repository of QoL weights to assist cost-effectiveness analysis.[12,13] The other alternative is to use population-based approaches, with the caveat that these measures also need validation in dermatology populations.

Cost-Benefit Analysis

WTP is the preference-based measure that is incorporated into cost-benefit analyses. Similar to utilities, WTP can capture aspects of health care that patients maybe consider important but are not necessarily captured within the conventional effectiveness measures.[14,15] A cost-benefit analysis ties in all relevant costs and benefits. Both the costs and benefits are expressed in monetary terms to determine the value of an intervention. The overall value of an intervention can be calculated by subtracting the cost of an intervention from the benefit (or WTP) amount.

Cost-effectiveness analysis has gained greater acceptance in health care than cost-benefit analysis because the benefit in the latter type of analysis is expressed in dollar terms and thus favors that the wealthy would then benefit more than poor individuals.[16,17] However, cost-benefit analyses are potentially advantageous because of their basis in dollar amounts because disparate comparisons may be made, including between health care and spending on other goods, such as housing or education.[16] Cost-effectiveness analysis requires that the benefits of compared interventions be measured in the same units.

In addition, as monetary measures, WTP may be added to conventional calculations that are included in cost-of-illness studies. It has been argued that without including WTP measures, cost-of-illness calculations (that include direct costs as well as loss of productivity) actually underestimate the true economic burden of disease.[15]

UTILITIES IN DERMATOLOGY

The concept of utilities was introduced to the dermatology community in 2004.[12] A catalog of dermatology utilities obtained from direct patient interviews was presented for 236 subjects from Grady Hospital in Atlanta Georgia, Stanford; medical center in Palo Alto, California; and Parkland Hospital in Dallas, Texas. The utility values ranged from 0.64 for bullous disorders to 1.0 for alopecia, cosmetic concerns, and urticaria. In this article, utilities were presented for 17 diagnostic categories in dermatology.[12] Diagnostic categories with a utility less than 0.95 (arbitrarily defined here as remarkable because they have a utility less than 0.95) were bullous disorders, 0.64 (N = 2); lymphoma, 0.82 (N = 6); pruritus and related conditions, 0.915 (N = 9); papulosquamous disorders, 0.919 (N = 13); ulcers, 0.923 (N = 4); infection or infestation, 0.933 (N = 35); dermatitis, 0.939 (N = 52); acneiform eruptions, 0.940 (N = 30); and sarcoid, 0.949 (N = 1). Utilities of specific diagnoses that were remarkable (arbitrarily defined again here as remarkable because they have a utility less than 0.95) were mycosis fungoides, 0.867 (N = 5); prurigo nodularis, 0.943 (N = 5); psoriasis, 0.907 (N = 11); condyloma, 0.706 (N = 5); atopic dermatitis, 0.890 (N = 5); contact dermatitis, 0.898 (N = 10); and acne vulgaris, 0.938 (N = 28).

This article[12] also puts the utilities in a clinical context by comparing dermatologic diseases with other health conditions. For comparison, the investigators point out that metastatic prostate cancer has a mean utility of 0.58 determined by a gambler automated graphical tool.[18] They also comment that breast cancer has a utility of 0.89, derived from verbal interviews.[19]

Littenberg and colleagues[13] also present dermatology utilities for 6 diagnoses, whereby utilities were elicited by the standard gamble method using a paper questionnaire.

Melanoma, nonmelanoma skin cancer, acne, keratoses, and nevi all have a utility value greater than 0.975. Psoriasis (the lowest utility value in this study) also had a high-appearing utility value of 0.925.

Utilities that have been gathered by direct assessment of patients with dermatologic diseases are mostly high. This has been referred to as the ceiling effect because most cutaneous conditions are considered minor and tend to cluster toward the upper end of the utility scale.[4] Because many dermatologic conditions are considered minor health states, they may lend themselves more to WTP.

WTP IN DERMATOLOGY

WTP is in the very early stages of exploration in dermatology. Qureshi and colleagues[20] examined preferences for telemedicine compared with in-person visits by using WTP comparisons. Their results suggest that patients (73% of their sample) prefer telemedicine if it expedites their access to care and that they are willing to pay about $25 for this expedited approach. When the time to access a physician in person or by telemedicine was held constant, 19% of the subjects preferred telemedicine, and more than half of this group was willing to pay a median of $25 for telemedicine.

There have been a few prior studies from Europe and the United States, looking at WTP values to assess burden in specific skin diseases that have had varying methodologies. The largest of these studies was from Germany.[21] In this study, 1023 patients with vitiligo completed a national postal survey asking them 2 close-ended questions with ranges of amounts that one would be willing to pay in a 1-time payment and in monthly payments to be completely cured from their disease. They also were asked to name an unrestricted amount for a 1-time payment for a cure. The following WTP amounts were all converted to US dollar amounts. The average unrestricted 1-time investment amount was $10,134. The range responses for 1-time cure amounts were greater than $688 in 9.8% of respondents, up to $1377 in 23%, up to $6885 in 29%, and greater than $6885 in 32%. The range responses for monthly payments to be cured of their disease were up to $69 in 33%, up to $207 in 35%, and greater than $207 in 32%. The investigators showed that the Dermatology Quality of Life Index, QoL instrument, and WTP were related (ie, scores were not independent of one another by a χ^2 test). The investigators also found that middle-aged patients showed a higher WTP than elderly patients, but differences in income were not addressed in this study.

Another study evaluated utilities and WTP in 366 patients from Sweden[22] with psoriasis and atopic dermatitis. The investigators found a weak correlation (r = −0.133, P<.05) between time trade-off utilities and WTP as assessed by the dichotomous choice method. In their dichotomous choice method, respondents rejected both choices or rejected 1 of the 2 choices. The prices were varied in subsamples, and the mean WTP was estimated by logistic regression analysis. The mean monthly WTP for a cure for psoriasis was $190; and this amount was $146 for atopic dermatitis (converted to US dollars).

Another study from Germany assessed 25 patients with port wine stains (24 of them on the face and 1 on the head and neck) who completed WTP and time trade-off utility questionnaires.[23] The responses of 23 patients to the WTP component revealed that on average, these patients had a WTP of 11.8% of their monthly income for an imaginary treatment that relieve them from all the problems and complaints related to their disease. The time trade-off component of this study used a methodology that is completely different from the method previously described.[2] The time trade-off in this study asked about the time one would be willing to spend on the treatment. The investigators concluded that the patients understood the methodologies and provided meaningful responses.[23]

There was a small study involving patients with onychomycosis in the United States.[11] In this study, 44 participants completed self-administered surveys at baseline and 1 month later to assess test-retest reliability. (One month was selected to avoid any impact of the treatment in influencing responses.) The survey asked respondents to indicate a dollar range amount they would be willing to pay for a 1-time treatment with an 85% cure rate and no side effects. The WTP responses were as follows: 48% would pay $0 to $50, 27% would pay $51 to $100, 5% would pay $101 to $150, 7% would pay $151 to $200, and 11% would pay $201 to $300. Fifty-five percent of subjects reported the same WTP on the initial test and the retest. The quadratic-weighted (Fleiss-Cohen) statistic showed moderate agreement (κ = 0.50, P<.01). Thus, WTP in onychomycosis had moderate pretest and posttest reliability. In terms of the annual income test and retest amounts, 71% of patients reported the same annual income category (κ = 0.72, P<.01). Based on these results, the investigators suggest that WTP has a potential role in onychomycosis.

DIFFERENCES BETWEEN UTILITIES AND WTP

An ongoing area of work is the evaluation of the relationship between health status and utilities and WTP. By nature, these instruments measure different entities. Accordingly, the correlation between them has not been found to be strong in prior research.[22] As a methodology, whereby responses are expressed in monetary terms, WTP is, by nature, different from a utility. Although both are preference-based measures, they are different currencies. The amount of time that individuals would be willing to give from their life may not be consistent with the amount of money they would be willing to pay. People feel differently about time traded from their lives and expenditure amounts.

It is possible that WTP has applicability where utilities do not. Relevance seems most likely for diseases that are mild and acute and are less of a burden in terms of QoL. In the setting of these more minor conditions, the conceptualization of paying out-of-pocket for a treatment or cure may be more straightforward than in severe or more chronic conditions.[24] As commented earlier, many dermatologic diseases having little to no burden that can be captured by the time trade-off method, likely because individuals would rather live with a minor health state than take any time at all from their lives. However, in these more minor health states, it is quite possible that WTP has a more relevant role. WTP may allow minor differences in burden in these less severe conditions to be distinguished from one another.

We have some experience with assessing the correlation between WTP and time trade-off utilities using data from the McCombs and Chen's catalog paper.[4] The sample of 254 patients answered questions on WTP for a cure (a 1-time treatment to eliminate the disease) and control (a daily treatment required to suppress symptoms of the disease) as well as provided time trade-off–derived utilities. Our results are presented in the section that follows.

WTP AND TIME TRADE-OFF UTILITY CORRELATION IN DERMATOLOGY

For our sample of 254 patients, there was a weak statistically significant correlation between WTP control with time trade-off utility ($r = -0.17$, $P = .008$) and WTP cure with time trade-off utility ($r = -0.14$, $P = .030$). When Spearman correlation coefficients were examined by income groups (non-Medicaid and Medicaid), we found that the non-Medicaid group had correlations between WTP and time trade-off utilities that were stronger ($r = -0.26$, $P<.05$) than when the sample was considered as a whole. Further, when the Medicaid group was considered separately, there were insignificant correlations between WTP control and cure and time trade-off utilities.

We repeated the analyses for one diagnostic group, in case the low correlation was because of the heterogeneity of diagnoses. The acne diagnosis group included the greatest number of patients, and we found a moderate correlation between WTP control ($r = 0.57$) and cure ($r = 0.49$) and time trade-off utility values ($P<.01$ for both). When the non-Medicaid acne group was considered separately, the Spearman correlation coefficients indicated slightly stronger correlations between WTP control ($r = 0.61$) and control ($r = 0.53$) with time trade-off utility scores ($P<.01$ for both).

We explored the relationship between WTP and utilities in acne patients, while adjusting for Medicaid status, disease severity, and educational level in a generalized linear model. We found that, after adjustments, the utility value had a significant effect ($P<.05$) on both WTP control and cure amounts,

such that an increase in 0.01 in the utility was associated with significant decreases in the WTP cure and WTP control amounts. Medicaid status did not have a significant role in our model, although 24 of the 30 patients were not eligible for Medicaid, limiting the comparison in this model. In addition, the severity of the acne did not seem to have a significant effect in our model. We found a trend ($P = .1$) that those who had completed college or graduate level education (N = 19) were willing to pay more than those who had not completed these higher levels of education (N = 11).

These data indicate that WTP and utilities may be correlated but understandably not strongly for either income group, given that the former is expressed in monetary terms, whereas the latter is a measurement in life-years traded for a better health state, and these measures are qualitatively different. Perhaps this difference is particularly apparent for people in lower income groups, but this would need further investigation.

We also found that when considered separately, the acne group had a stronger correlation between WTP and utilities than the rest of the sample after adjusting for Medicaid status, severity, and education. This preliminary evidence suggests that either WTP may be more relevant in certain diseases or WTP is best summarized across 1 disease.

SUMMARY

Utilities and WTP are preference-based measures. They aim to capture the burden of skin diseases. By nature, utilities and WTP are very different measures. Accordingly, they are not well correlated for all diseases.

Both preference-based measures have a potentially significant role in decision making for their incorporation in cost-effectiveness analysis and cost-benefit analysis. In addition, they may be used at the bedside or in clinics as tools to provide additional information on the degree to which a disease is affecting a patient. This may have a role in considering the potential value that a given treatment may provide.

Both measures have limitations. WTP is limited in the sense that it may be difficult to conceptualize for individuals in certain income categories or with certain diseases that are chronic or so severe that imagining paying large sums of money for the treatment would be difficult. Utilities are limited in the iterative process that is required to empirically elicit data; proxy measures have yet to be validated in dermatology populations. The use of preference-based measures in dermatology is still new. Further work in this area is warranted.

REFERENCES

1. Goldstein MK, Tsevat J. Assessing desirability of outcome states for medical decision making and cost-effectiveness analysis. In: Lynn J, Max MB, editors. Symptom research: methods and opportunities. Bethesda (MD): National Institutes of Health; 2003. p. 1–14, Chapter 24.
2. Dolan P, Gudex C, Kind P, et al. Valuing health states: a comparison of methods. J Health Econ 1996;15(2): 209–31.
3. van Osch SM, Wakker PP, van den Hout WB, et al. Correcting biases in standard gamble and time tradeoff utilities. Med Decis Making 2004;24(5): 511–7.
4. McCombs K, Chen SC. Patient preference quality of life measures in dermatology. Dermatol Ther 2007; 20(2):102–9.
5. Lidgren M, Wilking N, Jonsson B, et al. Health related quality of life in different states of breast cancer. Qual Life Res 2007;16:1073–81.
6. Zethraeus N, Johannesson M. A comparison of patient and social tariff values derived from the time trade-off method. Health Econ 1999;8:541–5.
7. DeLong LK, Kini S, McIlwain M, et al. Comparison of interview based and EuroQoL derived utilities among patients with chronic pruritus. J Invest Dermatol 2008;128:S82.
8. Thomas DR. Psychosocial effects of acne. J Cutan Med Surg 2004;8:3–5.
9. Shuster S, Fisher GH, Harris E, et al. The effect of skin disease on self image. Br J Dermatol 1978;99: 18–9.
10. Ongenae K, Beelaert L, van Geel N, et al. Psychosocial effects of vitiligo. J Eur Acad Dermatol Venereol 2006;20:1–8.
11. Cham PM, Chen SC, Grill JP, et al. Reliability of self-reported willingness-to-pay and annual income in patients treated for toenail onychomycosis. Br J Dermatol 2007;156(5):922–8.
12. Chen SC, Bayoumi AM, Soon SL, et al. A catalog of dermatology utilities: a measure of the burden of skin diseases. J Investig Dermatol Symp Proc 2004;9(2):160–8.
13. Littenberg B, Partilo S, Licata A, et al. Paper Standard Gamble: the reliability of a paper questionnaire to assess utility. Med Decis Making 2003;23(6):480–8.
14. Drummond MF, Jefferson TO. Guidelines for authors and peer reviewers of economic submissions to the BMJ. The BMJ Economic Evaluation Working Party. BMJ 1996;313(7052):275–83.
15. Thompson MS. Willingness to pay and accept risks to cure chronic disease. Am J Public Health 1986; 76(4):392–6.
16. Gold MR, Siegel JE, Russell LB, et al. Cost-effectiveness in health and medicine. New York: Oxford University Press; 1996. p. 425.
17. Drummond MF, O'Brien BJ, Stoddart GL, et al. Methods for the economic evaluation of health care programmes. 3rd edition. Oxford (United Kingdom): Oxford University Press; 2005.
18. Krahn MD, Mahoney JE, Eckman MH, et al. Screening for prostate cancer. A decision analytic view. JAMA 1994;272(10):773–80.
19. Grann VR, Panageas KS, Whang W, et al. Decision analysis of prophylactic mastectomy and oophorectomy in BRCA1-positive or BRCA2-positive patients. J Clin Oncol 1998;16(3):979–85.
20. Qureshi AA, Brandling-Bennett HA, Wittenberg E, et al. Willingness-to-pay stated preferences for telemedicine versus in-person visits in patients with a history of psoriasis or melanoma. Telemed J E Health 2006;12(6):639–43.
21. Radtke MA, Schafer I, Gajur A, et al. Willingness-to-pay and quality of life in patients with vitiligo. Br J Dermatol 2009;161(1):134–9.
22. Lundberg L, Johannesson M, Silverdahl M, et al. Quality of life, health-state utilities and willingness to pay in patients with psoriasis and atopic eczema. Br J Dermatol 1999;141(6):1067–75.
23. Schiffner R, Brunnberg S, Hohenleutner U, et al. Willingness to pay and time trade-off: useful utility indicators for the assessment of quality of life and patient satisfaction in patients with port wine stains. Br J Dermatol 2002;146(3):440–7.
24. Bala MV, Zarkin GA. Are QALYs an appropriate measure for valuing morbidity in acute diseases? Health Econ 2000;9(2):177–80.

The Skindex Instruments to Measure the Effects of Skin Disease on Quality of Life

Mary-Margaret Chren, MD*

KEYWORDS

- Quality of life • Patient-reported outcomes
- Outcomes research • Skin diseases

In practicing dermatology one soon realizes that the severity of most skin diseases is not easily assessed and communicated. Most skin conditions cannot be followed by laboratory values, and typically patients survive with (rather than die from) their diseases. Also, one quickly learns that the visible extent of disease often does not correlate with the degree to which patients are disturbed by it; patients with minimal clinical involvement may be highly distressed, but others with extensive involvement may not be bothered. The severity of a skin disease is related both to its clinical extent (using clinimetric measures) and its effects on patients' quality of life (using psychometric measures).

This article describes how the author and her colleagues designed and worked with a measure of the effects of skin disease on quality of life, called Skindex. The article reviews the development of the two versions of Skindex, discusses their measurement properties and interpretability, and gives examples of how they have been used and adapted for dermatologic research internationally. Specifically discussed are studies of quality of life in patients with nonmelanoma skin cancer (NMSC), to illustrate how Skindex has been used to understand quality of life and to compare effectiveness of different treatments for this highly prevalent condition.

DEVELOPMENT OF SKINDEX

When we began to develop Skindex, we were greatly informed by the previous work of Finlay and coworkers[1,2] on measuring disability from skin disease. Our goal was to develop an instrument to measure comprehensively the effects of skin disease on health-related quality of life, and we specifically designed the instrument to be able to discriminate between patients with different effects and to detect changes in patients over time.[3] An incremental strategy was followed that began with a hypothesis: based on a literature review of previous clinical and psychologic studies and substantial input from patients and clinicians, we constructed a comprehensive conceptual framework for the ways in which we hypothesized skin diseases affected patients. Survey items were composed to measure all domains in the framework, and then the hypothesis was tested by examining the validity of the items in a series of psychometric tests using the responses of a large sample of patients.

Funding Support: This work was supported by grant K24 AR052667 from the National Institute of Arthritis and Musculoskeletal and Skin Diseases, National Institutes of Health.

Disclosure: The author has nothing to disclose.

Department of Dermatology, University of California at San Francisco, San Francisco, CA, USA

* Mt. Zion Cancer Research Building, 2340 Sutter Street, Room N412, Box 0808, San Francisco, CA 94143–0808.
E-mail address: chrenm@derm.ucsf.edu

Dermatol Clin 30 (2012) 231–236
doi:10.1016/j.det.2011.11.003
0733-8635/12/$ – see front matter Published by Elsevier Inc.

Original Conceptual Framework

We proposed that skin diseases affect patients in either psychosocial or physical ways. We suggested that psychosocial effects could be cognitive (beliefs about self or others); social; or emotional. Subdimensions of emotional effects include depression, fear, embarrassment, and anger. Physical effects are either discomfort or limitations in physical functioning. This original hypothesized framework is depicted in **Fig. 1**.

Item Composition and Prototype Skindex

The team consisted of two psychometricians, and using conventional principles we composed 65 items to assess the dimensions in the conceptual framework. This draft survey was pilot-tested and ambiguous and redundant items were changed or deleted, which left a 61-item prototype version of Skindex. The measurement properties of this trial version were tested in a series of studies that demonstrated it to be reliable and to have substantial evidence of validity as a measure of the effects of skin disease on quality of life.[4]

Refinement into Skindex-29

We wanted to improve the ability of the prototype Skindex to discriminate among patients with likely different degrees of quality-of-life effect, and to be more sensitive to even modest changes in patients' experiences over time. We also wanted to shorten the instrument to make it more useful in research and clinical settings. To accomplish these goals, the performance of each item was assessed, using not only qualitative judgments but also based on a priori criteria for suboptimal item performance, including reproducibility, discriminant validity, complexity, ambiguity, response distribution, and item-total correlation. The factors, or themes, that explained the variability in responses to the psychometrically soundest items were analyzed, which permitted us to test and refine the theorized model for the effects of skin

disease on quality of life. Finally, we composed new items that we judged would improve discriminative and evaluative capability of the instrument.

This sequential process generated a refined conceptual framework. We now propose that the effects of skin disease on quality of life can be understood in three domains: (1) symptoms, (2) emotions, and (3) functioning (**Fig. 2**). The analyses yielded a 29-item version of Skindex that remained reliable and valid, but that had reduced respondent burden, and improved discriminative and evaluative capability.[5]

Skindex-29 inquires about how often (never, rarely, sometimes, often, all the time) during the previous 4 weeks the patient experienced the effect described in each item. Seven items address the symptoms domain, 10 items the emotional domain, and 12 items the functioning domain. All responses are transformed to a linear scale of 100, varying from 0 (no effect) to 100 (effect experienced all the time). Skindex scores are reported as three scale scores, corresponding to the three domains; a scale score is the average of a patient's responses to items in a given domain.

Construction of Skindex-16

Longitudinal research studies often require waves of data collection with lengthy survey instruments to assess multiple aspects of patients' experience. We sought to develop a version of Skindex that would remain accurate and responsive as a measure of skin-related quality of life, but that would be brief (contained on one page). Also, we wanted to assess not only how often patients have a particular experience, but how much they are bothered by it. Thus, Skindex-29 was used as the substrate for a series of studies that developed a different, single-page version, Skindex-16. We used item analyses similar to those described previously to select only those items that performed well according to the criteria, and eliminated items to which most patients responded "never." New items were composed to address

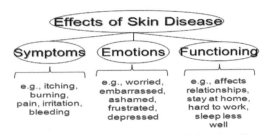

Fig. 1. Original hypothesized conceptual framework for the effects of skin disease on the quality of life of affected patients.

Fig. 2. Refined conceptual framework for the effects of skin disease on the quality of life of affected patients.

aspects of quality of life that patients mentioned often in their qualitative responses but that had not been addressed in Skindex-29. This process generated a new instrument, which fits on a single page. The header inquires "During the past x weeks, how often have you been bothered by…" The response choices are on a continuous bipolar scale with seven boxes anchored by the words "never bothered" and "always bothered" at each end. As with the parent instrument, scores vary from 0 (no effect) to 100 (effect experienced all the time), and responses are aggregated in symptoms (four items), emotions (seven items), and functioning scales (five items). The performance of this new instrument, Skindex-16, was tested in more than 500 patients, and it was reliable, retained substantial evidence of validity, and was responsive to clinical change.[6]

CHOOSING BETWEEN SKINDEX-29 AND SKINDEX-16

The Skindex instruments are copyrighted to ensure standardization in their use and scoring; permission to use either version is obtained through the non-profit MAPI research trust (http://www.mapi-trust.org/). Investigators often inquire about which of the two versions they should use for their studies. This decision typically depends on the research question being addressed. Because it is longer, Skindex-29 is more comprehensive, and it might be more suitable if the goal of a project is to investigate and understand the effects of a given condition on quality of life. Also, because Skindex-29 is older and has been used more broadly in clinical research, typical scores of patients with different skin conditions are widely available and can be compared with those of patients with the disease in question. For example, we were interested in learning more about quality-of-life effects from vulvodynia, a highly painful vulvar condition that is poorly understood. We used Skindex-29 in a large sample of women and determined that those with vulvodynia were substantially more likely than those with other vulvar conditions to have feelings of depression, anger, and frustration, and to report that the vulvodynia affected broad aspects of their social and physical functioning.[7]

Skindex-16, however, consists of the items that had the best performance characteristics in the longer instrument, and additional items that are not in Skindex-29, but that address aspects of skin disease that many patients had mentioned in response to qualitative research (eg, bother from the persistence or reoccurrence of the skin condition). Also, Skindex-16 measures bother rather than frequency of experience, which we reasoned may more directly assess effects on patients' quality of life. Finally, because it has been refined into a single page, Skindex-16 is useful for studies in which respondent burden is a concern. For example, we have used Skindex-16 in waves of data collection over 10 years in a longitudinal study of more than 1500 patients with NMSC, as part of research to document and compare outcomes after therapy, as described later.

INTERPRETATION OF SCORES

To use quality-of-life measures to study disease and improve patient care, one needs to know not only raw scores, but also what the scores mean with respect to severity of effect and comparison with other patients.[8] Because the Skindex instruments are generic in the sense that they can be used in patients with skin disease of any sort, valuable information can be obtained by comparisons of mean scores of groups of patients with certain diseases. **Table 1** contains mean Skindex scores in unselected groups of patients with a variety of skin conditions.

Table 1
Mean Skindex scores in patients with different dermatologic diagnoses

Diagnosis	Skindex-29 Scores[a]				Skindex-16 Scores[a]			
	No.	Symptoms	Emotions	Functioning	No.	Symptoms	Emotions	Functioning
Eczematous dermatitis	102	48 ± 23	41 ± 27	26 ± 26	84	42 ± 31	52 ± 30	24 ± 29
Psoriasis	44	42 ± 21	39 ± 27	23 ± 27	27	49 ± 29	68 ± 25	39 ± 33
Acne vulgaris	63	30 ± 19	41 ± 25	16 ± 16	38	31 ± 24	75 ± 23	38 ± 30
Warts	24	23 ± 18	22 ± 16	6 ± 13	33	23 ± 23	48 ± 31	24 ± 31
Other benign growths	76	22 ± 20	21 ± 21	9 ± 17	56	15 ± 20	34 ± 29	12 ± 21

[a] Mean ± SD.

In addition to these comparisons, distribution-based and anchor-based methods have been used to aid interpretation of Skindex-29 scores.[8] Using mixture analyses to assess whether the distribution of responses could be clustered into statistically distinct categories based on degree of quality-of-life effect, Nijsten and colleagues[9] demonstrated five distinct categories for the symptoms scale, and four for the emotions and functioning scales. For example, for the symptoms scale, the cutoff value for "very little" effect was less than or equal to 3, "mild" effect 4 to 10, "moderate" effect 11 to 25, "severe" effect 26 to 49, and "extremely severe" effect greater than or equal to 50. Using an anchor-based method, Prinsen and colleagues[10] determined these cut-off Skindex-29 scores for severe effect: symptoms greater than or equal to 52, emotions greater than or equal to 39, and functioning greater than or equal to 37. Similar studies to aid interpretation of Skindex-16 scores have not yet been performed.

USING SKINDEX IN RESEARCH STUDIES AND IN CLINIC
Understanding Quality of Life in Dermatologic Conditions

Skindex has been used to study the effects of a wide variety of skin conditions on patients' lives, and in addition to answering research questions these investigations can lead to new insights to inform patient care. For example, even controlling for clinical severity, the quality of life of older patients ($\geq$40 years) with acne vulgaris is more affected than that of younger patients.[11] Patients with cutaneous lymphoma experience many quality-of-life effects, including skin sensitivity and annoyance about the disease, worry that it could worsen, and effects on sexual life.[12] Similar quality-of-life assessments have been made in patients with psoriasis,[13] dermatitis,[14] alopecia,[15] and urticaria,[16] among others.

Clinical Trials

Because it was developed to be responsive to changes in quality of life, Skindex can be used as an outcomes measure in clinical trials. Examples of this use include studies of therapies for psoriasis,[17,18] acne vulgaris,[19] and atopic dermatitis.[20]

Cultural Adaptation and Translations of Skindex

Skindex has been translated into several languages, typically using adaptations of conventional guidelines for ensuring cultural equivalence in quality-of-life instruments.[21] A good example is the development of the Spanish version of Skindex-29 in which a step-wise process was used to forward-translate, back-translate, pilot test, refine, and evaluate the measurement properties of the adapted version.[22] For certain expressions a simple translation was not sufficient; for example, further consideration was necessary to determine the best translations for "embarrassed" and "ashamed," which is typical of linguistic issues in other translations.[23]

Quality-of-Life Instruments Based on Skindex

Skindex is a generic instrument in the sense that it is intended to be used by patients with any skin condition. It has been used as a basis for several more specific instruments or modules to measure quality of life in particular populations or in patients with certain diagnoses. For example, variations of Skindex have been developed for patients with leg ulcers,[24] onychomycosis,[25] scalp disorders,[26] and for teenagers.[27]

Outcomes Research and Comparative Effectiveness of Therapies

Because quality-of-life is a central outcome of nonfatal conditions, such as most skin diseases, Skindex can be used to assess how patients progress over time or after therapies. For example, we have used Skindex-16 to document the effects of NMSC and its treatments on quality of life over time, as part of a prospective cohort study of a large sample of patients with this common tumor.

We determined the skin-related quality of life of 633 consecutive patients with NMSC diagnosed in 1999 and 2000 and treated with the three major treatments used in the United States: (1) electrodessication and curettage (ED&C), (2) excision, or (3) Mohs surgery.[28] Scores for the symptoms, emotions, and functioning subscales of Skindex-16 in the three treatment groups before therapy are contained in **Table 2**. Compared with

Table 2
Skindex-16 scores (mean ± SD) before treatment of 633 patients with nonmelanoma skin cancer

Skindex Subscale	Treatment Groups		
	ED&C	Excision	Mohs Surgery
Symptoms	20 (24)	22 (23)	22 (24)
Emotions	33 (28)	39 (30)	46 (27)
Functioning	12 (22)	15 (25)	14 (21)

Skindex-16 scores of patients with inflammatory dermatologic conditions (see **Table 1**), the scores of these patients with NMSC were relatively low, indicating that overall the tumors have less effect on quality of life than the effects of psoriasis, eczematous dermatitis, or acne vulgaris. There was no significant difference in the treatment groups in mean symptoms or functioning scores, but the mean emotions score of patients whose tumors were ultimately treated with Mohs surgery were higher than mean emotions scores of those treated with the other two treatments ($P<.0001$). After treatment, in analyses that adjusted for differences in treatment groups, the scores of patients treated with excision or Mohs surgery improved in all three Skindex domains, but patients treated with ED&C had no change in tumor-related quality of life (**Table 3**).

We were also interested in determining whether characteristics of the patients, tumors, or care were associated with better skin-related quality of life after treatment for NMSC.[29] We found that the strongest independent predictor of quality of life after treatment was quality of life before treatment. Fewer comorbid illnesses and better mental health status were also independent predictors. Tumor characteristics, however, did not predict quality of life. These results may improve clinical care by permitting clinicians to recognize patients at higher risk for poor quality-of-life outcomes.

FUTURE DIRECTIONS

The development of quality-of-life measures is a dynamic process. The interpretation of Skindex-29 and Skindex-16 scores will be enhanced as they are used and studied more widely. The instruments were developed using classical test theory methods, and the application of newer psychometric techniques, such as item response theory and computerized adaptive testing, may improve their measurement properties.[30] As tools to measure complex aspects of health become more commonplace in dermatology, investigators, clinicians, and other stakeholders may develop a consensus about features that should be present in widely accepted measures of disease severity[31]; these features will likely include at least some measure of patients' experience, such as symptoms or quality of life. Features to be included in an ideal quality-of-life measure could be defined using similar consensus techniques, and perhaps it will be possible to develop a core set of questions and metrics or repositories of items that perform well. Finally, because the patient report is a "vital sign" for dermatologic disease,[32] an exciting development would be testing whether for selected subgroups of patients the inclusion in the clinic of quantitative measures of patient reports (eg, Skindex) can improve care.

SUMMARY

Skindex-29 and Skindex-16 are validated measures of the effects of skin diseases on quality of life that are suitable for use in research about patients' experiences of illness and its treatment. This article reviews the development of Skindex and its use in a variety of clinical research studies.

REFERENCES

1. Finlay AY, Kelly SE. Psoriasis: an index of disability. Clin Exp Dermatol 1987;12:8–11.
2. Finlay AY, Khan GK. Dermatology life quality index (DLQI): a simple practical measure for routine clinical use. Clin Exp Dermatol 1994;19:210–6.
3. Kirshner B, Guyatt G. A methodological framework for assessing health indices. J Chronic Dis 1985; 38(1):27–36.
4. Chren MM, Lasek RJ, Quinn LM, et al. Skindex, a quality-of-life measure for patients with skin disease: reliability, validity, and responsiveness. J Invest Dermatol 1996;107:707–13.
5. Chren MM, Lasek RJ, Flocke SA, et al. Improved discriminative and evaluative capability of a refined version of Skindex, a quality-of-life instrument for patients with skin diseases. Arch Dermatol 1997; 133(11):1433–40.
6. Chren MM, Lasek RJ, Sahay AP, et al. Measurement properties of Skindex-16, A brief quality-of-life measure for patients with skin diseases. J Cutan Med Surg 2001;5(2):105–10.
7. Ponte M, Klemperer E, Sahay A, et al. Effects of vulvodynia on quality of life. J Am Acad Dermatol 2009; 60(1):70–6.
8. Chren M. Interpretation of quality-of-life scores. J Invest Dermatol 2011, in press.

Table 3
Improvement in Skindex-16 scores of 633 patients after treatment of nonmelanoma skin cancer

Treatment Group	Adjusted Change Score, Mean		
	Symptoms	Emotions	Functioning
ED&C	−3	−5	2
Excision	−10[a]	−19[a]	−3[a]
Mohs surgery	−10[a]	−22[a]	−5[a]

[a] $P<.05$ for difference before and after treatment.

9. Nijsten T, Sampogna F, Abeni D. Categorization of Skindex-29 scores using mixture analysis. Dermatology 2009;218(2):151–4.

10. Prinsen CA, Lindeboom R, Sprangers MA, et al. Health-related quality of life assessment in dermatology: interpretation of Skindex-29 scores using patient-based anchors. J Invest Dermatol 2010;130:1318–22.

11. Lasek RJ, Chren MM. Acne vulgaris and the quality of life of adult dermatology patients. Arch Dermatol 1998;134(4):454–8.

12. Sampogna F, Frontani M, Baliva G, et al. Quality of life and psychological distress in patients with cutaneous lymphoma. Br J Dermatol 2009;160(4):815–22.

13. De Korte J, Mombers FM, Sprangers MA, et al. The suitability of quality-of-life questionnaires for psoriasis research: a systematic literature review. Arch Dermatol 2002;138(9):1221–7 [discussion: 1227].

14. Zug KA, Aaron DM, Mackenzie T. Baseline quality of life as measured by Skindex-16+5 in patients presenting to a referral center for patch testing. Dermatitis 2009;20(1):21–8.

15. Reid EE, Haley AC, Borovicka JH, et al. Clinical severity does not reliably predict quality of life in women with alopecia areata, telogen effluvium, or androgenic alopecia. J Am Acad Dermatol 2011, in press.

16. Maurer M, Ortonne JP, Zuberbier T. Chronic urticaria: a patient survey on quality-of-life, treatment usage and doctor-patient relation. Allergy 2009;64(4):581–8.

17. Ortonne JP, Ganslandt C, Tan J, et al. Quality of life in patients with scalp psoriasis treated with calcipotriol/betamethasone dipropionate scalp formulation: a randomized controlled trial. J Eur Acad Dermatol Venereol 2009;23(8):919–26.

18. de Korte J, van der Valk PG, Sprangers MA, et al. A comparison of twice-daily calcipotriol ointment with once-daily short-contact dithranol cream therapy: quality-of-life outcomes of a randomized controlled trial of supervised treatment of psoriasis in a day-care setting. Br J Dermatol 2008;158(2): 375–81.

19. Hayashi N, Kawashima M. Efficacy of oral antibiotics on acne vulgaris and their effects on quality of life: a multicenter randomized controlled trial using minocycline, roxithromycin and faropenem. J Dermatol 2011;38(2):111–9.

20. Gambichler T, Othlinghaus N, Tomi NS, et al. Medium-dose ultraviolet (UV) A1 vs. narrowband UVB phototherapy in atopic eczema: a randomized crossover study. Br J Dermatol 2009; 160(3):652–8.

21. Guillemin F, Bombardier C, Beaton D. Cross-cultural adaptation of health-related quality of life measures: literature review and proposed guidelines. J Clin Epidemiol 1993;46(12):1417–32.

22. Jones-Caballero M, Penas PF, Garcia-Diez A, et al. The Spanish version of Skindex-29. Cultural adaptation and preliminary evidence of validity and equivalence with the original American version. Int J Dermatol 2000;39:907–12.

23. Higaki Y, Kawamoto K, Kamo T, et al. The Japanese version of Skindex-16: a brief quality-of-life measure for patients with skin diseases. J Dermatol 2002; 29(11):693–8.

24. Hareendran A, Doll H, Wild DJ, et al. The venous leg ulcer quality of life (VLU-QoL) questionnaire: development and psychometric validation. Wound Repair Regen 2007;15(4):465–73.

25. Warshaw EM, Foster JK, Cham PM, et al. NailQoL: a quality-of-life instrument for onychomycosis. Int J Dermatol 2007;46(12):1279–86.

26. Chen SC, Yeung J, Chren MM. Scalpdex: a quality-of-life instrument for scalp dermatitis. Arch Dermatol 2002;138(6):803–7.

27. Smidt AC, Lai JS, Cella D, et al. Development and validation of Skindex-Teen, a quality-of-life instrument for adolescents with skin disease. Arch Dermatol 2010;146(8):865–9.

28. Chren MM, Sahay AP, Bertenthal DS, et al. Quality-of-life outcomes of treatments for cutaneous basal cell carcinoma and squamous cell carcinoma. J Invest Dermatol 2007;127(6):1351–7.

29. Chen T, Bertenthal D, Sahay A, et al. Predictors of skin-related quality of life after treatment of cutaneous basal cell carcinoma and squamous cell carcinoma. Arch Dermatol 2007;143(11):1386–92.

30. Nijsten TE, Sampogna F, Chren MM, et al. Testing and reducing skindex-29 using Rasch analysis: Skindex-17. J Invest Dermatol 2006;126(6):1244–50.

31. Schmitt J, Langan S, Stamm T, et al. Core outcome domains for controlled trials and clinical recordkeeping in eczema: international multiperspective Delphi consensus process. J Invest Dermatol 2011;131(3): 623–30.

32. Chren MM. Measurement of vital signs for skin diseases. J Invest Dermatol 2005;125(4):viii–viix.

A Review of the Use of the Dermatology Life Quality Index as a Criterion in Clinical Guidelines and Health Technology Assessments in Psoriasis and Chronic Hand Eczema

Mohammad K.A. Basra, DDSc, MD[a],*,
Mahbub M.U. Chowdhury, FRCP[b], Emma V. Smith, MRCP[b],
Nick Freemantle, PhD[c], Vincent Piguet, MD, PhD[a],*

KEYWORDS

- Chronic hand eczema • Psoriasis • Quality of life
- Dermatology Life Quality Index (DLQI)

Skin diseases are very common in the community and although most are not life threatening, many are chronic and incurable. Skin diseases significantly affect patients' quality of life (QOL), due to several issues including chronic, disabling, and disfiguring nature, with symptoms such as discomfort and additional associated stigma. These effects on patients may not be captured using traditional biomedical outcome measures, and hence QOL assessment has become an important end point in clinical trials in addition to traditional clinical outcomes. Moreover, QOL is increasingly being incorporated into routine clinical practice, patient service evaluation, and policy making and for health resource allocation. The use of QOL and other patient-reported outcomes have become a regulatory requirement for the pharmaceutical industry in supporting labeling claims.[1]

The Dermatology Life Quality Index (DLQI) was developed in 1994,[2] and today is the most commonly

Funding Statement: Manuscript development was supported by unconditional funding from Basilea Pharmaceutica International Ltd., Basel.

Disclosures: None (M.K.A.B.); received educational grants and consultancy fees from Basilea (M.M.U.C.); none (E.V.S.); received funding for research and consulting from Pfizer, Basilea, MSD (N.F.); received educational grants and/or consulting fees from Pfizer, GSK, Abbott, Basilea, MSD/Schering, Janssen (V.P.).

[a] Department of Dermatology and Wound Healing, Cardiff University School of Medicine, Heath Park, Cardiff, CF14 4XN, Wales, UK
[b] Department of Dermatology, Welsh Institute of Dermatology, University Hospital of Wales, Heath Park, Cardiff, CF14 4XW, Wales, UK
[c] Department of Primary Care and Population Health, University College London Medical School (Royal Free Campus), Rowland Hill Street, London, NW3 2PF, UK
* Corresponding author.
E-mail addresses: BasraMK@cardiff.ac.uk; PiguetV@cardiff.ac.uk

Dermatol Clin 30 (2012) 237–244
doi:10.1016/j.det.2011.11.002

used dermatology-specific QOL measure in clinical trials of skin diseases.[3,4] The DLQI has been used in more than 36 skin diseases (inflammatory, noninflammatory, and skin cancers) in more than 32 countries and is available in more than 55 international language versions.[5] The DLQI has been shown to be easy to use in clinical practice because of its simplicity and brevity,[6] with an average completion time of approximately 2 minutes.[7] It consists of 10 questions concerning dermatologic patients' perception of the impact of skin diseases on different aspects of their QOL over the last week. The items of the DLQI encompass aspects such as symptoms and feelings, daily activities, leisure, work or school, personal relationships, and the side effects of treatment. Each item is scored on a 4-point scale: not at all/not relevant, a little, a lot, and very much. Scores of individual items (0–3) are added to yield a total score (0–30); higher scores mean greater impairment of a patient's QOL. In 2005, Hongbo and colleagues[8] introduced the much needed banding of the DLQI scores to facilitate the clinical interpretation of scores. According to this banding system, a DLQI score of 0 and 1 means no impact on a patient's QOL whereas a score of 2 to 5, 6 to 10, 11 to 20, and 21 to 30 indicates a small, moderate, large, and an extremely large effect on patient's QOL, respectively. Psychometrically, the DLQI has been shown to be a strong instrument regarding its internal consistency, reproducibility, validity,[6,9,10] and sensitivity to change.[11] The DLQI has been used in descriptive and evaluative studies in various countries,[5] and has also been incorporated into various treatment guidelines[12] as well as cost-of-illness[13] and cost-effectiveness analysis studies.[14,15]

This nonsystematic review gives an overview of the use of the DLQI as an outcome in clinical research and Health Technology Assessment in psoriasis and chronic hand eczema (CHE) with particular emphasis on determining the severity of these 2 conditions based on DLQI scores.

LITERATURE SEARCH STRATEGY

The review involved a comprehensive search of literature in electronic databases, including Ovid, MEDLINE, EMBASE, PubMed, Google Scholar, and the Cochrane Library, from 1994 to the present using search terms such as quality of life, DLQI, psoriasis, hand dermatitis, and CHE. The references of articles were also hand-searched.

CLINICAL USE OF THE DLQI IN PSORIASIS

Psoriasis is a chronic immune-mediated inflammatory skin disease characterized by scaly red plaques. The incidence of psoriasis in European countries has been estimated to be 1.5% to 2%.[16] This disfiguring skin condition not only significantly affects sufferers' QOL[17,18] but also is associated with loss in productivity[19] and substantial economic burden on society.[20] The impact of psoriasis on patients' lives has been found to be comparable to the impact of many chronic systemic illnesses, such as heart diseases, diabetes, cancer, depression, and chronic respiratory conditions.[21] The latest evidence suggests that psoriasis should be considered a systemic illness because of its frequent association with comorbidities, such as metabolic syndrome, cardiovascular diseases, arthritis, and psychiatric diseases.[22,23]

Conventionally, severity of psoriasis has been based on the magnitude and extent of physical signs and/or total body surface area (BSA) affected, as is reflected by the commonly used objective disease severity tool, Psoriasis Area and Severity Index (PASI).[24] However, PASI and other similar objective tools do not capture the actual severity of the disease from the patients' perspective and the impact on their lives that may be much greater than the visible severity measured by these tools.[25] Nevertheless, because of the unavailability of a universal tool that could assess the impact on patients based on both physical severity and QOL impairment, the PASI has become the most widely used disease severity outcome measure in clinical trials.

Introduction of the "rule of tens" was an effort to define the concept of psoriasis severity in relationship to QOL in simple terms.[26] According to this rule, psoriasis should be considered severe if a patient's DLQI score or BSA or PASI is more than 10. These 3 parameters have also been used to define the treatment goals for psoriasis therapy in clinical trials. A DLQI score of 0 or 1 has been suggested as a treatment goal after 10 to 16 weeks of antipsoriasis therapy, whereas a DLQI score reduction of at least 5 points (the minimal clinically important difference of the DLQI) is required to demonstrate the minimum efficacy achieved by the therapy.[27] Similarly, the British Association of Dermatologists (BAD) has defined the treatment response as a minimum of a 5-point reduction in the DLQI scores along with 50% PASI reduction.[12] Although in a review of randomized controlled trials of biologics the improvement in the DLQI scores was shown to be paralleled by a similar PASI improvement,[28] the DLQI may be better than PASI at capturing information regarding treatment benefit from patients' perspective and should therefore be given more weight.[27,29]

Based on the rule of tens definition of severe psoriasis, a DLQI score of more than 10 has been adopted as an essential eligibility criterion in both

Table 1
BAD guidelines for biologics in psoriasis

	Criteria	Other	Assessment of Response (wk)	Criteria for Adequate Response
Infliximab	Severe plaque psoriasis PASI ≥10 and DLQI >10	At least one of 1. Phototherapy/ standard systemics[a]	14 (license)	PASI 75 from baseline or PASI 50 and 5-point reduction in DLQI
Etanercept	Severe plaque psoriasis PASI ≥10 and DLQI >10	contraindicated or risk of toxicity 2. Intolerance of standard systemics	12	PASI 75 from baseline or PASI 50 and 5-point reduction in DLQI
Adalimumab	Severe plaque psoriasis PASI ≥10 and DLQI >10	3. Unresponsive to standard systemics 4. Comorbidity precluding	16	PASI 75 from baseline or PASI 50 and 5-point reduction in DLQI
Ustekinumab	Severe plaque psoriasis PASI ≥10 and DLQI >10	systemic use 5. Severe, unstable, life-threatening disease	28 (license)	PASI 75 from baseline or PASI 50 and 5-point reduction in DLQI

[a] Cyclosporine (2.5 mg/kg once daily; up to 5 mg/kg once daily); and in men, and women not at risk of pregnancy, methotrexate (single dose [oral, subcutaneous intramuscular] of 15 mg weekly; maximum 25 mg weekly) and acitretin (25–50 mg daily).

the BAD (**Table 1**) and National Institute for Health and Clinical Excellence (NICE, **Table 2**) guidelines for biological intervention of psoriasis.[12,30] Although the BAD guidelines require a minimum DLQI score of more than 10 consistently for all licensed biologics, the NICE guidelines for infliximab require a DLQI score of more than 18 (and PASI of 20 or more) and more than 10 for the rest of licensed biologics. The guidelines for biological intervention in some other countries such as Italy have similar criteria to those in the BAD guidelines.[31] According to the European Dermatology Expert Group, which has given recommendations for the use of etanercept for psoriasis, moderate

Table 2
NICE guidance for biologics in psoriasis

	Criteria	Other	Assessment of Response (wk)	Criteria for Adequate Response
Infliximab	Very severe plaque psoriasis PASI ≥20 and DLQI >18	Failure to respond/ intolerant of/ contraindication to standard systemic therapies[a]	10	PASI 75 from baseline or PASI 50 and 5-point reduction in DLQI
Etanercept	Severe plaque psoriasis PASI ≥10 and DLQI >10		12	PASI 75 from baseline or PASI 50 and 5-point reduction in DLQI
Adalimumab	Severe plaque psoriasis PASI ≥10 and DLQI >10		16	PASI 75 from baseline or PASI 50 and 5-point reduction in DLQI
Ustekinumab	Severe plaque psoriasis PASI ≥10 and DLQI >10		16	PASI 75 from baseline or PASI 50 and 5-point reduction in DLQI

[a] Cyclosporine, methotrexate, or psoralen UV-A.

to severe psoriasis has been defined by a PASI of 10 or a BSA of 10, or a DLQI score of 10.[32]

CLINICAL USE OF THE DLQI IN CHE

CHE is a debilitating condition affecting up to 15% of northern Europeans at some point during their lifetime, and 0.5% to 0.7% of the population are severely affected.[33,34] It can be psychologically distressing, disfiguring, and also has considerable social stigma attached. CHE may be detrimental to patients' QOL and may significantly affect sick leave and employment prospects of patients.[33]

The DLQI has been used to evaluate the impact of CHE on the QOL of patients and to assess correlation with other measures establishing the validity of the DLQI in CHE.[35] Agner and colleagues[36] found a median DLQI score of 8 in patients with hand eczema, and there was a significant correlation with disease severity measured by the Hand Eczema Severity Index (P<.001). Cvetkovski and colleagues[37] found a mean DLQI score of 7.8 in Danish patients with severe disease, and there was a clear correlation with the severity of hand eczema. However, a Dutch study (mean DLQI score = 9.7) suggested a lack of correlation with patient-scored severity and clinical severity scores in this context.[38] An analysis of 100 patients with occupational hand dermatitis suggested that additional generic tools such as the 36-Item Short-Form Health Survey may be better at detecting the impact on mental health and gender differences.[39] Furthermore, high DLQI scores were associated with prolonged sick leave and unemployment in patients with occupational hand eczema.[37]

Most of the studies in CHE using the DLQI are epidemiologic, and the only major drug study that has used the tool was a phase II trial looking at oral alitretinoin.[40] A total of 319 patients unresponsive to at least 4 weeks of topical steroids and with moderate to severe CHE were randomized to 3 different doses of alitretinoin or placebo, of which only 51.4% of patients in both treatment and placebo groups completed DLQI questionnaires. Median change in score from baseline was −3 for the alitretinoin group (doses of 20 and 40 mg) and −2 in the placebo group. The reduction was not statistically significant, possibly because of the lack of statistical power in the study.[41] A subsequent analysis based on these data showed that DLQI scores were significantly different by Physicians Global Assessment (PGA) group (ie, 15.1 for PGA severe and 1.7 for PGA clear/almost clear in this sample, on average). These scores were used to impute the EuroQoL-5D (EQ-5D) for each PGA group and inform the economic analysis in a later single-technology appraisal of alitretinoin (**Table 3**).[41]

From the phase II alitretinoin trial, the side effects of the drug did not seem to affect the QOL because the treated patients had greater reduction in DLQI score, yet reported more adverse effects (53% in the 40-mg group, 35% in the placebo group).[40] However, the DLQI score reduction did not reach significance, and the side effects were only presented if complained of by more than 3% of the patients in any group.

HEALTH ECONOMIC USE OF DLQI IN HEALTH TECHNOLOGY APPRAISAL OF NEW DERMATOLOGY TREATMENTS

Provision of evidence on the effects of health care treatments on the QOL is gaining importance. The view of the regulatory agencies in indicating the

Table 3
From PGA to DLQI and utility in CHE patients

PGA	Change in DLQI from PGA Severe	P Value	95% Confidence Interval	DLQI[a]	Utility[b]
Severe	0	<.0001	(12.20, 17.96)	15.08	0.582
Moderate	−5.3	<.0001	(−7.86, −2.73)	9.78	0.713
Mild	−9.15	<.0001	(−11.92, −6.37)	5.93	0.809
Almost clear	−12.03	<.0001	(−14.67, −9.40)	1.74	0.913
Clear	−14.65	<.0001	(−18.01, −11.30)		

An analysis of data for 162 patients (Freemantle et al,[42] 2009/Ruzicka et al,[40] 2004) was performed, using a generalized mixed model, including treatment group and PGA score at 3 months as fixed effects, with investigational center included as a random effect.
  [a] Baseline DLQI score (Intercept value): 15.08 (P<.0001, 95% confidence interval 12.20, 17.96). Test of overall PGA effect: degrees of freedom = 4 denominator degrees of freedom = 126. F-statistic = 30.88, P<.0001.
  [b] DLQI scores were converted into EQ-5D scores using the following algorithm: EQ-5D utility score = 0.956 − (0.0248 × DLQI Total Score) (Woolacott et al,[43] 2006).

importance of patient-reported outcomes (PROs), and the response from industry in using QOL measures, such as the DLQI, is entirely logical. In the United Kingdom the NICE has developed a framework for the evaluation of the relative cost-effectiveness of different treatments based on notional threshold values of the cost per quality-adjusted life-year (QALY).[44] The basic principles involve the comparison of the costs and benefits (as measured by QALYs) of different treatment options, which usually involves the comparison of a new treatment with the existing standard of care. For the evaluation of alitretinoin in the treatment of severe hand eczema, the comparison with standard care presented particular problems because the research evidence for the alternative therapies was limited and there was no comparative evidence.[41] There was also no direct estimation of the effects of alitretinoin to derive a health utility index necessary to calculate a QALY. Health utility is a measure with a maximum of 1 (for optimal health status), in which the value of 0 is equivalent to the status of death, and negative values (for states judged to be less preferable than death) are possible. Generic instruments, such as the EQ-5D,[45] are frequently used to elicit health utilities directly from the population in clinical trials, but unfortunately no such measure was used in the phase II trial of alitretinoin.[40]

To overcome the limitation of direct elicitation of health utility from the trials, a published algorithm was used to translate results from the DLQI to health utilities using longitudinal data from the alitretinoin phase II trial.[40] Deriving health utilities for the NICE model was based on 2 stages: the analysis of phase II data to gain association between PGA and DLQI, and the application of the mapping equation used to calculate EQ-5D based on the data on psoriasis.[43] The results of this mapping process are described in **Table 3**. Thus, a subject with severe PGA has an estimated DLQI of 15.1 and a health utility index of 0.582. If that health utility index was to be maintained for 1 year, the subject would accrue 0.582 QALY. This analysis furnished an estimate of the cost per QALY of alitretinoin compared with best supportive care of approximately £13,000, and suggested that alitretinoin was both less costly and more effective than psoralen UV-A and cyclosporine.[41] While noting the indirect estimation of health utility through the DLQI, the NICE Appraisal Committee judged that the economic case had been made for the use of alitretinoin in patients with a DLQI of 15 or more.[41] corresponding to the score of patients with severe PGA in the phase II trial sample.

Although arguably the best that can be done with the available data, the approach is open to some criticism. Psoriasis is usually considered a more serious condition because it is so obvious, well publicized, and can be on the whole body. Consistent with this view, the utility gain of 0.33 in the alitretinoin NICE submission was not initially accepted by the committee. However, despite the potential uncertainties of the method, the utility gains were ultimately accepted through a process of consultation with stakeholders, which may have been influenced by patient testimony. There seemed to be an acceptance that not only did skin disease on the hands have a disproportionate effect on QOL because of the link with manual dexterity, ability to work, and so forth, but also clearance of skin is a far more relevant outcome for patients than partial improvement, which may be achievable on other treatments.

DISCUSSION

Psoriasis and CHE are skin conditions that have a profound detrimental effect on the QOL of those affected. Apart from the physical symptoms, the impact of psoriasis on QOL seems to be dominated by the disfigurement caused, which is manifested in terms of psychological distress.[46] By contrast, CHE seems to affect more directly an individual's ability to work and his or her productivity, with difficulty in pursuing normal daily activities, frequent sick leave, and even job loss in some instances.[47,48] This problem implies that these aspects should be given proper emphasis when measuring the overall severity and impact of these skin conditions from the patient's perspective, which may be achieved by combining the traditional QOL measures such as the DLQI with relevant measures of psychological status and/or utility measures.

The clinical severity of skin disease and psoriasis in particular does not always correlate with the impact on patients' QOL assessed by, for example, the DLQI.[49,50] Similarly, the correlation between BSA affected in psoriasis and the DLQI scores has been found to be low.[51] Moreover, the DLQI scores and not the severity of psoriasis has been shown to be associated with loss of work productivity,[52] disadvantages for employment, and greater use of health care resources.[51] In the case of CHE the location of lesions seems particularly relevant, and hand involvement in contact dermatitis was found to be the key predictor of high DLQI scores.[48] CHE is also one example in which a strong association could be seen between high degree of severity of hand eczema and low QOL using the DLQI.[36,37]

Despite the widespread use of the DLQI, it is important to realize that a generic dermatology-specific QOL measure such as the DLQI may not be sufficient to capture the unique constellation of specific skin conditions such as CHE. For example, the number of work impairment–related items in the DLQI is underrepresented. Moreover, some items may become redundant in CHE, for example, choice of clothes item. This fact is well demonstrated in studies of CHE in which a score of DLQI even for severe hand disease has been less than 10. For example, in a Danish study the mean DLQI for all CHE patients was found to be 5.5 and only 7.8 for severe disease.[37] Regarding psoriasis, a DLQI score in the same range as for severe CHE (ie, 7.8) as found in this study would not be considered severe disease unless it was more than 10.[26] This result implies that the degree of QOL impairment measured by the DLQI for different skin conditions such as psoriasis versus CHE may not be an accurate representation of the magnitude of actual QOL impairment caused by these individual conditions. Ideally, to have a comprehensive assessment of QOL impairment caused by CHE, a CHE-specific measure should be used as an adjunct to the DLQI.

In contrast to psoriasis, with extensive evidence of its impact on patients' QOL, there is a paucity of literature regarding the impact of CHE on QOL especially using the DLQI. Correspondingly, the amount of data on clinical efficacy of different treatments used regarding the improvement in patients' QOL and health state utilities is much more extensive for psoriasis in comparison with the very limited evidence for CHE treatments. This gap in the literature has the potential to adversely affect the way treatment guidelines are formulated.

With the advent of expensive drugs in dermatology such as biologics, there is more pressure on the pharmaceutical industry to demonstrate efficacy and cost effectiveness. Efficacy may be demonstrated by improvement in both the severity of disease and patients' QOL. Cost effectiveness may be measured in terms of direct cost reduction (eg, reduced hospital stays, shorter duration of treatment) and indirectly by improvement in patients' QOL and enhanced productivity (eg, time off work). Although several studies have been performed to assess the cost effectiveness of various psoriasis treatments, especially biologics,[14,15,53] there are limited data on cost effectiveness of treatments used in CHE and, in particular, for alitretinoin.[41,54] Because of the lack of adequate evidence and in particular preference-based QOL data, the cost-effectiveness analysis in the recent NICE single-technology appraisal for the use of alitretinoin in CHE had to rely on a mapping exercise to link the DLQI to the EQ-5D.[41] This technique has also been used in other studies to convert the DLQI values to EQ-5D utility weights using an algorithm for cost-effectiveness analysis of biologics in psoriasis.[43] However, it should be noted that utility estimates from these mapping exercises have yet to be validated against empirically derived utilities.

Developing economic models, particularly in areas where there has been relatively little pharmacologic development in recent years for comparator treatments, can often involve making the best of the data that are available. Mapping approaches are used commonly to overcome missing data but are clearly less useful than direct elicitation of QOL in relevant randomized trials. Health policy makers are in the difficult position of having to come to concrete decisions regarding reimbursement for health technologies with incomplete information. This situation can lead to specific judgments (such as the DLQI severity criteria used by NICE for alitretinoin compared with biologics for psoriasis) in which the limited methods available are used to try and achieve access to treatment in patients for whom it should prove worthwhile and cost effective, while avoiding excess resource consumption by limiting use in subjects for whom the outcome is less likely to be cost effective.

SUMMARY

Both psoriasis and CHE can have a significant, yet distinct impact on patients' QOL. The use of QOL measures such as the DLQI in addition to disease severity measures in clinical trials has greatly influenced the way guidelines have been developed for various treatments used in these 2 common skin conditions. Incorporating generic QOL instruments into these trials to measure utility would facilitate economic appraisal, widen the influence of eventual guidelines to the overall health care system, and better inform value judgments about how limited health care resources should be allocated between competing disease areas. Moreover, to avoid methodological controversies and the use of different formulations of the cost-effectiveness and cost-utility models by health economists and analysts, clinical trials should be conducted with the aim of presenting results in a standard format to facilitate comparison.

ACKNOWLEDGMENTS

Writing support and coordination were provided by Elizabeth Balman (WG Consulting Healthcare Ltd).

REFERENCES

1. Patrick DL, Burke LB, Powers JH, et al. Patient-reported outcomes to support medical product

labeling claims: FDA perspective. Value Health 2007;10(Suppl 2):s125–37.

2. Finlay AY, Khan GK. Dermatology Life Quality Index (DLQI)—a simple practical measure for routine clinical use. Clin Exp Dermatol 1994;19:210–6.

3. Both H, Essink-Bot ML, Busschbach J, et al. Critical review of generic and dermatology-specific health-related quality of life instruments. J Invest Dermatol 2007;127:2726–39.

4. Le Cleach L, Chassany O, Levy A, et al. Poor reporting of quality of life outcomes in dermatology randomized controlled clinical trials. Dermatology 2008;216:46–55.

5. Basra MK, Fenech R, Gatt RM, et al. The Dermatology Life Quality Index 1994-2007: a comprehensive review of validation data and clinical results. Br J Dermatol 2008;159:997–1035.

6. Bronsard V, Paul C, Prey S, et al. What are the best outcome measures for assessing quality of life in plaque type psoriasis? A systematic review of the literature. J Eur Acad Dermatol Venereol 2010; 24(Suppl 2):17–22.

7. Loo WJ, Diba VC, Chawla M, et al. Dermatology Life Quality Index: influence of an illustrated version. Br J Dermatol 2003;148:279–84.

8. Hongbo Y, Thomas CL, Harrison MA, et al. Translating the science of quality of life into practice: what do Dermatology Life Quality Index scores mean? J Invest Dermatol 2005;125:659–64.

9. Badia X, Mascaro JM, Lozano R. Measuring health-related quality of life in patients with mild to moderate eczema and psoriasis: clinical validity, reliability and sensitivity to change of the DLQI. Br J Dermatol 1999;141:698–702.

10. Hahn HB, Catherine A, Melfi CA, et al. Use of the Dermatology Life Quality Index (DLQI) in a midwestern US urban clinic. J Am Acad Dermatol 2001;45: 44–8.

11. Mazzotti E, Picardi A, Sampogna F, et al. Sensitivity of the Dermatology Life Quality Index to clinical change in patients with psoriasis. Br J Dermatol 2003;149:318–22.

12. Smith CH, Anstey AV, Barker JN, et al. British Association of Dermatologists' guidelines for biologic interventions for psoriasis 2009. Br J Dermatol 2009;161:987–1019.

13. Colombo G, Altomare G, Peris K, et al. Moderate and severe plaque psoriasis: cost-of-illness study in Italy. Ther Clin Risk Manag 2008;4:559–68.

14. Heinen-Kammerer T, Daiel D, Stratmann L, et al. Cost-effectiveness of psoriasis therapy with etanercept in Germany. J Dtsch Dermatol Ges 2007;5:762–9.

15. Nelson AA, Pearce DJ, Fleischer AB, et al. Cost-effectiveness of biologic treatments for psoriasis based on subjective and objective efficacy measures assessed over a 12-week treatment period. J Am Acad Dermatol 2008;58:125–35.

16. Nevitt GJ, Hutchinson PE. Psoriasis in the community: prevalence, severity and patients' beliefs and attitudes towards the disease. Br J Dermatol 1996;135:533–7.

17. Choi J, Koo JY. Quality of life issues in psoriasis. J Am Acad Dermatol 2003;49:S57–61.

18. Krueger G, Koo J, Lebwohl M, et al. The impact of psoriasis on quality of life: results of a 1998 Psoriasis Foundation patient-membership survey. Arch Dermatol 2001;137:280–4.

19. Schoffski O, Augustin M, Prinz J, et al. Costs and quality of life in patients with moderate to severe plaque-type psoriasis in Germany: a multi-center study. J Dtsch Dermatol Ges 2007;5:209–18.

20. Fowler JF, Duh MS, Rovba L, et al. The impact of psoriasis on health care costs and patient work loss. J Am Acad Dermatol 2008;59:772–80.

21. Rapp SR, Feldman SR, Exum ML, et al. Psoriasis causes as much disability as other major medical diseases. J Am Acad Dermatol 1999;41:401–7.

22. Augustin M, Reich K, Glaeske G, et al. Comorbidity and age-related prevalence of psoriasis—analysis of health insurance data in Germany. Acta Derm Venereol 2010;90:147–51.

23. Davidovici BB, Sattar N, Jörg PC, et al. Psoriasis and systemic inflammatory diseases: potential mechanistic links between skin disease and comorbid conditions. J Invest Dermatol 2010; 130:1785–96.

24. Fredriksson T, Pettersson U. Severe psoriasis—oral therapy with a new retinoid. Dermatologica 1978; 157:238–44.

25. Heydendael VM, de Borgie CA, Spuls PI, et al. The burden of psoriasis is not determined by disease severity only. J Investig Dermatol Symp Proc 2004; 9:131–5.

26. Finlay AY. Current severe psoriasis and the rule of tens. Br J Dermatol 2005;152:861–7.

27. Reich K, Mrowietz U. Treatment goals in psoriasis. J Dtsch Dermatol Ges 2007;5:566–74.

28. Katugampola RP, Lewis VJ, Finlay AY. The Dermatology Life Quality Index: assessing the efficacy of biological therapies for psoriasis. Br J Dermatol 2007;156:945–50.

29. Feldman SR, Gordon KB, Bala M, et al. Infliximab treatment results in significant improvement in the quality of life of patients with severe psoriasis: a double-blind placebo-controlled trial. Br J Dermatol 2005;152:954–60.

30. NICE. National Institute for Health and Clinical Excellence: full guidance on adalimumab for the treatment of psoriasis. TA146. London (UK): National Institute for Health and Clinical Excellence; 2008. Available at: www.nice.org.uk/TA146. Accessed November 18, 2011.

31. Marchesoni A, Altomare G, Matucci-Cerinic M, et al. An Italian shared dermatological and rheumatological proposal for the use of biological agents in

psoriatic disease. J Eur Acad Dermatol Venereol 2010;24:578–86.

32. Boehncke WH, Brasie RA, Barker J, et al. Recommendations for the use of etanercept in psoriasis: a European Dermatology Expert Group consensus. J Eur Acad Dermatol Venereol 2006;20:988–98.

33. Thyssen JP, Johansen JD, Linneberg A, et al. The epidemiology of hand eczema in the general population—prevalence and main findings. Contact Dermatitis 2010;62(2):75–87.

34. Diepgen TL, Agner T, Aberer W, et al. Management of chronic hand eczema. Contact Dermatitis 2007; 57:203–10.

35. Reilly MC, Lavin PT, Kahler KH, et al. Validation of the Dermatology Life Quality Index and the Work Productivity and Activity Impairment—chronic hand dermatitis questionnaire in chronic hand dermatitis. J Am Acad Dermatol 2003;48:128–30.

36. Agner T, Anderson KE, Brandao FM, et al. Hand eczema severity and quality of life: a cross-sectional, multicentre study of hand eczema patients. Contact Dermatitis 2008;59:43–7.

37. Cvetkovski RS, Zachariae R, Jensen H, et al. Quality of life and depression in a population of occupational hand eczema patients. Contact Dermatitis 2006;54:106–11.

38. van Coevorden AM, van Sonderen E, Bouma J, et al. Assessment of severity of hand eczema: discrepancies between patient and physician related scores. Br J Dermatol 2006;155:1217–22.

39. Wallenhammar LM, Nufjall M, Lindberg M, et al. Health-related quality of life and hand eczema— a comparison of two instruments, including factor analysis. J Invest Dermatol 2004;122:1381–9.

40. Ruzicka T, Larsen FG, Galewicz D, et al. Oral alitretinoin (9-cis-retinoic acid) therapy for chronic hand dermatitis in patients refractory to standard therapy. Arch Dermatol 2004;140:1453–9.

41. Rodgers M, Griffin S, Paulden M, et al. Alitretinoin for severe chronic hand eczema: a NICE single technology appraisal. Pharmacoeconomics 2010;28: 351–62.

42. Freemantle N, Aldridge R, Stanley G. Quality of life in chronic hand eczema as measured by the Dermatology Life Quality Index. Poster presented at the 12th Annual European Congress of the International Society for Pharmacoeconomic and Outcomes Research. Paris (France), October 24–27, 2009. [Abstract published in Value Health 2009:12(7): A459.]

43. Woolacott N, Hawkins N, Mason A, et al. Etanercept and efalizumab for the treatment of psoriasis: a systematic review. Health Technol Assess 2006;10:1–233.

44. NICE. Available at: http://www.nice.org.uk/media/419/27/EPMethodsGuidePublicConsultation.pdf. Accessed July 02, 2011.

45. EuroQoL group. EuroQoL—a new facility for the measurement of health-related quality of life. Health Policy 1990;16:199–208.

46. Ramsey B, O'Reagan M. A survey of the social and psychological effects of psoriasis. Br J Dermatol 1988;188:195–201.

47. Cvetkovski RS, Rothman KG, Olsen J, et al. Relation between diagnosis on severity, sick leave and loss of job among patients with occupational hand eczema. Br J Dermatol 2005;152:93–8.

48. Holness DL. Results of a quality of life questionnaire in a patch test clinic population. Contact Dermatitis 2001;44:80–4.

49. Jayaprakasam A, Darvay A, Osborne G, et al. Comparison of assessments of severity and quality of life in cutaneous disease. Clin Exp Dermatol 2002;27:306–8.

50. Sampogna F, Sera F, Abeni D. Measures of clinical severity, quality of life and psychological distress in patients with psoriasis: a cluster analysis. J Invest Dermatol 2004;122:602–7.

51. Sato R, Milligan G, Molta C, et al. Health-related quality of life and healthcare resource use in European patients with plaque psoriasis: an association independent of observed disease severity. Clin Exp Dermatol 2010;36:24–8.

52. Schmitt JM, Ford DE. Work limitations and productivity loss are associated with health-related quality of life but not with clinical severity in patients with psoriasis. Dermatology 2006;213:102–10.

53. Lloyd A, Reeves P, Conway P, et al. Economic evaluation of etanercept in the management of chronic plaque psoriasis. Br J Dermatol 2009; 160:380–6.

54. Blank PR, Blank AA, Szucs T. Cost-effectiveness of oral alitretinoin in patients with severe chronic hand eczema—a long term analysis from a Swiss perspective. BMC Dermatol 2010;10:4.

Health-Related Quality of Life in Patients with Melanoma: Overview of Instruments and Outcomes

Janice N. Cormier, MD, MPH*, Kate D. Cromwell, MS,
Merrick I. Ross, MD

KEYWORDS

- Health-related quality of life • Melanoma
- Quality-of-life instruments • Patient-reported outcomes

Quality of life (QOL) has increasingly been recognized as an important patient-reported outcome measure that can facilitate patient-doctor communication, reveal symptoms that should be addressed, and influence medical decision making. QOL is a multidimensional construct encompassing physical, functional, emotional, and social and family well-being.[1] Physical well-being, in this context, refers to symptoms related to disease (eg, pain, nausea, and fatigue) and the side effects of treatment. Functional well-being refers to an individual's ability to perform activities of daily living (eg, walking, bathing, and dressing oneself) and perform one's societal role. Emotional well-being refers to coping ability and reflects the experience of feelings ranging from enjoyment to distress. Social and family well-being reflects the quality of relationships with family and friends as well as the degree of a measure of social interaction.[2] This article focuses on health-related QOL, which is a component of overall QOL. To simplify terminology, QOL is used to mean health-related QOL throughout the rest of this article.

Longitudinal assessment of QOL can provide essential information on the impact of a disease and its treatment.[3] In several studies, QOL has been demonstrated to be an independent predictor of survival and response to therapy in patients with cancer.[4–8] In a study on patients with melanoma, baseline QOL was a predictor of survival in patients with advanced melanoma who received chemotherapy.[5] In a study on patients with metastatic melanoma, patients who were optimistic about their expected survival or who minimized the impact of cancer on their daily lives were found to live longer.[9] Evaluation of QOL outcomes may also facilitate clinical decision making when differences between the survival expectations associated with the various treatment options are anticipated to be modest.[10,11]

Many QOL instruments exist and have been used in patients with cancer. These instruments are generally classified using 3 categories: generic, disease specific, and symptom or event specific.[12–19] Most QOL instruments include items or questions inquiring about both symptoms and function.[20] Despite an increase in the incidence of melanoma, studies examining QOL in patients with melanoma are uncommon in the literature.[21] This review examines the body of literature pertaining to the assessment of QOL in patients with melanoma regarding the various instruments used and the melanoma-specific findings. An

Department of Surgical Oncology, Unit 444, The University of Texas MD Anderson Cancer Center, 1400 Holcombe Boulevard, Houston, TX 77030-4009, USA
* Corresponding author.
E-mail address: jcormier@mdanderson.org

Dermatol Clin 30 (2012) 245–254
doi:10.1016/j.det.2011.11.011

QOL INSTRUMENTS
Generic Instruments

Generic QOL instruments are general health measures used in a wide variety of clinical settings and diseases, which allow for comparison of scores across a variety of different illnesses.[21,22] One of the most widely used generic QOL instruments is the Medical Outcome Study Short-Form Health Survey (SF-36),[15,23] which is reviewed elsewhere in this issue. The SF-36 is the most commonly administered generic QOL instrument and has been used in more than 1000 studies to date.[15,23–33] As a result, typical SF-36 scores have been established for a variety of medical conditions and permit valuable comparisons of QOL across diseases. There are no cancer-specific items,[34] and in the application of the SF-36 to melanoma several interesting findings have been elucidated, which are detailed subsequently in the systematic review.

Disease-Specific Instruments

Disease-specific instruments include items that focus on specific symptoms frequently associated with particular illnesses; these instruments can be very specific (eg, for melanoma) or more general (eg, cancer specific or skin disease specific).

Cancer-specific instruments
Several cancer-specific instruments have been shown to be more sensitive and responsive measures of QOL than generic QOL instruments in patients with cancer; several cancer-specific instruments have been developed for various anatomic sites and types of malignancy. The Functional Assessment of Cancer Therapy Scale—General (FACT-G) and the European Organization for Research and Treatment of Cancer Quality of Life Questionnaire (EORTC QLQ-C30) are 2 of the most widely used cancer-specific QOL measures. The FACT-G is a 33-item questionnaire that was validated in a 4-phase trial involving patients and oncologists.[35] This instrument evaluates physical, functional, social, and emotional well-being as well as the patient-doctor relationship, and takes an average of 5 minutes to complete. Scores obtained from the FACT-G can vary according to tumor stage.[36] The EORTC-QLQ-C30 includes items pertaining to general, physical, and psychological health, and the ability to complete normal activities of daily living.[37] The first generation of this instrument was developed in 1987 and modified in 1993 with a reduction in the number of items from 36 to 30; the EORTC-QLQ-C30 has a reported completion time of 10 to 12 minutes.[16]

Melanoma-specific instruments
Patients with cancer experience disease-related issues that often affect their QOL, similar to patients with most other chronic conditions, which questions the applicability of generic QOL measures for patients with cancer in clinical trials or investigative settings, because generic instruments may not be responsive to QOL changes specific to cancer.[22] In response to this problem, cancer site–specific or tumor-specific QOL instruments have been developed and are widely used for most malignancies, including breast cancer, colon cancer, and lung cancer.[10,38,39]

An identified lack of melanoma-specific QOL instruments led to the development of melanoma-based modules for both the FACT-G[36] and the EORTC-QLQ-C30.[16] These instruments have been validated in patients with melanoma and have been shown to be responsive and sensitive to change.[37,40–43] The melanoma module for the FACT-G has been developed and validated as an independent tool and an add-on to the FACT-G; when the FACT-G and the melanoma module are administered together, they constitute the FACT-M. The FACT-M has been shown to be responsive and sensitive in patients with melanoma at all stages of disease.[12,44] The melanoma module consists of 16 items related to melanoma and an additional 8 items pertaining to the surgical treatment of melanoma.[21] These items fall within the domains of physical, social, and emotional well-being.[12] The melanoma module of the EORTC-QLQ-C30 is designed for patients only with advanced (stage IV) melanoma. This module consists of 13 items and evaluates disease-specific symptoms related to disease treatment and progression (Table 1).[41]

Skin disease–specific instruments
Several instruments have been developed for the assessment of QOL in patients with a variety of dermatologic conditions. These include Skindex and the Dermatology Life Quality Index (DLQI) (Table 2). Skindex was created to capture skin-related emotional, symptom, and functional issues,[13] and has been applied to quantify the differences in QOL between immediately before and after dermatologic surgery. Skindex has multiple versions that range from 16 to 61 items.[13,45,46] The 29-item Skindex has been used in patients with melanoma and other skin malignancies more often than in patients with other skin conditions. The DLQI has 10 items.[32] In addition to being shorter than the Skindex, the DLQI has a family version that is used to

Table 1
Reported QOL outcomes in patients with melanoma from studies using cancer-specific QOL instruments

Instrument	Description	Cronbach Alpha	Test-Retest Reliability	Melanoma-Specific Findings
FACT-G	33 items Designed for all types of malignancies	0.89[36]	0.92[36]	Treatment influences QOL[37] Fatigue is the most common symptom during treatment[69]
EORTC-QLQ-C30	30 items 5 functional scales: physical, role, cognitive, social, and emotional 3 symptom scales: fatigue, pain, nausea and vomiting	0.54–0.86[16]	NA	Decreases in QOL correlate with increases in physical symptoms[41] Survey not sensitive to variations in QOL based on different course of treatment[43] Amount of supportive care received correlates with QOL[41] Complete lymph node dissection associated with lower QOL than sentinel lymph node biopsy[40] Emotional functioning, fatigue and insomnia, and overall global health status decline during diagnostic process and treatment[80]

Abbreviation: NA, not available.

assess the effect of the dermatologic condition of interest on other family members.[14] This measure has most commonly been used in patients with non-metastatic skin cancer or other benign dermatologic diseases, such as eczema or psoriasis.[47]

Symptom Assessment Tools

A wide variety of symptom assessment tools have been developed; these are also called state-specific QOL measures. Symptom assessment tools have been designed to evaluate the event-specific impact of a symptom on a patient's reported QOL. Symptom assessment instruments are beneficial in identifying specific symptoms rather than assessing overall QOL.[48] In some circumstances, identifying the most relevant symptom to be assessed may be challenging, and certain symptom assessment tools may not indicate distress when a patient is experiencing other adverse symptoms. Symptom assessments may only be valuable in certain clinical settings or used in combination with additional instruments; instrument choice is critical in accurately assessing QOL.[49]

Two of the most widely used cancer-related symptom assessment tools are the MD Anderson Symptom Inventory (MDASI) and the Memorial

Table 2
Reported QOL outcomes in patients with melanoma from studies using skin-specific QOL instruments

Instrument	Description	Cronbach Alpha	Test-Retest Reliability	Melanoma-Specific Findings
Skindex	61 items; also shorter versions with 36, 29, and 17 items 3 domains: emotional, social, and appearance	0.76–0.86[13]	0.68–0.90[13]	Reported outcomes influenced by cytokine patterns[71]
DLQI	10 items Impact of chronic skin diseases[14] Family version available that measures impact of the skin disease on patient's family	0.92[81]	0.95[14]	Follow-up schedule does not affect QOL[70]

Symptom Assessment Scale (MSAC). The MDASI is a 19-item measure that evaluates symptoms, such as pain, fatigue, lack of appetite, and other symptoms that interfere with activities of daily living.[50] The MSAC evaluates physical and psychological symptoms and has been shown to be a predictor of survival.[51,52] Although the use of these 2 instruments has not been documented in patients with melanoma, they are widely used as symptom assessment tools in other types of cancer.

Symptom assessment tools that have been used in published studies of patients with melanoma include the Horowitz Impact of Event Scale, the Hospital Anxiety and Depression Scale, Ways of Coping Checklist, Brief Symptom Inventory, and the Rotterdam Symptom Checklist **(Table 3)**.[34,53,54] The Horowitz Impact of Event Scale measures the postevent stress response to clinically significant events, such as a cancer diagnosis.[54] The Hospital Anxiety and Depression Scale quantifies inpatient anxiety or depression in nonpalliative cancer settings.[19] The Ways of Coping Checklist is designed to evaluate various methods commonly used for coping with a significant illness.[34] The Brief Symptom Inventory was designed to evaluate the psychological symptom status of patients in both psychiatric and more general medical settings.[17] Unlike other symptom inventories, the Brief Symptom Inventory is designed to measure several dimensions of psychological distress and may be a valuable tool for use in diagnostic settings.[55] The Rotterdam Symptom Checklist is a 38-item checklist that assesses psychological measures, activities of daily living, and primary symptoms of illness.[56] This checklist has been proved to be valid in multiple oncologic settings.[24,57–60]

METHODS

To assess the current body of published literature specifically related to the assessment of QOL in patients with melanoma, a systematic literature search was performed. Several databases (MEDLINE, Current Contents [which includes databases including Clinical Medicine, Social and Behavioral Sciences, Health, and Psychosocial Instruments], Cancerlit, and the Cochrane Library) were examined for articles published from 1966 through 2011 using the following search terms: quality of life, melanoma, psychosocial, well-being, and health-related quality of life. The bibliographies in identified articles were also reviewed to identify other potentially relevant articles. Articles were selected from the following criteria: (1) written in English, (2) at least 20% of patients in the study

population had a diagnosis of melanoma, and (3) measures of QOL were the primary or secondary outcomes of the study. All types of studies were considered, including clinical trials (randomized or nonrandomized), prospective cohort studies, and cross-sectional studies. Publications were excluded if study results could not be obtained from the abstract or the article. The QOL instruments used in the study were classified as generic, disease specific (ie, cancer, melanoma, or skin disease), or symptom assessment. The findings related to melanoma were abstracted and summarized.

MELANOMA-SPECIFIC FINDINGS
Generic Instruments

Generic instruments were the most commonly used QOL assessment tool in the studies of patients with melanoma.[21] Results of studies using the SF-36 indicate that gender, age, and comorbidity had the highest association with the physical and mental components of the survey, when used on patients with melanoma.[30,61] These studies found that patients with melanoma reported overall QOL better than that of patients with congestive heart failure and about equal to that of patients with renal cell carcinoma.[26] Patients with melanoma had medium to high distress, and this distress improved if patients received a cognitive-behavioral intervention.[62] The distress among patients with local and regional disease (stages I–III) was positively correlated with state and trait anxiety, escape-avoidance coping, and accepting-responsibility coping; there was no variation of distress by gender or disease stage.[34] Gender was a significant predictor of QOL: women reported lower overall QOL than men.[63] In addition, patients in a phase I trial who reported strong social support at treatment initiation reported lower distress and higher mental health 1 month into treatment.[64] SF-36 scores have also been shown to be associated with treatment; for example, patients who underwent more extensive operations reported lower overall QOL scores.[31] In addition, SF-36 scores have been shown to provide important information pertaining to postmelanoma surveillance; patients show similar anxiety whether follow-up appointments are scheduled with a general practitioner or an oncologist.[65]

Cancer-Specific Instruments

In studies using cancer-specific instruments, QOL scores for patients with melanoma have been reported to be similar to those of a general population of healthy adults.[66] The EORTC-QLQ-C30 was found to be sensitive to changes in QOL during the

Table 3
Reported QOL outcomes in patients with melanoma from studies using symptom assessment tools

Instrument	Description	Cronbach Alpha	Test-Retest Reliability	Melanoma-Specific Findings
Horowitz Impact of Event Scale	15 items Assesses posttraumatic stress related to significant events such as a cancer diagnosis[54]	0.86[82]	0.87[82]	Diagnosis and progression shown to produce acute and long-term posttraumatic response in patients and families[53]
Hospital Anxiety and Depression Scale	14 items Assesses anxiety and depression[54]	0.86–0.89[83]	0.86–0.91[84]	Higher anxiety than depression reported for hospitalized cancer-related surgery[61] Correlates with out-of-hospital QOL[41,61,72] Performs best in nonpalliative cancer settings[19]
Ways of Coping Checklist	66 items 8 scales (confrontive coping, distancing, self-control, seeking social support, accepting responsibility, escape avoidance, problem solving, positive reappraisal) Measures coping and if coping mechanisms increase distress[34]	NA	NA	High active coping and low depressive coping were predictors of perceived support for patients in regular melanoma follow-up[85] Social support was the strongest health-enhancing factor[73] Women had more psychological symptoms and coping methods[73]
Brief Symptom Inventory	53 items Measures emotional distress	0.75–0.89[86]	0.90[17]	Significant levels of distress noted with significant variability in findings (29% reported moderate to high levels)[34]
Rotterdam Symptom Checklist	38 items 3 sections: psychological, medical, and activities of daily living[87]	0.89[60]	NA	Psychological or physical well-being were not associated with melanoma survival[74] Most common symptoms included worrying, fatigue, lethargy, and muscle soreness[73]

Abbreviation: NA, not available.

course of chemotherapy treatment of melanoma.[33] Decreased EORTC-QLQ-C30 scores represent a decline in health status before and during treatment with certain agents (fotemustine) but not with other agents (dacarbazine).[67] When used alone, the EORTC-QLQ-C30 did not discriminate among the stages of disease[16] but was sensitive to changes throughout the course of melanoma treatment.[68] Patients with melanoma commonly indicated that fatigue was the most significant symptom during the course of their treatment.[69] Few studies have been published using the FACT-G alone in patients with melanoma. In one report, FACT-G scores reflected the type of treatment, which influenced patient-reported QOL.[37]

Melanoma-Specific Instruments

The FACT-M has been shown to distinguish between disease stages: there is a significant decline in QOL scores between patients with early-stage melanoma and patients with advanced (stages III or IV) melanoma (see **Table 1**).[12,21] In addition, use of this instrument revealed that patients with early stages of disease were often more concerned with the cosmetic aspects of treatment, whereas patients with more advanced disease were focused on the mortality and morbidity (such as lymphedema) associated with treatment.[12]

Among patients with distant metastatic melanoma, the melanoma module of the EORTC-QLQ-C30 showed that the ability to complete activities of daily living deteriorated over the first 9 weeks of treatment and continued to decline throughout the course of treatment.[41] The most commonly reported dysfunction among patients with advanced-stage disease undergoing chemotherapy was decline in neurologic sensory function, and as treatment progressed, more patients reported significant pain during rest, movement, or both.[41]

Skin-Specific Instruments

The DLQI and the Skindex are widely used in patients with nonmelanoma skin cancer but have been used in only a few studies of patients with melanoma (see **Table 2**). In patients with melanoma, both instruments have been shown to be valuable for quantifying the effect of illness on physical appearance and body image. Studies using the DLQI have indicated that women have a lower QOL immediately after surgery but a greater improvement in QOL over time. The DLQI has also been administered to evaluate the impact of postmelanoma surveillance, which reportedly did not influence QOL.[70] Studies with the Skindex have indicated that QOL outcomes may be influenced by cytokine patterns.[71]

Symptom Assessment Instruments

Melanoma-specific findings in studies that used symptom assessment tools are summarized in **Table 3**. In studies of patients with melanoma to whom the State-Trait Anxiety Inventory Checklist measure was administered, the findings indicated that patients with melanoma did not present with significant anxiety during the diagnostic process.[34] Melanoma-specific findings from assessments using the Hospital Anxiety and Depression Scale have shown that patients have more anxiety than depression when hospitalized for cancer-related surgery.[61] In addition, scores from the Hospital Anxiety and Depression Scale have been found to correlate with QOL when a patient is out of the hospital.[41,61,72]

In patients with melanoma evaluated with the Ways of Coping Checklist, social support has been identified as the most health-enhancing component of the coping process.[73] When used to measure QOL among patients with melanoma, this instrument has shown that there are significant differences in coping methods according to gender.[73]

The psychological and physical subscale scores of the Rotterdam Symptom Checklist have not been predictive of postmelanoma survival.[74] When the Rotterdam Symptom Checklist is administered across several research protocols involving patients with melanoma, the most commonly identified symptoms were fatigue, lethargy, and muscle soreness.[73]

The Brief Symptom Inventory demonstrates wide variability in distress among patients with melanoma with non–stage IV disease.[34] However, one of the primary disadvantages of the Brief Symptom Inventory is the significant respondent burden due to the high number of items, which often results in patient frustration and missing data.[75]

Patients with melanoma and their families assessed with the Horowitz Impact of Event Scale were shown to have both acute and long-term posttraumatic stress responses to their diagnosis and progression of disease.[53]

SUMMARY

Despite the increasing burden of melanoma as a public health problem, there have been few studies examining QOL in patients with melanoma. QOL is generally evaluated regarding several domains, most commonly including physical, social, functional, emotional, and social well-being.[1] The assessment of QOL is critical, particularly in oncology trials, because self-assessed QOL has been demonstrated to be an independent predictor of survival among patients with various types of cancer.[4,6,76,77] In addition, QOL outcomes may be of primary concern regarding clinical decision making in clinical trials where survival differences are modest.[10,11] A wide variety of QOL instruments are available, many of which have been used to assess patients with melanoma.[24] In addition to generic and cancer-specific QOL instruments, skin disease–specific instruments have been used to quantify changes during the course of melanoma diagnosis, treatment, and surveillance.[33,41,47,54,66,71,73,74]

Given that overall QOL assessment requires information about multiple psychosocial domains, QOL research often uses a combination of instruments that are administered longitudinally.[32] Longitudinal analysis of QOL is important because in many patients, QOL fluctuates throughout the course of the disease.[20] The results of these longitudinal assessments indicating changes over time may be most meaningful in helping patients and clinicians make treatment decisions and conduct effective disease management.[24] In selecting the proper instruments for QOL assessment, it is important to consider the burden for the respondent; longer instruments may be biased by patient fatigue or missing responses.[78]

It is often difficult to capture disease-specific issues even with the administration of a combination of instruments. For example, in patients with melanoma, issues such as lymphedema and postsurgical scarring would not likely be assessed with most available QOL instruments.[21] The FACT-M was developed to address melanoma-specific issues related to QOL for patients with all stages of melanoma.

Physicians should select QOL instruments based on the specific QOL outcome they wish to measure and the anticipated outcomes. It is critical to review the full QOL questionnaire to ensure that the items are appropriate for the setting intended. Physicians should also be aware of the length of the questionnaire and the burden on the respondents, who must complete the questionnaire repeatedly.[21] Given that QOL is an important component of overall health and a predictor of postmelanoma survival, routine clinical assessment of QOL should be considered for all patients undergoing treatment.[9,79]

ACKNOWLEDGMENTS

The authors would like to acknowledge Stephanie Deming for her editorial assistance.

REFERENCES

1. Cella DF, Tulsky DS. Quality of life in cancer: definition, purpose, and method of measurement. Cancer Invest 1993;11(3):327–36.
2. Cella D, Nowinski CJ. Measuring quality of life in chronic illness: the functional assessment of chronic illness therapy measurement system. Arch Phys Med Rehabil 2002;83(12 Suppl 2):S10–7.
3. Langenhoff BS, Krabbe PF, Wobbes T, et al. Quality of life as an outcome measure in surgical oncology. Br J Surg 2001;88(5):643–52.
4. Coates A, Gebski V, Signorini D, et al. Prognostic value of quality-of-life scores during chemotherapy for advanced breast cancer. Australian New Zealand Breast Cancer Trials Group. J Clin Oncol 1992;10(12):1833–8.
5. Coates A, Thomson D, McLeod GR, et al. Prognostic value of quality of life scores in a trial of chemotherapy with or without interferon in patients with metastatic malignant melanoma. Eur J Cancer 1993;29(12):1731–4.
6. Roychowdhury DF, Hayden A, Liepa AM. Health-related quality-of-life parameters as independent prognostic factors in advanced or metastatic bladder cancer. J Clin Oncol 2003;21(4):673–8.
7. Maisey NR, Norman A, Watson M, et al. Baseline quality of life predicts survival in patients with advanced colorectal cancer. Eur J Cancer 2002; 38(10):1351–7.
8. Jerkeman M, Kaasa S, Hjermstad M, et al. Health-related quality of life and its potential prognostic implications in patients with aggressive lymphoma: a Nordic Lymphoma Group Trial. Med Oncol 2001; 18(1):85–94.
9. Butow PN, Coates AS, Dunn SM. Psychosocial predictors of survival in metastatic melanoma. J Clin Oncol 1999;17(7):2256–63.
10. Brady MJ, Cella DF, Mo F, et al. Reliability and validity of the functional assessment of cancer therapy-breast quality-of-life instrument. J Clin Oncol 1997; 15(3):974–86.
11. Yellen SB, Cella DF, Webster K, et al. Measuring fatigue and other anemia-related symptoms with the Functional Assessment of Cancer Therapy (FACT) measurement system. J Pain Symptom Manage 1997;13(2):63–74.
12. Cormier JN, Ross MI, Gershenwald JE, et al. Prospective assessment of the reliability, validity, and sensitivity to change of the Functional Assessment of Cancer Therapy-Melanoma questionnaire. Cancer 2008; 112(10):2249–57.
13. Chen M, Lasek R, Quinn L, et al. Skindex, a quality-of-life measure for patients with skin disease: reliability, validity and responsiveness. J Invest Dermatol 1996;107(5):707–13.
14. Finlay AY, Khan GK. Dermatology Life Quality Index (DLQI)—a simple practical measure for routine clinical use. Clin Exp Dermatol 1994;19(3):210–6.
15. McHorney CA, Ware JE Jr, Lu JF, et al. The MOS 36-item Short-Form Health Survey (SF-36): III. Tests of data quality, scaling assumptions, and reliability across diverse patient groups. Med Care 1994; 32(1):40–66.
16. Aaronson NK, Ahmedzai S, Bergman B, et al. The European Organization for Research and Treatment of Cancer QLQ-C30: a quality-of-life instrument for use in international clinical trials in oncology. J Natl Cancer Inst 1993;85(5):365–76.
17. Derogatis LR, Meliasaratos N. The Brief Symptom Inventory: an introductory report. Psychol Med 1983;13(3):595–605.
18. Sundin EC, Horowitz MJ. Horowitz's Impact of Event Scale evaluation of 20 years of use. Psychosom Med 2003;65(5):870–6.
19. Mitchell AJ, Meader N, Symonds P. Diagnostic validity of the Hospital Anxiety and Depression Scale (HADS) in cancer and palliative settings: a meta-analysis. J Affect Disord 2010;126(3):335–48.

20. Lipscomb J, Gotay CC, Snyder C. Outcomes assessment in cancer. New York: Cambridge University Press; 2005.

21. Cormier JN, Askew RL. Assessment of patient-reported outcomes in patients with melanoma. Surg Oncol Clin N Am 2011;20(1):201–13.

22. Sprangers MA. Quality-of-life assessment in oncology. Achievements and challenges. Acta Oncol 2002; 41(3):229–37.

23. McHorney CA, Ware JE Jr, Raczek AE. The MOS 36-Item Short-Form Health Survey (SF-36): II. Psychometric and clinical tests of validity in measuring physical and mental health constructs. Med Care 1993;31(3):247–63.

24. Cornish D, Holterhues C, van de Poll-Franse LV, et al. A systematic review of health-related quality of life in cutaneous melanoma. Ann Oncol 2009; 20(Suppl 6):vi51–8.

25. Ware JE Jr. SF-36 health survey update. Spine (Phila Pa 1976) 2000;25(24):3130–9.

26. Cohen L, Parker PA, Sterner J, et al. Quality of life in patients with malignant melanoma participating in a phase I trial of an autologous tumour-derived vaccine. Melanoma Res 2002;12(5):505–11.

27. Melia BM, Moy CS, McCaffrey L. Quality of life in patients with choroidal melanoma: a pilot study. Ophthalmic Epidemiol 1999;6(1):19–28.

28. Mols F, Holterhues C, Nijsten T, et al. Personality is associated with health status and impact of cancer among melanoma survivors. Eur J Cancer 2010; 46(3):573–80.

29. Kendall AR, Mahue-Giangreco M, Carpenter CL, et al. Influence of exercise activity on quality of life in long-term breast cancer survivors. Qual Life Res 2005;14(2):361–71.

30. Holterhues C, Cornish D, van de Poll-Franse LV, et al. Impact of melanoma on patients' lives among 562 survivors: a Dutch population-based study. Arch Dermatol 2011;147(2):177–85.

31. Noorda EM, van Kreij RH, Vrouenraets BC, et al. The health-related quality of life of long-term survivors of melanoma treated with isolated limb perfusion. Eur J Surg Oncol 2007;33(6):776–82.

32. Both H, Essink-Bot ML, Busschbach J, et al. Critical review of generic and dermatology-specific health-related quality of life instruments. J Invest Dermatol 2007;127(12):2726–39.

33. Cashin RP, Lui P, Machado M, et al. Advanced cutaneous malignant melanoma: a systematic review of economic and quality-of-life studies. Value Health 2008;11(2):259–71.

34. Trask PC, Paterson AG, Hayasaka S, et al. Psychosocial characteristics of individuals with non-stage IV melanoma. J Clin Oncol 2001; 19(11):2844–50.

35. Fallowfield L. Quality of life: a new perspective for cancer patients. Nat Rev Cancer 2002;2(11):873–9.

36. Cella DF, Tulsky DS, Gray G, et al. The Functional Assessment of Cancer Therapy Scale: development and validation of the general measure. J Clin Oncol 1993;11(3):570–9.

37. Rataj D, Jankowiak B, Krajewska-Kulak E, et al. Quality-of-life evaluation in an interferon therapy after radical surgery in cutaneous melanoma patients. Cancer Nurs 2005;28(3):172–8.

38. Cella DF, Bonomi AE, Lloyd SR, et al. Reliability and validity of the Functional Assessment of Cancer Therapy-Lung (FACT-L) quality of life instrument. Lung Cancer 1995;12(3):199–220.

39. Ward WL, Hahn EA, Mo F, et al. Reliability and validity of the Functional Assessment of Cancer Therapy-Colorectal (FACT-C) quality of life instrument. Qual Life Res 1999;8(3):181–95.

40. de Vries M, Hoekstra HJ, Hoekstra-Weebers JE. Quality of life after axillary or groin sentinel lymph node biopsy, with or without completion lymph node dissection, in patients with cutaneous melanoma. Ann Surg Oncol 2009;16(10):2840–7.

41. Sigurdardottir V, Bolund C, Sullivan M. Quality of life evaluation by the EORTC questionnaire technique in patients with generalized malignant melanoma on chemotherapy. Acta Oncol 1996;35(2):149–58.

42. Sigurdardottir V, Brandberg Y, Sullivan M. Criterion-based validation of the EORTC QLQ-C36 in advanced melanoma: the CIPS questionnaire and proxy raters. Qual Life Res 1996;5(3):375–86.

43. Young AM, Marsden J, Goodman A, et al. Prospective randomized comparison of dacarbazine (DTIC) versus DTIC plus interferon-alpha (IFN-alpha) in metastatic melanoma. Clin Oncol (R Coll Radiol) 2001;13(6):458–65.

44. Cormier JN, Davidson L, Xing Y, et al. Measuring quality of life in patients with melanoma: development of the FACT-melanoma subscale. J Support Oncol 2005;3(2):139–45.

45. Chren MM, Lasek RJ, Flocke SA, et al. Improved discriminative and evaluative capability of a refined version of Skindex, a quality-of-life instrument for patients with skin diseases. Arch Dermatol 1997; 133(11):1433.

46. Chren MM, Lasek RJ, Sahay AP, et al. Measurement properties of Skindex-16: a brief quality-of-life measure for patients with skin diseases. J Cutan Med Surg 2001;5(2):105–10.

47. Burdon-Jones D, Thomas P, Baker R. Quality of life issues in nonmetastatic skin cancer. Br J Dermatol 2010;162(1):147–51.

48. Kirkova J, Davis MP, Walsh D, et al. Cancer symptom assessment instruments: a systematic review. J Clin Oncol 2006;24(9):1459–73.

49. Osoba D. A taxonomy of the uses of health-related quality-of-life instruments in cancer care and the clinical meaningfulness of the results. Med Care 2002;40(Suppl 6):III31–8.

50. Cleeland CS, Mendoza TR, Wang XS, et al. Assessing symptom distress in cancer patients: the M.D. Anderson Symptom Inventory. Cancer 2000;89(7): 1634–46.

51. Portenoy RK, Thaler HT, Kornblith AB, et al. The Memorial Symptom Assessment Scale: an instrument for the evaluation of symptom prevalence, characteristics and distress. Eur J Cancer 1994; 30(9):1326–36.

52. Chang VT, Thaler HT, Polyak TA, et al. Quality of life and survival: the role of multidimensional symptom assessment. Cancer 1998;83(1):173–9.

53. Kelly B, Raphael B, Smithers M, et al. Psychological responses to malignant melanoma. An investigation of traumatic stress reactions to life-threatening illness. Gen Hosp Psychiatry 1995;17(2):126–34.

54. Bergenmar M, Mansson-Brahme E, Hansson J, et al. Surgical resection margins do not influence health related quality of life or emotional distress in patients with cutaneous melanoma: results of a prospective randomised trial. Scand J Plast Reconstr Surg Hand Surg 2010;44(3):146–55.

55. Baider L, Kaplan De-Nour A. Psychological distress and intrusive thoughts in cancer patients. J Nerv Ment Dis 1997;185(5):346–8.

56. de Haes JC, van Knippenberg FC, Neijt JP. Measuring psychological and physical distress in cancer patients: structure and application of the Rotterdam Symptom Checklist. Br J Cancer 1990; 62(6):1034–8.

57. Eiser C, Havermans T, Craft A, et al. Validity of the Rotterdam Symptom Checklist in paediatric oncology. Med Pediatr Oncol 1997;28(6):451–4.

58. de Haes JC, Olschewski M. Quality of life assessment in a cross-cultural context: use of the Rotterdam Symptom Checklist in a multinational randomised trial comparing CMF and Zoladex (Goserlin) treatment in early breast cancer. Ann Oncol 1998;9(7):745–50.

59. Tchen N, Soubeyran P, Eghbali H, et al. Quality of life in patients with aggressive non-Hodgkin's lymphoma. Validation of the medical outcomes study short form 20 and the Rotterdam symptom checklist in older patients. Crit Rev Oncol Hematol 2002; 43(3):219–26.

60. Stein KD, Denniston M, Baker F, et al. Validation of a modified Rotterdam Symptom Checklist for use with cancer patients in the United States. J Pain Symptom Manage 2003;26(5):975–89.

61. Newton-Bishop JA, Nolan C, Turner F, et al. A quality-of-life study in high-risk (thickness > = or 2 mm) cutaneous melanoma patients in a randomized trial of 1-cm versus 3-cm surgical excision margins. J Investig Dermatol Symp Proc 2004;9(2): 152–9.

62. Trask PC, Paterson AG, Griffith KA, et al. Cognitive-behavioral intervention for distress in patients with melanoma: comparison with standard medical care and impact on quality of life. Cancer 2003;98(4): 854–64.

63. Baider L, Perry S, Sison A, et al. The role of psychological variables in a group of melanoma patients. An Israeli sample. Psychosomatics 1997; 38(1):45–53.

64. Devine D, Parker PA, Fouladi RT, et al. The association between social support, intrusive thoughts, avoidance, and adjustment following an experimental cancer treatment. Psychooncology 2003; 12(5):453–62.

65. Murchie P, Nicolson MC, Hannaford PC, et al. Patient satisfaction with GP-led melanoma follow-up: a randomised controlled trial. Br J Cancer 2010;102(10): 1447–55.

66. Schlesinger-Raab A, Schubert-Fritschle G, Hein R, et al. Quality of life in localised malignant melanoma. Ann Oncol 2010;21(12):2428–35.

67. Avril MF, Aamdal S, Grob JJ, et al. Fotemustine compared with dacarbazine in patients with disseminated malignant melanoma: a phase III study. J Clin Oncol 2004;22(6):1118–25.

68. Kiebert GM, Jonas DL, Middleton MR. Health-related quality of life in patients with advanced metastatic melanoma: results of a randomized phase III study comparing temozolomide with dacarbazine. Cancer Invest 2003;21(6):821–9.

69. Redeker NS, Lev EL, Ruggiero J. Insomnia, fatigue, anxiety, depression, and quality of life of cancer patients undergoing chemotherapy. Sch Inq Nurs Pract 2000;14(4):275–90 [discussion: 291–8].

70. Schiffner O, Wilde J, Schiffner-Rohe W, et al. Difference between real and perceived power of dermoscopical methods for detection of malignant melanoma. Eur J Dermatol 2003;13(3):288–98.

71. Amerio P, Gambi F, Larlori C, et al. Stress, behaviour and immune function: psychological, psychopathological characteristics and cytokine pattern in melanoma patients. Exp Dermatol 2007;16(4): 347–83.

72. Skarstein J, Aass N, Fossa SD, et al. Anxiety and depression in cancer patients: relation between the Hospital Anxiety and Depression Scale and the European Organization for Research and Treatment of Cancer Core Quality of Life Questionnaire. J Psychosom Res 2000;49(1):27–34.

73. Lehto US, Ojanen M, Kellokumpu-Lehtinen P. Predictors of quality of life in newly diagnosed melanoma and breast cancer patients. Ann Oncol 2005; 16(5):805–16.

74. Lehto US, Ojanen M, Dyba T, et al. Baseline psychosocial predictors of survival in localized melanoma. J Psychosom Res 2007;63(1):9–15.

75. Fayers PM, Hays RD. Assessing quality of life in clinical trials: methods and practice. 2nd edition. New York: Oxford University Press; 2004.

76. Fang FM, Liu YT, Tang Y, et al. Quality of life as a survival predictor for patients with advanced head and neck carcinoma treated with radiotherapy. Cancer 2004;100(2):425–32.

77. Fang FM, Tsai WL, Chiu HC, et al. Quality of life as a survival predictor for esophageal squamous cell carcinoma treated with radiotherapy. Int J Radiat Oncol Biol Phys 2004;58(5):1394–404.

78. Clauser SB, Ganz PA, Lipscomb J, et al. Patient-reported outcomes assessment in cancer trials: evaluating and enhancing the payoff to decision making. J Clin Oncol 2007;25(32):5049–50.

79. Brown JE, Butow PN, Culjak G, et al. Psychosocial predictors of outcome: time to relapse and survival in patients with early stage melanoma. Br J Cancer 2000;83(11):1448–53.

80. Al-Shakhli H, Harcourt D, Kenealy J. Psychological distress surrounding diagnosis of malignant and nonmalignant skin lesions at a pigmented lesion clinic. J Plast Reconstr Aesthet Surg 2006;59(5):479–86.

81. Morgan M, McCreedy R, Simpson J, et al. Dermatology quality of life scales—a measure of the impact of skin diseases. Br J Dermatol 1997;136(2):202–6.

82. Sundin EC, Horowitz MJ. Impact of event scale: psychometric properties. Br J Psychiatry 2002;180: 205–9.

83. Olsson I, Mykletun A, Dahl AA. The Hospital Anxiety and Depression Rating Scale: a cross-sectional study of psychometrics and case finding abilities in general practice. BMC Psychiatry 2005;5:46.

84. Spinhoven P, Ormel J, Sloekers PP, et al. A validation study of the Hospital Anxiety and Depression Scale (HADS) in different groups of Dutch subjects. Psychol Med 1997;27(2):363–70.

85. Sollner W, Zschocke I, Zingg-Schir M, et al. Interactive patterns of social support and individual coping strategies in melanoma patients and their correlations with adjustment to illness. Psychosomatics 1999;40(3):239–50.

86. Boulet J, Boss MW. Reliability and validity of the Brief Symptom Inventory. Psychological Assessment 1991;3:433–7.

87. Moinpour CM, Feigl P, Metch B, et al. Quality of life end points in cancer clinical trials: review and recommendations. J Natl Cancer Inst 1989;81(7): 485–95.

Quality-of-Life Issues in Vitiligo

Sulochana S. Bhandarkar, MD[a],*, Roopal V. Kundu, MD[b]

KEYWORDS

• Vitiligo • Quality of life • Color • Dermatology

Vitiligo, a cutaneous disease prevalent since ancient times, continues to affect millions worldwide.[1] The historical confusion of this disease with leprosy in ancient Indian texts has contributed to the stigmatization associated with vitiligo.[2] Despite the burden of vitiligo and its associated psychosocial comorbidities, it is unfortunately often categorized as a harmless cosmetic disorder. Skin color plays a major role in an individual's perception of health, wealth, worth, and desirability. Pigmentary disfigurements caused by vitiligo can considerably influence social interactions.[1] The authors highlight the significant negative effects vitiligo imposes on different parameters of quality of life (QoL).

EPIDEMIOLOGY

Vitiligo is amongst the most important acquired depigmentation disorders with an average worldwide prevalence of 0.5% to 2.0%,[3] with specific countries, such as India, reporting prevalence rates of up to 4.0% to 8.8%.[4,5] The disease can develop at any age; however, in half of all individuals with vitiligo, onset occurs between the ages of 10 and 30 years.[6] A positive family history is present in 7.7% to 50.0% of patients.[5] The mean age of onset tends to be earlier in those with a positive family history.

SKIN TYPE

Although vitiligo equally affects people across all races and ethnicities, there is generally a more negative impact on QoL with darker skin types.

However, this is not universally true. Porter and Beuf[7] administered questionnaires focused on patient's emotional reaction toward vitiligo; they distributed the Coopersmith Self-Esteem Inventory tool and stigmatization questionnaire among 158 subjects with vitiligo, 60% white and 40% black. Blacks and whites did not differ in degree of disturbance by the disorder.

Research from different countries indirectly helps to better understand the implications of skin phototype and ethnicity on vitiligo. Most of these studies originate from Western countries and the Middle East, with surprisingly fewer from India where vitiligo was once considered 1 of the top 3 major medical problems in India.[4]

QoL research from Western European countries such as the Netherlands indicate that subjects with darker skin types (skin type IV–VI) showed more health-related QoL (HRQL) impairment using a generic QoL measuring tool (36-Item Dutch Short form [SF-36]) and a dermatology-specific HRQL tool (Skindex-29) compared with their lighter-skinned counterparts. Linthorst Homan and colleagues[1] reported that most individuals with an impaired QoL were immigrants, originally from Suriname, India, Morocco, Turkey, Curacao, Indonesia, China, or Afghanistan, who generally have darker skin types. The Netherlands Institute for Pigmented Disorders also reported on subjects with universal vitiligo (a rare type of extensive generalized vitiligo with more than 80% body surface area [BSA] depigmentation) or generalized vitiligo (the most common form of vitiligo characterized by symmetric widespread distribution of depigmented macules) again using the

a Department of Dermatology, School of Medicine, Emory University, 1315 Clifton Road, Atlanta, GA 30322, USA
b Department of Dermatology, Northwestern Center for Ethnic Skin, Feinberg School of Medicine, Northwestern University, 676 North Saint Clair Street, Suite 1600, Chicago, IL 60611, USA
* Corresponding author.
E-mail address: ssbhand@emory.edu

Dermatol Clin 30 (2012) 255–268
doi:10.1016/j.det.2011.11.013
0733-8635/12/$ – see front matter © 2012 Elsevier Inc. All rights reserved.

SF-36 and the Skindex-29. A greater number of individuals with skin phototype I to III with both generalized and universal vitiligo were included than those with skin phototype IV to VI. Statistically significant poorer physical QoL (physical function and bodily pain) was demonstrated in subjects with universal vitiligo when compared with age- and sex-matched subjects with generalized vitiligo.[8] These studies emphasize that several different parameters, such as ethnicity, skin phototype, and extent of disease involvement, can predict negative effects of vitiligo on QoL. A study from Italy including 181 subjects with vitiligo (80% skin type III, 13% skin type II, and 7% skin type IV) showed higher prevalence of probable depression or anxiety (39%) and alexithymia (24%) than the general population (10%). These subjects also had many HRQL problems such as worry of the disease getting worse (60%), anger (37%), embarrassment (34%), feeling depressed (31%), having social life affected (28%), and shame (28%).[3]

Kruger and colleagues[9] enrolled 71 vitiligo subjects, with the majority being skin type III (N = 55), 4 with skin type II, 8 with skin type V, and 2 with skin type IV and VI. The mean Dermatology Quality and Life Index (DLQI) was 7.8 compared with a mean DLQI of 10.67 in a study originating from India that included data from 141 subjects with vitiligo.[10] Although skin types were not specified, it has been suggested that most were likely of darker phenotype (IV–VI).[4] Studies from the Middle East also with a population predominantly of darker phenotypes show similar results. Dolatshahi and colleagues[11] reported significantly higher mean DLQI scores in individuals with skin type V (20.67) than in those with skin type II (5.21), III (8.34), and IV (8.07).

Surprisingly few studies have evaluated QoL in vitiligo in a diverse population with varying skin types as in the United States. A study on pigmentary disorders and their impact on QoL included 140 subjects out of which only 1 had vitiligo.[12] Multiple reviews written on vitiligo discuss the devastating psychosocial consequences on skin of color subjects[13] and try to incorporate psychological intervention in treatment.[14] A disease-specific HRQL instrument for vitiligo is currently being developed.[15] During validation of this instrument, several factors were found to be associated with worse HRQL: female gender, having dark brown or black hair, being single, and self-identifying as Asian. Moreover, age, number of areas of the body affected, and skin type all directly correlated with HRQL (Kundu, personal observation, 2011).

These studies indicate that subjects with darker phenotype have a relative worse HRQL impairment, but subjects with lighter phenotype are still negatively affected.

AGE

About 50% of affected individuals develop vitiligo before age 20 years, although some studies show that vitiligo can have a bimodal age of onset, with children developing the disease between the ages of 1 and 10 years and adults between 20 and 50 years.[1] Childhood, particularly adolescence, is characterized by rapid psychological and social development, coupled with emotional vulnerability. Negative experiences due to disfiguring diseases such as vitiligo can affect childhood psychological and emotional development.[16] Studies have also shown that stress can be related to vitiligo onset and exacerbation in up to 57% of children.[17] It has been shown that negative experiences from childhood vitiligo seem to be associated with HRQL impairment in young adults with vitiligo.[16] A study from Istanbul, Turkey,[17] showed that vitiligo relates to severity of depression in children, and location of vitiligo on legs, genitals, and arms had a negative effect on HRQL in adolescents as measured by the Pediatric Quality of Life inventory (PedsQL), parent (PedsQL-P) and child (PedsQL-C) versions. This study concluded that location of lesions is a significant factor that leads to HRQL impairment, probably because of its effects on identity development.

MARITAL STATUS

The effect of marital status on vitiligo has not been extensively studied and varies according to country of origin probably because of difference in social norms. A unique study from China[18] focused exclusively on marital QoL in 101 subjects with vitiligo compared with 126 controls. The DLQI and SF-36 tools, along with the ENRICH (Evaluating and Nurturing Relationship Issues, Communication and Happiness) tool, were used. The ENRICH provides scores for spousal evaluation of marital relationship in 12 categories (only 9 selected for this study), with higher scores indicating more positive outcome. Subjects with vitiligo showed statistically significant worse and less stable relationships compared with controls in many categories: satisfaction (33.87 vs 36.83, $P = .003$), personality issues (32.54 vs 35.59, $P<.001$), communication (32.67 vs 34.69, $P = .020$), leisure activity (31.67 vs 33.70, $P<.001$), sexual relationship (32.02 vs 34.56, $P<.001$), family and friends (33.93 vs 35.85, $P = .004$), and egalitarian roles (30.73 vs 32.24, $P = .037$).

Most other studies that comment on marital status originate in the Middle East. A study comparing DLQI amongst married and single subjects in Iran showed married subjects had a higher (greater QoL impact) DLQI (9.22) than single subjects (6.91). This is one of the few studies that showed a significant relationship between mean DLQI score and marital status ($P = .033$).[11] Further analyses of the data showed that the higher DLQI scores were mainly in married women than in single women.[11] This finding was proposed to be influenced by a unique law that supports Iranian men to be able to file for divorce without any alimony if their wives did not disclose their vitiligo before marriage. Another study performed in Iran using the modified Persian version of DLQI also found a significant ($P = .002$) higher HRQL impairment in married subjects.[19] In contrast to these studies, a study performed in Saudi Arabia showed that married subjects had less HRQL impairment than single subjects,[20] which was proposed to be because of the inherent stability and security of marriage in this local culture.

LOCATION OF VITILIGO: EXPOSED VERSUS UNEXPOSED

Several studies have some conclusive evidence regarding anatomic location of vitiligo and its effect on HRQL, whereas few others state no difference. The UK-based Vitiligo Society questionnaire study,[18,21] which had 520 respondents, showed that in 80% vitiligo affected hands and in 76% the face was affected. These respondents considered hand and face vitiligo to be most disfiguring. Of those with vitiligo, 58.6% also described that genital skin (generally considered unexposed skin) was affected, and this was associated with fear because it was mistakenly believed to be associated with sexually transmitted disease and cancer. Sampogna and colleagues[3] reported that subjects with vitiligo patches on the feet, legs, and arms had worse HRQL than those with no localization on those body parts using the Skindex-29. In contrast, presence of localization of vitiligo on hands and genitalia did not seem to affect HRQL.

A large questionnaire-based study of 1023 subjects with vitiligo using DLQI along with a generic HRQL questionnaire (Nondisease-Specific European Quality of Life tool [EuroQoL]) showed significantly worse HRQL in those with visible lesions ($P<.001$).[6] A study performed to study DLQI scores based on location of disease (face/head/neck, hands, arms, trunk, genital area, legs, and feet) showed that vitiligo on face/head/neck substantially affects the DLQI,

independent of extent of disease.[22] In a study of children (8–18 years old) with vitiligo, there were mixed results. Involvement of genitals (classically unexposed) and feet (exposed) had a negative effect on HRQL, and this difference was more noted in girls. In contrast, localization of lesions on the head/face/neck (exposed) gave relatively better HRQL scores for girls (PedsQL-C total $Z = -2.18$) but worse scores for boys (PedsQL-C total $Z = -2.58$) using pediatric-specific QoL tools.[17]

Several studies have showed no association of worsening HRQL and location of vitiligo patches. An Iranian study of 100 subjects with vitiligo showed no statistical association between visibility of lesions and DLQI ($P = .486$),[11] although 90% of their respondents had lesions on exposed areas of their body. A study involving 119 subjects with vitiligo[23] had grouped body site location as uncovered: head, face, neck, and hands; seasonally uncovered: arms, legs, and feet; and occasionally uncovered: trunk and genitals. Although no association between body sites grouped and DLQI was found, they noted a significant association with number of locations and increasing DLQI score ($P<.001$).

GENDER

Vitiligo affects men and women equally, although some studies suggest that women have more adverse effects on HRQL than their male counterparts.[1] This trend in women is in line with the greater psychosocial impact found in various other dermatologic conditions such as psoriasis, atopic dermatitis, and urticaria.[24] Furthermore, in some geographic regions, women have been found to have higher cosmetic concerns than men.[1] In the Indian culture, vitiligo in women can have severe social consequences, even affecting their ability to find a partner.[4] However, a study from India shows that despite women with vitiligo facing graver social consequences, vitiligo can negatively affect men on the same scale as women.[10] In certain Muslim regions of the world, women with vitiligo tend to be more negatively affected in their general and psychological health than men.[25] Other studies suggest that men can be just as affected as women,[26] although there is usually less HRQL impairment in men.[3] A study from Iran[25] as well as Saudi Arabia[20] shows significantly less QoL issues in men than women, and this could be explained based on cultural and religious differences in these countries, but another study also from Iran using the Persian version of DLQI found no difference in HRQL in men and women with vitiligo.[19]

Although most studies in Western countries do not show a gender difference in HRQL impairment,[26,27] there are a few that show similar results as from the Middle East. Studies from Germany showed higher DLQI scores in women (7.5) than men (5.5),[6] and those from Belgium showed similar higher DLQI scores in women (6.45) than men (3.13).[23] Studies from the Netherlands[1] and Italy[3] using Skindex-29 showed that women reported more emotional problems and higher mean scores than men.

CURRENT TOOLS FOR MEASUREMENT OF QoL IN VITILIGO

There are several generic instruments and dermatology-specific HRQL tools that have been used in vitiligo. Generic instruments to measure HRQL are useful in comparing impact among different diseases, but disease-specific instruments are more sensitive to disease-specific issues. This is an unmet need in vitiligo, although a vitiligo-specific instrument to measure HRQL is currently being developed and validated (**Table 1**).[15]

Dermatology-Specific QoL Tools

DLQI
Finlay and Khan[28] are credited with developing the first instrument, the DLQI (see article elsewhere in this issue), to measure the effects of dermatologic conditions on the quality of patients' lives, as described in greater detail in the overview article by Kini and colleagues in this compendium. The investigators demonstrated that this tool can be used to assess levels of disability and thereby help with targeting interventions. Six dimensions are included: symptoms and feelings, daily activities, leisure, work and school, personal relationships, and treatment. The DLQI score ranges from 0 to 30. The higher the score, the worse the QoL expressed, which has been clinically interpreted in bands of DLQI scores (0–1: no effect on HRQL, 2–5: small effect, 6–10: moderate effect, 11–20: very large effect, and 21–30: extremely large effect). A comprehensive review of DLQI over 13 years published by Basra and colleagues[29] acknowledges that DLQI is one of the most widely used dermatology-specific QoL instruments and has been used for 32 different skin conditions, including vitiligo.

DLQI was first used and validated for vitiligo by Kent and al-Abadie.[27] Kent and al-Abadie[27] compared the DLQI scores with validated tools, such as the 12-Item General Health Questionnaire (GHQ-12) and Rosenberg Self-Esteem Scale, and found concordant results. Their study evaluated 614 subjects with vitiligo who belonged to the UK Vitiligo Society. The mean DLQI was 4.82, with no difference between men and women

or relationship status. Scores correlated with perceived stigma, extent of body involvement, and age. Moreover, this study showed the correlation between DLQI and perceived stigma and poor self-esteem, revealing a role of psychological intervention during treatment.

The DLQI was subsequently used to measure HRQL in subjects with vitiligo across many continents. A study from India conducted by Parsad and colleagues[10] compared DLQI in subjects with vitiligo before (10.67) and after (7.06) successful treatment. Research from European countries, such as France, used the DLQI along with various other tools for psychological assessment: the perceived disease severity scale, the French adaptation of the revised NEO (Neuroticism-Extroversion-Openness) personality inventory, and a French adaptation by Vallieres and Vallerand of the Rosenberg Self-Esteem Scale. These assessments also indicate that vitiligo has a moderate effect on HRQL.[26] Their mean DLQI was 7.17, comparable to that in other European studies. However, the studies demonstrated lower DLQI, indicating better QoL impact, when compared with studies from Iran (8.16)[11] or India (10.67).[9]

In Belgium, Ongenae and colleagues[23] used DLQI to compare vitiligo (4.95) with psoriasis (6.26). Vitiligo caused equally disabling social and emotional consequences as psoriasis. Further research by Ongenae and colleagues[22] showed significant improvement in DLQI from 7.3 before camouflage to 5.9 (P = .006) with use of cosmetic camouflage.

A very interesting and unique study done in Germany used mailed questionnaires and reached 1023 subjects. The investigators used DLQI and EuroQoL (a generic QoL tool) and also included willingness to pay (WTP), which is known to assess burden of disease. They found a statistically significant correlation between WTP and DLQI scores ($P<.0001$). Specifically, subjects who were middle aged, had longer duration of disease, or had a larger affected BSA had a higher WTP.[6]

Modified DLQI
DLQI has been translated into several other languages and used for QoL studies in other dermatologic diseases besides vitiligo.[30,31] However, these translations have also been beneficial to study vitiligo. The Persian version of DLQI was the first such translated tool used for vitiligo that was developed using the forward-backward translation procedure. The validity and reliability of the translated version was studied in 70 Iranian subjects with vitiligo. Similar to other vitiligo studies, the mean DLQI was 7.05. The investigators concluded that the Persian version is a reliable and valid instrument to measure HRQL in Iranian subjects with vitiligo.[19]

The validated Persian version of DLQI was then used by a different group on 83 subjects with vitiligo. Their mean DLQI of 7.4 was slightly higher than the first Persian DLQI study in which higher mean DLQI was seen in women (8.6) than men (5.8).[32]

Tjioe and colleagues[33] modified the original DLQI to suit their retrospective study design and included a few additional questions about general well-being and cosmetic camouflage. Their study had a different scoring pattern, with a score of 1 or 2 indicating an improvement in HRQL, score of 0 implying no change, and a score of −1 or −2 indicating deterioration of HRQL. Their analyzed data from 30 subjects who responded to treatment with narrowband UV-B (NBUVB) phototherapy showed that nearly 70% showed improvement in HRQL after up to 4 years of treatment.

Skindex-29

Chren and colleagues[34,35] developed the Skindex (see article elsewhere in this issue) as a measure of HRQL in patients with skin disease, as detailed in Kini's overview and Chren's Skindex article in this issue. This questionnaire comprised 3 subscales (symptoms, emotions, and functioning) and has 5 response possibilities ranging from "Never" to "All the Time." Scale and global scores are calculated on a 100-point scale, with lower scales indicating a better QoL.

Sampogna and colleagues[36] used Skindex-29 along with GHQ-12 to prove an association between poorer HRQL and psychiatric morbidity with different dermatologic conditions. The GHQ-12 is a self-administered instrument designed to detect minor nonpsychotic psychiatric disorders.[37] This study found more HRQL impairment in symptomatic dermatologic diseases such as psoriasis and dermatitis than in asymptomatic disease such as vitiligo or benign nevi. The same investigator administered the Skindex-29 and GHQ-12 along with the 20-Item Toronto Alexithymia Scale (TAS-20) to 181 subjects with vitiligo.[3] The TAS-20 is a valid and reliable tool used to detect alexithymia (difficulty in recognizing and expressing feelings).[38] Their study showed a prevalence of 39% with probable depression or anxiety and 24% with difficulty in recognizing or expressing feelings, implying that a higher percentage of depression and alexithymia exists among subjects with vitiligo (compared with 10% prevalence of both in the general population), with these subjects also reporting a worse HRQL.

Other versions of Skindex-29

As with the DLQI, the Skindex has been translated into a variety of other languages and used in vitiligo studies. The Korean version of Skindex-29 has been used by Kim and colleagues[39] who compared 133 subjects with vitiligo with 112 subjects with mild dermatologic diseases such as eczematous dermatitis, localized alopecia, warts, nevi, and superficial fungal infections. Although the global Skindex-29 score in subjects with vitiligo (30.7) did not show a statistically significant difference from control subjects (27.4), both the functional (27.8 vs 21.3) and emotional (42.8 vs 32.1) scale scores were significantly higher in female subjects with vitiligo than that in female control subjects. A positive correlation in functional scale was also seen in subjects who had a longer duration of disease or multiple visits to clinics or had tried different therapeutic modalities. Subjects who thought their condition was intractable and those who had a perception of worse severity than as assessed by a physician also had higher Skindex scores on function, emotion, and global scales. The modified translated Korean version of Skindex-29[39] was also used in assessing vitiligo HRQL in Korean adolescents with emphasis on their psychological adaptation using tools such as the Piers-Harris Self-Concept scale (a self-reporting instrument designed to measure the concept of self in children and adolescents), the Center for Epidemiologic Studies Depression scale (a self-rated measurement of depressive symptoms during the previous week), and the Revised Children's Manifest Anxiety Scale (a scale that focuses on anxiety scores as well as subscale scores of worry, oversensitivity, physiologic factors, and concentration).[40] Skindex-29 was modified toward adolescent use by changing item 28 to "My skin condition affects me when going out with boyfriends or girlfriends." Choi and colleagues[40] surveyed 57 adolescent subjects with vitiligo. Worse HRQL was reported by those with facial involvement, longer duration of disease, and prior treatment history and by subjects who perceived their disease as moderate or severe. Overall HRQL had a significant negative correlation with overall self-concept. Popularity, physical appearance, behavior, happiness, and satisfaction correlated highly with impaired HRQL. This study demonstrated that in adolescents functional and emotional HRQL are closely related to subjective assessment of severity, chronicity of disease, and psychiatric morbidity rather than clinical severity of the condition itself.

Other Tools Used to Measure QoL in Subjects with Vitiligo

DLQI and Skindex-29 are the most popular tools used to assess QoL in subjects with vitiligo, but

Table 1
Different dermatology-specific and dermatology-nonspecific tools used to measure HRQL in subjects with vitiligo

Study (PMID)	HRQL Tool	Country of Study	Type of Scale	Scoring Method	Final Score (Mean When Provided)
Linthorst Homan et al,[1] 2009 (19577331)	1. Medical Outcomes Study, SF -36 2. Skindex-29	The Netherlands	1. 36 items, 8 subscales, and 2 summary scores 2. 3 subscales, 5 point scoring system on Likert-type scale	1. Minimum score, 0; maximum score, 100; higher scores = better HRQL 2. 3 subscales: symptoms, emotions, and functioning; 5 response possibilities: never to all the time Minimum score, 0; maximum score, 100; higher score = worse HRQL	1. PCS, 54.0; MCS, 46.3 2. Emotion, 35.9; function, 16.7; symptom, 13.9
Sampogna et al,[3] 2008 (18565189)	Skindex-29	Italy	See ref[1]	See ref[1]	Emotion: 28.7 (men), 41.1 (women); function: 17.3 (men), 24.7 (women)
Radtke et al,[6] 2009 (19298268)	1. DLQI (German version) 2. EuroQOL	Germany	1. 10-item 4-point scale 2. 5 items for first part, visual analog scale for second part	1. Minimum score, 0; maximum score, 30; higher score = worse HRQL 2. For first part, 3-point scale; for visual analog scale: maximum score of 100 and worst imaginable health state with score of 0	1. DLQI: 7.0 2. EuroQoL: 83.6

Study	Instrument	Country	Description	Scoring	Results
Linthorst Homan et al,[8] 2008 (18711089)	1. Modified Skindex-29 (Dutch version) 2. SF-36	The Netherlands	1. See ref[1] 2. See ref[1]	1. See ref[1] 2. See ref[1]	1. Universal, 24.7; generalized, 21.7 2. Universal PCS, 48; generalized PCS, 52.4
Kruger et al,[9] 2011 (21240455)	DLQI	UK and Germany	See ref[6]	See ref[6]	DLQI: 7.8
Parsad et al,[10] 2003 (12588405)	DLQI	India	See ref[6]	No minimum or maximum score reported	DLQI: 10.67
Dolatshahi et al,[11] 2008 (19177700)	DLQI	Iran	See ref[6]	See ref[6]	DLQI: 8.18
Linthorst Homan,[16] 2008 (18717679)	1. Skindex-29 2. SF-36	The Netherlands	1. See ref[1] 2. See ref[1]	1. See ref[1] 2. See ref[1]	1. No mean provided 2. SF-36; PCS: 54.9
Bilgic et al,[17] 2011 (21198786)	Pediatric QoL Inventory, Parent and Child Versions (PedsQL-P and PedsQL-C)	Turkey	2 subscale scores: psychosocial and physical health and a total score	Scored on a 5-point Likert-type scale; higher score = better HRQL	PedsQL-P: 8–12 y: 73.30 13–18 y: 73.48 PedsQL-C: 8–12 y: 78.59 13–18 y: 76.47
Aghaei et al,[19] 2004 (15294022)	Modified DLQI (Persian version)	Iran	See ref[6]	See ref[6]	DLQI: 7.05
Al-Mubarak et al,[20] 2011 (21572679)	Validated Arabic questionnaire	Saudi Arabia	41 questions, 4 scales	Higher score = worse HRQL	Score: 17.1
Ongenae et al,[22] 2005 (15942213)	DLQI	Belgium	See ref[6]	See ref[6]	DLQI: 6.9
Ongenae et al,[23] 2005 (15948977)	DLQI	Belgium	See ref[6]	See ref[6]	DLQI: 4.95
Borimnejad et al,[25] 2006 (16860271)	Modified DLQI (Persian version)	Iran	17-item 4-point scale	1. Very much 2. A lot 3. A little 4. Not at all Minimum score: 17; maximum score: 68	Modified DLQI (men): 51.6; modified DLQI (women): 42.9
Kostopoulou,[26] 2009 (19298280)	DLQI (French version)	France	See ref[6]	See ref[6]	DLQI: 7.17

(continued on next page)

Table 1
(continued)

Study (PMID)	HRQL Tool	Country of Study	Type of Scale	Scoring Method	Final Score (Mean When Provided)
Kent G & al-Abadie,[27] 1996 (9136149)	DLQI	UK	12-item 4-point scale	Minimum score, 0; maximum score, 36; higher score = worse HRQL.	DLQI: 4.82
Mashayekhi,[32] 2010 (20827019)	Modified DLQI (Persian version)	Iran	See ref[6]	See ref[6]	DLQI: 7.54
Kim do et al,[39] 2009 (19500179)	Modified Skindex-29 (Korean version)	Korea	See ref[1]	See ref[1]	Emotion, 42.8; function score, 27.8; symptom, 18.4
Choi et al,[40] 2010 (19807826)	Modified Skindex-29 (Korean version)	Korea	See ref[1]	See ref[1]	Emotion, 29.5; function, 18.6; symptom, 16.3
Hartmann et al,[47] 2008 (18779885)	DLQI	Germany	10 items, along with 2 additional items	See ref[6]	DLQI: 12.4
Agarwal et al,[48] 2005 (16029343)	DLQI	India	See ref[6]	See ref[6]	DLQI: 4
van Geel et al,[51] 2006 (16778422)	DLQI	Belgium	See ref[6]	See ref[6]	DLQI: 6.95
Sahni et al,[52] 2011 (21269348)	DLQI	India	See ref[6]	See ref[6]	DLQI Group A: 8.85 DLQI Group B: 11.42

Abbreviations: DLQI, Dermatology Quality and Life Index; EuroQoL, Nondisease-specific European Quality of Life tool; MCS, mental component score; PCS, physical component score; SF-36, 36-Item Dutch Short form.

the burden of vitiligo has been measured by using nondermatologic tools focusing on psychosocial aspects.

Illness Perception Questionnaire

The Illness Perception Questionnaire is a tool created to provide a theoretically derived measurement instrument suitable for any patient population. It has been used in cardiac disease, chronic fatigue syndrome, chronic pain, and psoriasis. This scale was modified to include only 4 subscales: cause, timeline, consequences, and cure/control. The cause subscale includes 10 items measuring personal ideas about the cause of vitiligo. The timeline subscale includes 3 items addressing perceptions about how long the disease will last. The consequences subscale includes 6 items concerned with the expected effects and outcomes of illness. The cure/control subscale includes 6 items that details the beliefs about recovery from or control of the condition.

An Iranian study done by Firooz and colleagues[41] used the Illness Perception Questionnaire to measure HRQL in vitiligo. This study included 80 subjects with vitiligo, and scoring was done based on 4 possible answers: strongly agree, agree, do not know, and disagree. Stress was believed to be a major factor in the onset of vitiligo in 62.5% of subjects. About 48.8% believed that their illness had a major consequence on their life, and 57.5% of subjects felt that vitiligo affected their self-esteem. There was no association found between self-esteem and clinical parameters such as duration of disease. Subjects who did have a longer duration of disease tended to believe that their disease was permanent, with 42.5% of subjects believing that even if their vitiligo cleared it would come back. Only 13.8% of subjects thought their disease would last for a short period. This study focused on cognitive appraisals held by subjects about their illness and concluded that accurate, accessible, and community-based education about natural history and treatment options for vitiligo might help in clearing some of the misconceptions associated with this disease. Earlier studies done on patients' beliefs about acne show that accurate knowledge about the disease is required to clear misconceptions that could have negative psychosocial impact and in turn effects on QoL.[42]

Feelings of Stigmatization Questionnaire

Kent and al-Abadie[27] found that the stigmatization experience accounted for 39% of the variance in the HRQL in subjects with vitiligo. Schmid-Ott and colleagues[43] wanted to measure this stigmatization experience by using the Questionnaire on Subject Experience with Skin Complaints (QES). Different dimensions of stigmatization were assessed using the Adjustment to Chronic Skin Disorders Questionnaire (ACS) and Sense of Coherence Questionnaire. Duration of illness and extent of skin involvement graded on a scale of 0 (no current symptoms or skin involvement) to 5 (most severe) were also included. The QES is a modified questionnaire from the original German version of Feelings of Stigmatization Questionnaire.[44] It consists of 6 scales: (1) interference of skin symptoms and self-esteem scale, (2) outward appearance and situation-caused retreat scale, (3) rejection and devaluation scale, (4) composure scale, (5) concealment scale, and (6) experienced refusal scale. Data using QES from 363 subjects showed a statistically significant difference between men and women on the QES outward appearance and situation-caused retreat ($P = .03$) and composure ($P<.001$) scales. Specifically, women retreated more frequently and were more worried than men. There are conflicting studies regarding location of vitiligo lesions and HRQL, but this study showed that subjects with visible vitiligo lesions had lower self-esteem and poorer capacity to cope. However, the investigators concluded that locality of lesions probably does not play a critical role in the stigmatization experience because the location of lesions likely leads to a tendency to avoid situations that would promote stigmatization. This study stressed the importance of psychological intervention and addressing the emotional aspects of vitiligo to reduce the stigmatization experience.

Participation scale

Pichaimuthu and colleagues[45] used the participation scale in a study performed in India, which measures the extent to which people participate in common social events. A total of 150 subjects with vitiligo and psoriasis were compared using 3 parameters: socioeconomic status, clinical profile, and participation scale. The participation scale has been used and validated in Nepal, India, and Brazil. It is an 18-item instrument graded on severity of participation restriction and covers several internationally classified participation domains of functioning, disability, and health. The instrument scale is scored from 0 to 90, with no restriction scored from 0 to 12, mild from 13 to 22, moderate from 23 to 32, severe from 33 to 52, and extreme from 53 to 90. Both subjects with vitiligo and psoriasis had restriction in their social and domestic life,[45] albeit subjects with psoriasis demonstrated more restriction, with 3.7% of subjects with psoriasis having extreme restriction compared with none of the subjects with vitiligo. Although the symptoms could explain the worse score amongst subjects with psoriasis, a limitation of the study was lack of matched subjects, with only 20% of subjects with vitiligo with more than 10% of BSA involvement, whereas 41.3% of subjects with psoriasis had more than 10% of BSA involvement.

Other psychosocial tools

Kostopoulou and colleagues[26] used data obtained from the assessment of objective clinical severity such as body percentage affected and a vitiligo staging score, along with personality characteristics such as anxiety, depression, and self-esteem traits. The investigators found that perceived severity of vitiligo was explained more by subjects' personality traits than by clinical objective data. In Belgium, study data from Italy where close to 80% of subjects were of skin type III showed that subjects with vitiligo reported a higher prevalence of both alexithymia (24%) and depression (39%) than the general population (prevalence of both estimated at 10% in white populations). The tools used for psychosocial assessment were a General Health Questionnaire and the TAS-20.[3]

IMPACT ON HRQL AFTER TREATMENT

In a very visible cutaneous disease such as vitiligo, the perception of disease is more important than clinical severity itself. Treatment responses should then be assessed by subjects' perception of response along with percentage of repigmentation. A very slight improvement in visibility of lesions can lead to a significant improvement in HRQL. The measurement of change in QoL after treatment remains a valuable tool when assessing treatment success.

Several studies have focused on change in HRQL after different forms of vitiligo treatment: (1) psychological interventions such as cognitive behavioral therapy (CBT)[46]; (2) medical modalities such as tacrolimus,[47] levamisole,[48] NBUVB phototherapy,[49] NBUVB versus broad-band UV-B in combination with topical calcipotriol,[50] and UV-A phototherapy[10]; and (3) surgical modalities such as noncultured epidermal cellular grafting[51] and noncultured melanocyte transplantation.[52]

Papadopoulos and colleagues[46] compared 2 matched groups with and without CBT and studied self-esteem, body image, and QoL before, during, and 5 months after treatment. Their studies indicated that CBT helped in coping and living with vitiligo.

The effects of phototherapy on QoL in subjects with vitiligo have been explored. Njoo and colleagues[49] measured the change in QoL in children with generalized vitiligo after successful treatment with NBUVB. A total of 51 children with vitiligo, age ranging between 4 and 16 years, with almost equal distribution of skin types II and III versus skin types IV and V were included. The response to treatment was followed up to 1 year. A validated Dutch version of Children's Dermatology Life Quality Index tool (CDLQI) was used to measure QoL before and after either by the parents or by the children themselves. Subjects with 26% to 75% repigmentation or more than 75% repigmentation showed significant decrease in CDLQI scores, indicating an improvement in their QoL after successful treatment. The investigators concluded that even moderate response to treatment led to satisfaction amongst subjects and parents because of reduced extent and visibility of lesions supporting the psychological benefits of treatment.

Tjioe and colleagues[33] retrospectively studied a smaller group of 30 adults who had been treated with NBUVB in the last 4 years for vitiligo. The investigators administered a nonvalidated modified version of DLQI to fit the retrospective nature of their study and added questions about general well-being and camouflage. The questionnaire had 14 questions and was scored on a Likert scale with positive numbers (1 or 2) indicating an improvement in HRQL and negative values (−1 and −2) indicating deterioration in HRQL. Maximum score for the questionnaire was 28 and minimum was −28 derived from summation of answers from all 14 questions. Seventy percent reported an improvement in QoL (score 1–20), and 26.7% reported a negative score (−1 to −12) indicating a worsening of HRQL. Treatment with phototherapy led to 23.3% of subjects noticing less influence of vitiligo on leisure activities after treatment, 13.3% had less problems with sports, and 6.7% had less problems with work or relationships. A greater number of subjects with vitiligo had to camouflage after phototherapy, and more time was spent on camouflaging as well (30% of subjects needed more time to camouflage after phototherapy compared with 10% who needed less time). This study concluded that long-term follow-up studies are required to evaluate effects on QoL a few years (in this study up to 4 years) after initial treatment.[33]

Another phototherapy study focused on 141 adults treated with oral or topical psoralen with UV-A (PUVA) along with combinations of topical PUVA, pulsed systemic corticosteroids, or oral levamisole. The investigators found that subjects with successful treatment (defined by lack of new lesions, stability of existing lesions, and >25% repigmentation of existing lesions at the end of 1 year) had lower mean DLQI (7.06, moderate effect) scores compared with mean DLQI (10.67, moderate to very large effect) scores before treatment and in subjects with treatment failure (13.12, very large effect).[10]

Kruger and colleagues[9] used 3 study instruments: DLQI, Beck Depression Inventory (BDI), and ASC in 167 subjects with vitiligo who were undergoing treatment with NBUVB-activated pseudocatalase (PC-KUS) for at least 1 year. Of these 167 subjects, 51 were already undergoing treatment with PC-KUS for at least 1 year and 116 subjects were initiating therapy. The mean baseline DLQI of the 116 subjects was 6.1 (moderate effect), which they compared with the 51 subjects on therapy (mean DLQI, 4.3; small effect). The ASC tool used 3 subscales: social anxieties/avoidance, helplessness, and anxious-depressive mood. The investigators also compared the treated versus untreated groups across these subscales: social anxiety/avoidance scale (34.6 vs 39.8, P = .032), anxious-depressive mood scale (18.0 vs 21.0, P = .012), and for helplessness (26.2 vs 28.1, P>.05). The BDI scores across treated versus untreated was 5.4 versus 7.7 (P>.05).

NONMEDICAL INTERVENTIONS

Kruger and colleagues[9] also focused on a nonmedical intervention: group climatotherapy at the Dead Sea. A total of 71 subjects with vitiligo and 42 healthy controls were evaluated after being at the Dead Sea for 20 days. Study instruments were DLQI, BDI, and ACS. Most subjects were of phototype III (N = 55). Mean DLQI scores of the whole group before climatotherapy was 7.8 and decreased to 1.9 at day 20 (decrease from moderate to small effect). The long-term effect was studied on those who returned to the Dead Sea after a year by including 33 of 71 subjects and 12 of 42 controls. Mean DLQI scores of the whole group before beginning treatment was 6.2 and decreased to 2.1 after 20 days of treatment (decreased from moderate to small effect). Social anxieties/avoidance decreased from a mean of 42.4 (day 1) to 36.2 (day 20) (P<.001). Anxious-depressive mood decreased from a mean score of 21.7 (day 1) to 19.2 (day 20) (P<.005), and helplessness decreased from a mean score of 29.1 (day 1) to 26.3 (day 20) (P<.005). BDI, used for measuring prevalence of depression and mild-moderate depression, was present in about 30% of subjects. Women had significantly higher BDI scores (mean 8.8) than men (mean 2.3) on day 1 compared with 6.79 versus 1.78 on day 20. The investigators concluded that a 20-day-long group climatotherapy at the Dead Sea leads to a dramatic improvement in QoL. Furthermore, subjects who returned after 1 year experienced a similar improvement after 20 days at the Dead Sea.

COSMETIC CAMOUFLAGE

Few studies have paid attention to the effects of cosmetic interventions on HRQL in vitiligo. Ongenae and colleagues[22] exclusively studied subjects with vitiligo attending a vitiligo meeting. A total of 86 subjects completed 2 questionnaires: DLQI and the stigmatization questionnaire before the use of any camouflage. The stigmatization questionnaire identifies 6 dimensions of stigma experience ([a] anticipation of rejection, [b] feelings of being flawed, [c] sensitivity to the opinions of others, [d] guilt and shame, [e] negative attitudes, and [f] secretiveness). Scoring was done from 0 to 5, corresponding with an increasing perception of stigmatization and the global score expressed as a percentage of maximal score obtained by summing up the 6 dimension scores. Of the 86 subjects, 78 responded and received a second questionnaire along with a camouflage sample matching their skin complexion. They were asked to return the second questionnaire after at least a 1-month use of the sample. Of the 78 subjects, 62 applied the camouflage sample as directed and returned the second questionnaire. The subjects used camouflage for a mean duration of 3.8 months, and the camouflage was mostly used on exposed locations such as face, hands, and neck. The mean DLQI score before camouflage was 7.3 and after use of camouflage was 5.9, which was statistically significant (P = .006) but may not be clinically significant because the score range for moderate effect on QOL is 6 to 10. The mean global stigmatization score was 38.4%, with anticipation of rejection present in 56% and guilt and shame in 58%. The investigators found a positive correlation between experience of being rejected and global stigmatization.

Although cosmetic camouflage moderately improved subjects' QoL, it did not influence the feeling of stigma. Kent and al-Abadie[27] suggested that although excellent cosmesis can be obtained, having to conceal the true condition may sustain the feeling of stigma and fear of rejection.

SURGICAL INTERVENTIONS

Several surgical interventions are used for recalcitrant vitiligo. van Geel and colleagues[51] used noncultured epidermal cell transplantation in 40 stable subjects with vitiligo and evaluated the repigmentation achieved with a digital image analysis system. The subjective evaluation was done only in half of the subjects (N = 20) by using DLQI before the intervention and after. The mean DLQI before starting treatment was 6.95 and decreased to 3.85 after treatment ($P = .013$, decrease from moderate to small effect). This group subsequently[53] used noncultured epidermal cellular grafting in a larger number (N = 87) of subjects with vitiligo and focused on parameters such as percentage repigmentation and color mismatch. About 87% of subjects mentioned a positive impact on their HRQL through a general questionnaire; however, no validated QoL tools were used. Better evidence for improvement in DLQI with noncultured melanocyte grafting was shown by Sahni and colleagues.[52] The investigators randomized 25 subjects with vitiligo to 2 groups: group A with noncultured melanocytes suspended in normal saline and group B with noncultured melanocytes suspended in their own serum. Their primary outcome was repigmentation achieved, and secondary outcome was improvement in DLQI. The mean DLQI of group A before treatment was 8.85 and decreased to 3.62 after treatment. The mean DLQI of group B before treatment was 11.42 and decreased to 2.17 after treatment. The mean reduction in DLQI was significantly greater in group B than in group A ($P = .005$).

SUMMARY

Many studies document significant effects of vitiligo on HRQL using general medical and dermatology-specific questionnaires. In vitiligo, impairments in HRQL are evidenced in measurements of self-esteem, body image, stigma, and anxiety, often to a greater degree than clinical severity. Commonly reported characteristics that are independent predictors of worse HRQL include having highly contrasting dark skin, not being Caucasian, being female, having more severe and extensive vitiligo, having prolonged duration of vitiligo, and failing treatment. Vitiligo also highlights potential cultural impact on the perception and QoL impact of skin diseases. Vitiligo significantly affects a person's HRQL, and the assessment of HRQL should be made in all subjects with vitiligo initially as well as through the course of treatment because patient satisfaction may not parallel clinical response parameters.

REFERENCES

1. Linthorst Homan MW, Spuls PI, de Korte J, et al. The burden of vitiligo: patient characteristics associated with quality of life. J Am Acad Dermatol 2009;61(3): 411–20.

2. Koranne RV, Sachdeva KG. Vitiligo. Int J Dermatol 1988;27(10):676–81.

3. Sampogna F, Raskovic D, Guerra L, et al. Identification of categories at risk for high quality of life impairment in patients with vitiligo. Br J Dermatol 2008; 159(2):351–9.

4. Parsad D, Dogra S, Kanwar AJ. Quality of life in patients with vitiligo. Health Qual Life Outcomes 2003;1:58.

5. Dwivedi M, Laddha NC, Shajil EM, et al. The ACE gene I/D polymorphism is not associated with generalized vitiligo susceptibility in Gujarat population. Pigment Cell Melanoma Res 2008;21(3):407–8.

6. Radtke MA, Schafer I, Gajur A, et al. Willingness-to-pay and quality of life in patients with vitiligo. Br J Dermatol 2009;161(1):134–9.

7. Porter JR, Beuf AH. Racial variation in reaction to physical stigma: a study of degree of disturbance by vitiligo among black and white patients. J Health Soc Behav 1991;32(2):192–204.

8. Linthorst Homan MW, Sprangers MA, de Korte J, et al. Characteristics of patients with universal vitiligo and health-related quality of life. Arch Dermatol 2008;144(8):1062–4.

9. Kruger C, Smythe JW, Spencer JD, et al. Significant immediate and long-term improvement in quality of life and disease coping in patients with vitiligo after group climatotherapy at the Dead Sea. Acta Derm Venereol 2011;91(2):152–9.

10. Parsad D, Pandhi R, Dogra S, et al. Dermatology Life Quality Index score in vitiligo and its impact on the treatment outcome. Br J Dermatol 2003;148(2): 373–4.

11. Dolatshahi M, Ghazi P, Feizy V, et al. Life quality assessment among patients with vitiligo: comparison of married and single patients in Iran. Indian J Dermatol Venereol Leprol 2008;74(6):700.

12. Taylor A, Pawaskar M, Taylor SL, et al. Prevalence of pigmentary disorders and their impact on quality of life: a prospective cohort study. J Cosmet Dermatol 2008;7(3):164–8.

13. Halder RM, Chappell JL. Vitiligo update. Semin Cutan Med Surg 2009;28(2):86–92.

14. Silvan M. The psychological aspects of vitiligo. Cutis 2004;73(3):163–7.

15. Borovicka JH, Lilly E, Lu P, et al. Development and validation of a vitiligo-specific health-related quality of life (VHRQoL) instrument. Annual American Academy of Dermatology Meeting. New Orleans (LA): J Amer Acad Dermatol; 2011.

16. Linthorst Homan MW, de Korte J, Grootenhuis MA, et al. Impact of childhood vitiligo on adult life. Br J Dermatol 2008;159(4):915–20.

17. Bilgic O, Bilgic A, Akis HK, et al. Depression, anxiety and health-related quality of life in children and adolescents with vitiligo. Clin Exp Dermatol 2011; 36(4):360–5.

18. Wang KY, Wang KH, Zhang ZP. Health-related quality of life and marital quality of vitiligo patients in China. J Eur Acad Dermatol Venereol 2011;25(4):429–35.

19. Aghaei S, Sodaifi M, Jafari P, et al. DLQI scores in vitiligo: reliability and validity of the Persian version. BMC Dermatol 2004;4:8.

20. Al-Mubarak L, Al-Mohanna H, Al-Issa A, et al. Quality of life in Saudi vitiligo patients. J Cutan Aesthet Surg 2011;4(1):33–7.

21. Talsania N, Lamb B, Bewley A. Vitiligo is more than skin deep: a survey of members of the Vitiligo Society. Clin Exp Dermatol 2010;35(7):736–9.

22. Ongenae K, Dierckxsens L, Brochez L, et al. Quality of life and stigmatization profile in a cohort of vitiligo patients and effect of the use of camouflage. Dermatology 2005;210(4):279–85.

23. Ongenae K, Van Geel N, De Schepper S, et al. Effect of vitiligo on self-reported health-related quality of life. Br J Dermatol 2005;152(6):1165–72.

24. Zachariae R, Zachariae C, Ibsen HH, et al. Psychological symptoms and quality of life of dermatology outpatients and hospitalized dermatology patients. Acta Derm Venereol 2004;84(3):205–12.

25. Borimnejad L, Parsa Yekta Z, Nikbakht-Nasrabadi A, et al. Quality of life with vitiligo: comparison of male and female muslim patients in Iran. Gend Med 2006; 3(2):124–30.

26. Kostopoulou P, Jouary T, Quintard B, et al. Objective vs. subjective factors in the psychological impact of vitiligo: the experience from a French referral centre. Br J Dermatol 2009;161(1):128–33.

27. Kent G, al-Abadie M. Factors affecting responses on Dermatology Life Quality Index items among vitiligo sufferers. Clin Exp Dermatol 1996;21(5):330–3.

28. Finlay AY, Khan GK. Dermatology Life Quality Index (DLQI)—a simple practical measure for routine clinical use. Clin Exp Dermatol 1994;19(3):210–6.

29. Basra MK, Fenech R, Gatt RM, et al. The Dermatology Life Quality Index 1994-2007: a comprehensive review of validation data and clinical results. Br J Dermatol 2008;159(5):997–1035.

30. de Tiedra AG, Mercadal J, Badia X, et al. A method to select an instrument for measurement of HR-QOL for cross-cultural adaptation applied to dermatology. Pharmacoeconomics 1998;14(4):405–22.

31. Schafer T, Staudt A, Ring J. German instrument for the assessment of quality of life in skin diseases (DIELH). Internal consistency, reliability, convergent and discriminant validity and responsiveness. Hautarzt 2001;52(7):624–8.

32. Mashayekhi V, Javidi Z, Kiafar B, et al. Quality of life in patients with vitiligo: a descriptive study on 83 patients attending a PUVA therapy unit in Imam Reza Hospital, Mashad. Indian J Dermatol Venereol Leprol 2010;76(5):592.

33. Tjioe M, Otero ME, van de Kerkhof PC, et al. Quality of life in vitiligo patients after treatment with long-term narrowband ultraviolet B phototherapy. J Eur Acad Dermatol Venereol 2005;19(1):56–60.

34. Chren MM, Lasek RJ, Quinn LM, et al. Skindex, a quality-of-life measure for patients with skin disease: reliability, validity, and responsiveness. J Invest Dermatol 1996;107(5):707–13.

35. Chren MM, Lasek RJ, Flocke SA, et al. Improved discriminative and evaluative capability of a refined version of Skindex, a quality-of-life instrument for patients with skin diseases. Arch Dermatol 1997; 133(11):1433–40.

36. Sampogna F, Picardi A, Chren MM, et al. Association between poorer quality of life and psychiatric morbidity in patients with different dermatological conditions. Psychosom Med 2004;66(4):620–4.

37. Bellantuono C, Fiorio R, Zanotelli R, et al. Psychiatric screening in general practice in Italy. A validity study of the GHQ (General Health Questionnaire). Soc Psychiatry 1987;22(2):113–7.

38. Taylor GJ, Ryan D, Bagby RM. Toward the development of a new self-report alexithymia scale. Psychother Psychosom 1985;44(4):191–9.

39. Kim do Y, Lee JW, Whang SH, et al. Quality of life for Korean patients with vitiligo: Skindex-29 and its correlation with clinical profiles. J Dermatol 2009; 36(6):317–22.

40. Choi S, Kim DY, Whang SH, et al. Quality of life and psychological adaptation of Korean adolescents with vitiligo. J Eur Acad Dermatol Venereol 2010; 24(5):524–9.

41. Firooz A, Bouzari N, Fallah N, et al. What patients with vitiligo believe about their condition. Int J Dermatol 2004;43(11):811–4.

42. Tan JK, Vasey K, Fung KY. Beliefs and perceptions of patients with acne. J Am Acad Dermatol 2001; 44(3):439–45.

43. Schmid-Ott G, Kunsebeck HW, Jecht E, et al. Stigmatization experience, coping and sense of coherence in vitiligo patients. J Eur Acad Dermatol Venereol 2007;21(4):456–61.

44. Schmid-Ott G, Jaeger B, Kuensebeck HW, et al. Dimensions of stigmatization in patients with psoriasis in a "Questionnaire on Experience with Skin Complaints". Dermatology 1996;193(4):304–10.

45. Pichaimuthu R, Ramaswamy P, Bikash K, et al. A measurement of the stigma among vitiligo and psoriasis patients in India. Indian J Dermatol Venereol Leprol 2011;77(3):300–6.

46. Papadopoulos L, Bor R, Legg C. Coping with the disfiguring effects of vitiligo: a preliminary investigation into the effects of cognitive-behavioural therapy. Br J Med Psychol 1999;72(Pt 3):385–96.

47. Hartmann A, Brocker EB, Hamm H. Occlusive treatment enhances efficacy of tacrolimus 0.1% ointment in adult patients with vitiligo: results of a placebo-controlled 12-month prospective study. Acta Derm Venereol 2008;88(5):474–9.

48. Agarwal S, Ramam M, Sharma VK, et al. A randomized placebo-controlled double-blind study of levamisole in the treatment of limited and slowly spreading vitiligo. Br J Dermatol 2005; 153(1):163–6.

49. Njoo MD, Bos JD, Westerhof W. Treatment of gener- alized vitiligo in children with narrow-band (TL-01) UVB radiation therapy. J Am Acad Dermatol 2000; 42(2 Pt 1):245–53.

50. Hartmann A, Lurz C, Hamm H, et al. Narrow-band UVB311 nm vs. broad-band UVB therapy in combi- nation with topical calcipotriol vs. placebo in vitiligo. Int J Dermatol 2005;44(9):736–42.

51. van Geel N, Ongenae K, Vander Haeghen Y, et al. Subjective and objective evaluation of noncultured epidermal cellular grafting for repigmenting vitiligo. Dermatology 2006;213(1):23–9.

52. Sahni K, Parsad D, Kanwar AJ, et al. Autologous noncultured melanocyte transplantation for stable vitiligo: can suspending autologous melanocytes in the patients' own serum improve repigmentation and patient satisfaction? Dermatol Surg 2011;37(2):176–82.

53. van Geel N, Wallaeys E, Goh BK, et al. Long term results of non cultured epidermal cellular grafting in vitiligo, halo nevi, piebaldism and nevus depigmen- tosus. Br J Dermatol 2010;163(6):1186–93.

Melasma Quality of Life Measures

Tiffany J. Lieu, BA, BS[a], Amit G. Pandya, MD[b],*

KEYWORDS

- Melasma • Quality of life • Translation • Outcome measures

Over the last 2 decades, multiple studies have demonstrated that skin diseases cause substantial physical and psychosocial distress. Assessing quality of life (QOL) is important in determining a treatment plan and its efficacy, particularly because health status may not correlate with severity of disease.[1,2] In the 1990s, QOL measures specific to dermatology, such as the Skindex[3] and Dermatology Life Quality Index[4] (DLQI), began to emerge, which documented the significant impact skin diseases can have on patients' QOL. More recently, QOL questionnaires specific for skin diseases have been developed because of their ability to more accurately assess a patient with a particular skin condition, such as the Cardiff Acne Disability Index,[5] Psoriasis Disability Index,[6] Quality of Life Index for Atopic Dermatitis,[7] Chronic Urticaria Quality of Life Questionnaire,[8] and Melasma Quality of Life scale (MELASQOL).[1]

The MELASQOL is a useful tool because melasma is asymptomatic but disfiguring, often leading to a significant effect on QOL.[1] Although initially developed in English, it has recently been translated into Spanish, Brazilian Portuguese, French, and Turkish. Development of a validated, translated, disease-specific QOL questionnaire is a complex process that is further discussed. Because melasma is a worldwide problem, it is important to develop the MELASQOL in other languages, although careful attention must be paid to cross-cultural adaptation and proper methods of translation to have an accurate tool. This article addresses these methods that could be useful to those desiring to develop the MELASQOL in other languages.

MELASMA

Melasma is a common disorder of acquired hyperpigmentation characterized by tan or brown macules and patches localized to photo-exposed areas of the face, particularly the malar areas, forehead, and chin. Melasma affects 8.8% of Latino women[9] and is more prevalent in women, with men comprising about 10% of all cases.[10] Melasma affects all races but is especially prevalent in those with darker skin types (Fitzpatrick skin types III to VI) and has been highly reported in patients of Hispanic, African American, Arab, South Asian, Southeast Asian, and East Asian descent.[11] The exact cause of melasma is unclear, but factors include genetic predisposition, ultraviolet light exposure, pregnancy, oral contraceptives, hormone replacement therapy, thyroid disease, cosmetics, and medications.[11] The lesions are usually asymptomatic but often have considerable emotional and psychological effects. The Melasma Area and Severity Index (MASI) is used to reliably measure the clinical severity of melasma and monitor changes after therapy.[12] However, the QOL of patients with melasma does not correlate well with the MASI score.[1,2] Hence, the psychological impact of melasma, with its disfiguring facial discoloration and chronic nature, has profound negative effects on patients' QOL, which is not captured by the MASI. In order to illustrate the

Funding support: none.

Conflicts of interest: The authors have nothing to disclose.

[a] University of Texas Southwestern Medical Center, 5323 Harry Hines Boulevard, Dallas, TX 75390-9190, USA

[b] Department of Dermatology, University of Texas Southwestern Medical Center, 5323 Harry Hines Boulevard, Dallas, TX 75390-9190, USA

* Corresponding author.

E-mail address: amit.pandya@utsouthwestern.edu

Dermatol Clin 30 (2012) 269–280

doi:10.1016/j.det.2011.11.009

full impact of melasma on a patient's life, several QOL instruments have been developed to address the various life domains that can be affected because of the presence of this disorder.

QOL INSTRUMENTS

Generic QOL measures, such as the internationally used 100-item World Health Organization Quality of Life Instrument[13] (WHOQOL) and its abbreviated version, the 26-item WHOQOL-BREF,[13] allow for comparison of health-related QOLs across all diseases. Like other nonspecific health-related QOL questionnaires, the WHOQOL-BREF can be used in a broad spectrum of patients, from those with hypertension to psoriasis to chronic obstructive pulmonary disease (COPD). To be applicable to such a diverse population, the WHOQOL-BREF covers several facets of life and equally weighs each of its items. For example, the instrument evaluates the physical life domain by assessing factors such as physical pain and mobility and their effects on daily life activities. For a patient with COPD, the disease often causes profound physical pain and decreased mobility, which negatively affect the physical aspect of QOL. However, psoriasis predominantly affects the skin, causing pruritus, scaling, bleeding, and infection, which typically do not cause the same type of restrictive physical symptoms that can detract from activities of daily life. These psoriasis-specific symptoms are disregarded in most of the WHOQOL-BREF items concerning physical QOL. Therefore, the WHOQOL-BREF, like other general health-related QOL questionnaires, fails to address many aspects of skin diseases even though the impact psoriasis has on QOL is comparable to heart disease, prompting the development of more suitable dermatology-specific questionnaires.[14]

Skin diseases have been shown to affect QOL to a similar extent as other chronic diseases. In children, generalized atopic dermatitis causes more QOL impairment than renal disease, cystic fibrosis, and asthma, and the effects of psoriasis and urticaria on QOL are worse than diabetes and epilepsy.[15] Adult psoriasis has been found to be more detrimental to QOL than angina and hypertension.[14] One study even determined that psoriasis caused worse physical and mental QOL than arthritis, cancer, myocardial infarction, and type II diabetes.[16] These findings further emphasize the importance of developing more accurate QOL tools for dermatologic conditions.

In 1994, Finlay and Khan[4] developed the DLQI, and Chren and colleagues[3] introduced the Skindex in 1996 and later the condensed Skindex-16,[17] both a great improvement from general health-related QOL questionnaires. For example, the Skindex-16 measures many aspects relevant to skin disease, including itching, burning or stinging, pain, irritation, persistence/recurrence, appearance, frustration, embarrassment, and depression.[17] However, the disease-specific Psoriasis Disability Index goes into more detail than the DLQI and Skindex by asking patients about their frequency of changing or washing clothes because of psoriasis, frequency of bathing due to psoriasis, and problems with psoriasis at the hairdresser.[6] Twenty-five percent of the Skindex-16 items concern physical symptoms, with the remaining 75% focusing on emotions and functioning,[17] yet most patients with melasma do not experience any physical distress. Today, there is a recognized need for QOL instruments that weigh the various life domains differently based on the unique features of a specific skin disease, as evidenced by the number of disease-specific QOL questionnaires available.

MELASQOL

Balkrishnan and colleagues[1] observed that little published information was available regarding the impact of melasma on daily life activities. In a pilot study of 50 women, melasma was associated with a significant impact on health-related QOL, with the strongest predictors of decreased QOL being increased disease severity, increased fear of negative evaluation, better perception of QOL without melasma, and lack of presence of concurrent rosacea or acne. Because of easy visible detection of melasma and its frustrating and often unsuccessful treatment, the investigators concluded that melasma had an undeniably greater psychosocial impact on QOL that needed to be explored and weighed more heavily in QOL instruments. Therefore, they sought to develop a QOL instrument for patients with melasma that accounted for the unique impact of the facial lesions on the psychological and social well-being of the individual while ignoring physical symptoms. To that end, the investigators devised the original MELASQOL in English to address the inadequacy of generic and dermatology QOL instruments for evaluating melasma. They randomly recruited 102 women by flyers or by referral from the Wake Forest University School of Medicine Dermatology Clinic in North Carolina. Women were eligible if they were older than 18 years, younger than 65 years, diagnosed with melasma by an investigator, and were able to complete the questionnaires. The investigators rated their melasma using the MASI instrument, and patients completed the Skindex-16, DLQI, a 7-item skin discoloration impact questionnaire created specifically for the study, and a 12-item Fear of Negative Evaluation questionnaire. The women also rated their perceived QOL on 8 aspects of their life with melasma and what they predicted it would be if they did not have melasma. Collection of these anonymous surveys in addition to patients' demographics and health practices occurred in 1 visit.

Balkrishnan and colleagues[1] chose 7 items from the Skindex-16 and 3 items from the skin discoloration questionnaire to form the new MELASQOL in an attempt to remove questions that had little correlation with melasma-specific health-related QOL, such as those concerned with physical discomfort. Items with the highest correlations with both Skindex-16 and the skin discoloration questionnaire were selected. The final 10-item questionnaire uses a Likert scale of 1 to 7 in which 1 signifies not bothered at all and 7 signifies bothered all the time (see **Box 1**). MELASQOL scores range from 7 to 70, a higher score signifying worse QOL. The mean MELASQOL score was 36, and the mean age was 39.7 years. Women in the

20- to 30-year age group had a significantly higher MELASQOL mean of 50.4 than other age groups. The questionnaire had a Cronbach α value of 0.95, reflecting very high internal consistency. Cronbach α is a coefficient of reliability used to assess the internal consistency of a psychometric scale, and a level greater than 0.70 is considered satisfactory.[18] Furthermore, the MELASQOL correlated highly with the Skindex-16, DLQI, and skin discoloration questionnaire.

Like the DLQI and Skindex-16, the MELASQOL only moderately correlated with the MASI, further demonstrating how melasma's impact on life quality is not merely based on disease severity. The MELASQOL discriminated better than the Skindex-16 among women with and without a history of psychiatric, psychological, or emotional problems. The new scale paralleled the Skindex-16, which was superior to the DLQI in discriminating among patient groups being treated with depigmenting creams or other methods or not being treated at all. The QOL domains most associated with lower QOL and higher MELASQOL scores, such as social life, leisure and recreation, and emotional well-being, were the same aspects patients perceived would improve the most if they were disease-free. The study was limited by the demographics of the patient population surrounding the academic medical center because most women were white married, and had at least a college education. As stated earlier, many patients with melasma do not fit into this demographic. Investigators acknowledged it would be beneficial to assess the discriminatory ability of the MELASQOL in monitoring improvement in QOL across different treatments. Overall, the MELASQOL is a valid objective instrument for measuring melasma's influence on QOL in the American English-speaking population.

To investigate the impact of treatment on QOL in patients with melasma and to evaluate the efficacy and safety of a triple combination cream combining fluocinolone acetonide 0.01%, hydroquinone 4.0%, and tretinoin 0.05% (Tri-Luma), Balkrishnan and colleagues[19] led a community-based trial at 393 centers in the United States. The Prospective Investigation Gauging Melasma Reduction with a New Treatment (PIGMENT) trial was an open-label phase IV study conducted on 1290 patients. Patients with melasma who were pregnant or nursing; could not avoid significant sun exposure; had recently taken any systemic medications that might confound results; had recently used any topicals, cosmetics, or procedures that could interfere with the cream; had sensitivities to any ingredients of the medication; had a history of alcohol or drug abuse; or had

---

Box 1
MELASQOL: English Version

On a scale of 1 (not bothered at all) to 7 (bothered all the time), the patient rates how she feels about:

1. The appearance of your skin condition

2. Frustration about your skin condition

3. Embarrassment about your skin condition

4. Feeling depressed about your skin condition

5. The effects of your skin condition on your interactions with other people (eg, interactions with family, friends, close relationship, and so forth.)

6. The effects of your skin condition on your desire to be with people

7. Your skin condition making it hard to show affection

8. Skin discoloration making you feel unattractive to others

9. Skin discoloration making you feel less vital or productive

10. Skin discoloration affecting your sense of freedom

All MELASQOLs are scored from 7 to 70, with a higher score indicating worse melasma-related health-related QOL.
Data from Ref.[1]

any skin conditions that could interfere with the trial were excluded. These criteria were used to ensure that only patients with chronic melasma were included. Ninety-six percent of patients were women, and, notably, 62.2% of patients were white, with only 15.8% of Hispanic origin, 10.1% African American, and 7.3% Asian. Patients applied the cream to lesions once nightly and were evaluated at 4 and 8 weeks by the MASI and an investigator's global assessment of improvement. At baseline and at 8 weeks, 1076 patients completed a comprehensive patient health questionnaire, including a skin discoloration impact evaluation questionnaire containing a few items that were later validated and included as part of the MELASQOL described previously. With a baseline mean MASI of 14.68, the trial demonstrated significant improvement of lesions at 4 weeks (mean MASI, 7.38) and even greater improvement at 8 weeks (mean MASI, 3.64) as measured by the mean MASI score across all races and Fitzpatrick skin types. Moderate to marked improvement in the investigator's global assessment was also reported. Responses to the QOL questionnaire showed improvement in areas pertaining to feeling self-conscious or scrutinized, feeling unattractive, using cosmetics to conceal lesions, and limiting social or leisure activities because of melasma, although a statistical quantification of this improvement was not presented. The trial also demonstrated that more than 50% of patients experienced significant improvement in QOL, as they felt less embarrassed, used fewer cosmetics, made fewer efforts to hide their skin, felt younger, and felt more attractive after treatment. Although the MELASQOL was not used in the PIGMENT trial, it was a large multicenter study that made an important step toward understanding melasma by following up patients undergoing treatment over time and characterizing the effects of melasma on QOL. Further studies should use the validated MELASQOL to evaluate its responsiveness, following patients for long-term effects, comparing multiple groups with different treatments, and sampling an even more diverse cross section of the population affected by melasma.

MELASMA IN LATINO MEN

Pichardo and colleagues[20] pooled data from 3 population studies of the prevalence of melasma in Latino men, which were collected by the Wake Forest University School of Medicine. The first study consisted of 25 male Latino poultry workers in North Carolina, the second cross-sectional study consisted of 55 male Latino farm workers in North Carolina, and the third longitudinal study comprised 300 male Latino farm workers. All patients completed a Mexican Spanish version of the DLQI to assess QOL, and demographic information such as age, nationality, and language spoken was collected. Diagnosis of melasma was made by direct examination by a dermatologist in the first 2 studies and by photographs evaluated by a dermatologist in the third study. Half of the participants were 30 years or younger. Ninety-two percent of the poultry workers were Guatemalan, and 96.3% and 98.7% of the cross-sectional and longitudinal farm workers, respectively, were Mexican. Ninety-two percent of the poultry workers spoke an indigenous language, whereas 87.3% of the longitudinal farm workers spoke only Spanish. Across all 3 studies, the prevalence of melasma was 14.5%. The melasma prevalence in the poultry worker study alone was 36%, and all these patients with melasma spoke an indigenous language. Patients older than 31 years had the highest prevalence of melasma at 70%, whereas melasma was not present in any of the workers aged 18 to 24 years. In the cross-sectional farm worker study, melasma was present in 7.4% of the participants, and all were of Mexican nationality. The prevalence was higher in those older than 31 years, but the condition was also present in those aged 18 to 24 years. In the longitudinal farm worker study, the prevalence of melasma was 14%, with all age groups affected, although, once again, the oldest age group (>31 years) had the highest prevalence. In this study, 50% of the men with melasma were Guatemalan, whereas 13.5% were Mexican. In addition, participants who spoke an indigenous language had a higher prevalence than those who spoke only Spanish (21.1% vs 13%).

In the poultry worker study, there was a statistically significant difference in the total DLQI between men with and without melasma. Men with melasma had a higher mean DLQI score of 7.5 than men without melasma at 2.8, indicating poorer QOL due to melasma. Latinos often associate melasma with ill health and poor nutrition. However, this correlation between melasma and QOL in Latino men could be confounded by other unknown shared demographic characteristics. Furthermore, the Mexican Spanish version of the DLQI may not have been appropriate for the primarily indigenous language–speaking participants in the first study. Further studies of the effect of melasma on QOL in Latino men should collect more demographic information, such as comorbidities and family history of melasma, to allow for improved comparison with other studies and to better characterize this minority group.

SPANISH MELASQOL

To address the increasing Latino population in the United States and its high prevalence of melasma, Dominguez and colleagues[2] adapted the MELASQOL to the Spanish language for use in multiple Spanish-speaking populations (see Box 2). The final Spanish-language MELASQOL (Sp-MELASQOL) was administered to 111 female patients with melasma recruited from a county hospital outpatient primary care clinic in Texas. Inclusion criteria consisted of female sex, melasma, at least 18 years of age, Hispanic origin, and the ability to read and understand Spanish. Exclusion criteria included pregnancy in the last 6 months, menopause, and history of bilateral oophorectomy to study patients with chronic melasma rather than those with transient melasma associated with pregnancy and those who might be on hormone replacement therapy. In addition to the Sp-MELASQOL and health-related QOL validation questionnaire used in the original MELASQOL, investigators collected demographics and medical

and psychiatric histories and determined patient MASI scores.

Using a final sample size of 99 participants with complete data, the mean age was 34 years and the majority were of Mexican descent, married, unemployed, and without a college education. All spoke Spanish as their primary language. The mean duration of melasma was 7 years. High correlation between the Sp-MELASQOL and the most affected QOL psychosocial domains determined by the QOL validation questionnaire demonstrated construct validity, and both questionnaires were determined to be highly internally reliable by Cronbach α (Cronbach $\alpha = 0.95$ and 0.91, respectively). Five of 8 health-related QOL domains showed statistically significant correlation with the Sp-MELASQOL, and the remaining 3 domains had similar correlation coefficients. Patients reported that the QOL domains most affected by melasma were emotional well-being, social life, physical health, and money matters, as measured by Cohen's D effect size,[21] whereas Balkrishnan and colleagues found that social life, leisure and recreation, and emotional well-being correlated most with higher MELASQOL scores. In the study by Dominguez and colleagues,[2] the women still perceived leisure and recreation, work, family life, and sexual relations to be substantially affected but at a lower rate than the domains listed earlier, showing the instrument's discriminant validity and uniqueness among items. Patients previously treated for melasma had significantly higher Sp-MELASQOL scores than untreated patients, although this group also scored higher on the MASI and had a longer duration of melasma. However, the study did not discriminate between different types of melasma treatments, such as folk medicine and home remedies. Patients with at least a seventh-grade education showed significantly better QOL than less educated patients, who reported a greater impact on the family life domain, social and sexual life, and emotional well-being. The lack of education in these patients, who often believe melasma is a result of undiagnosed liver or kidney disease, may explain their high rating of physical health as severely affected by melasma. Like Balkrishnan's study using the MELASQOL, the Sp-MELASQOL and MASI were only moderately correlated. Unlike the MELASQOL validation study, Dominguez and colleagues found no significant differences in groups divided by age or by coexisting medical or psychiatric conditions and similarly observed no differences in marital status and employment. The Sp-MELASQOL is a validated instrument that can be used in Spanish-speaking populations with melasma. Future studies should test the responsiveness

---

Box 2
MELASQOL: Spanish Version

Cuestionario de melasma

En una escala del 1 (nunca) al 7 (siempre) indique como se siente usted al respecto de lo siguiente (melasma significa paño, manchas, o máscara del embarazo):

1. Le molesta la apariencia de su melasma?
2. Siente frustración debido al melasma?
3. Se siente avergonzada de su melasma?
4. Se siente deprimida de su melasma?
5. Su melasma afecta sus relaciones con otras personas? (por ejemplo, relaciones con su familia, amigos, esposo, novio, etc.)
6. El melasma le afecta su deseo de estar con otras personas?
7. El melasma le dificulta mostrar afecto?
8. Su melasma le hace sentirse menos atractiva?
9. El melasma le afecta en su trabajo diario (por ejemplo, en casa o fuera de casa)?
10. Su melasma le afecta la manera en que usted expresa su libertad de ser? (por ejemplo, la libertad de salir a donde quisiera)

All MELASQOLs are scored from 7 to 70, with a higher score indicating worse melasma-related health-related QOL.
Data from Ref.[2]

of the questionnaire and its suitability for other Spanish-speaking populations, compare the results in men versus women, and collect more data regarding treatment methods and socioeconomic status.

TRANSLATION ISSUES

Multiple steps were taken by Dominguez and colleagues in translating a semantically equivalent melasma-specific QOL questionnaire to Spanish. The process of cross-cultural adaptation followed Guillemin and colleagues'[22] established guidelines and consisted of translation, back-translation, committee review, pretesting, and revision (see **Box 4**). Both nonmedical and medical Spanish speakers independently translated semantically equivalent Spanish versions of the MELASQOL, which were then reviewed by a committee including 2 of the investigators. Importantly, 4 unique back-translations by bilingual individuals were then reviewed by the original author of the MELASQOL, R. Balkrishnan. Any problematic items were newly translated and back translated again. The probe technique was used for pretesting with 25 female patients with melasma recruited from the aforementioned county hospital outpatient clinic in Texas. Every patient was requested to explain her understanding of each question and justify each answer. Any item that was difficult for more than one patient (>4%) was revised and back translated again. Corrected items were finally approved by R. Balkrishnan. To validate the new Sp-MELASQOL, a health-related QOL questionnaire was also similarly converted to Spanish.

Conversion to semantically equivalent Spanish presented several unforeseen translation issues. The format of the original MELASQOL questionnaire was changed from statements to questions because of awkward phrasing and syntax in Spanish (see **Boxes 1** and **2**). The term skin condition was replaced with melasma because the former may connote disease, which is more negatively received in Spanish-speaking cultures than English-speaking cultures. To cater to multiple Spanish-speaking populations from Mexico and Central and South America, melasma was also listed with the commonly used synonyms "paño," "manchas," and "máscara del embarazo." The most problematic items were questions 9 and 10. Question 9 described melasma's effect on making one feel less vital or productive, but in Spanish "vital" signifies "alive," so the item was altered to focus on the patient's ability to perform daily work both inside and outside the home. Item 10 was concerned with the patient's sense of freedom, an idea that has no true equivalent in Spanish. Therefore, the final translation included an example with item 10 to describe the ways melasma may affect the patient's comfort in going out in public, holding a specific job, or participating in specific activities that could bring more attention to their skin. In pretesting, patients did not fully understand item 1, so "Apariencia" was added to clarify how the appearance of melasma bothers the patient. These revisions required several repeated translations and back-translations, with final evaluation by the original investigator of the MELASQOL.

The problems faced by the developers of the Sp-MELASQOL and the methods used to solve them serve as good examples for those who would like to develop MELASQOL questionnaires in other languages. Close attention should be paid to syntax, context, cultural issues, folklore, and other items that may be unique to a language. Testing with affected patients followed by revision and back-translation to determine if the meaning of the question has changed are critical steps in development. Examples of activities and situations can be useful to further explain the meaning of a question.

BRAZILIAN PORTUGUESE MELASQOL

Cestari and colleagues[23] translated the MELASQOL to Brazilian Portuguese prior to a multicenter study in Brazil that validated the Brazilian Portuguese MELASQOL (MELASQOL-BP) and investigated the effect of a triple combination treatment on QOL of patients with melasma in Brazil. Similar to Dominguez and colleagues, the group followed previously established guidelines[22,24] and used 2 independent translators. They discussed the questionnaire with a multiprofession bilingual panel, pretested it on a sample of the target Brazilian Portuguese-speaking population, reviewed the questionnaire again with the panel, and back translated it to English. The investigators also consulted the original investigator of the MELASQOL before finalization (see **Box 3**). In the first phase of the study, 300 patients of both sexes, older than 18 years, and with moderate to severe melasma for more than 1 year were recruited at 10 sites across all 5 geographic regions of Brazil. The mean age was 42.5 years. All patients completed the validated Portuguese version of the WHOQOL-BREF and the MELASQOL-BP. Fifty-four percent of patients reported themselves as from a mixed racial background, 32.3% were white, 12.3% were black, and 1.3% were Asian. Most patients had skin types III to V. Fifteen eligible subjects from each site were randomly selected to participate in the second phase of the study assessing the impact of a triple

---

Box 3
MELASQOL: Brazilian Portuguese Version

Considerando a sua doença, melasma, como você se sente em relação a:

1. A aparência da sua pele
2. Frustração pela condição da sua pele
3. Constrangimento pela condição de sua pele
4. Sentindo-se depressivo pela condição da sua pele
5. Os efeitos da condição da sua pele no relacionamento com outras pessoas (por ex: interações com a família amigos, relacionamentos íntimos…)
6. Os efeitos da condição da sua pele sobre o seu desejo de estar com as pessoas
7. A condição da sua pele dificulta a demonstração de afeto
8. As manchas da pele fazem você não se sentir atraente para os outros
9. As manchas da pele fazem você se sentir menos importante ou produtivo
10. As manchas da pele afetam o seu senso de liberdade

All MELASQOLs are scored from 7 to 70, with a higher score indicating worse melasma-related health-related QOL.
Data from Ref.[23]

---

combination cream treatment on QOL. Inclusion criteria included absence of systemic disease requiring excluded drugs, negative pregnancy test result, and use of an effective nonhormonal contraceptive. Exclusion criteria included other skin conditions that may interfere with the evaluation of melasma, recent use of drugs or hormones that may affect melasma or the treatment, and excessive exposure to ultraviolet light. These criteria not only excluded any potential confounding factors but also ensured that patients with chronic melasma were enrolled rather than those with transient hormone-associated melasma because the former are the target of the MELASQOL-BP. One hundred thirty-nine patients (135 women, 4 men) applied the same formulation as the one studied in the PIGMENT trial (hydroquinone 4%, tretinoin 0.05%, fluocinolone acetonide 0.01%) daily for 8 weeks and were given sunscreen with sun protection factor 60 with instructions to apply it daily and to avoid sun exposure. Patients were evaluated at 4 and 8 weeks, completing both QOL questionnaires again at 8 weeks. Investigators used the MASI and investigator's global

assessment to quantify improvement and observed significant decreases in mean MASI scores from an initial 13.3 to 6.9 at 4 weeks and 4.1 at 8 weeks. Investigator's global assessment also showed that most patients had moderate or marked improvement or were almost clear at 4 and 8 weeks. However, clinical outcome was not associated with initial severity of melasma, skin color, or geographic region despite greater sun exposure in certain areas of the country. The mean MELASQOL-BP decreased significantly from 44.4 before treatment to 24.3 after treatment. The MELASQOL-BP was determined to be internally reliable by Cronbach α (Cronbach $\alpha = 0.919$) and showed significant inverse correlation to the WHOQOL-BREF, in which lower scores denote lower QOL. Values for individual domains of the WHOQOL-BREF were highest (signifying better QOL) for the environment domain, followed by the psychological domain, with lower scores in the social relations domain. The investigators stated that the discriminatory ability of the MELASQOL-BP was superior to the WHOQOL-BREF, although the data were not presented. In addition, QOL domains assessed by the MELASQOL-BP demonstrating major improvement were skin appearance (69.8% of pretreatment patients were bothered most or all of the time vs 10.1% of posttreatment patients), frustration, embarrassment, and relationships with other people.

The study by Cestari and colleagues has demonstrated significant improvement in the QOL of patients with melasma with treatment. Further revision of the MELASQOL-BP may help to improve patients' ability to understand the questionnaire, as 16.1% needed help in answering items. Including more demographics also helps to compare affected patients in Brazil with those included in the studies by Balkrishnan and colleagues and Dominguez and colleagues, for example, how socioeconomic and educational status affect QOL. As with all new outcome measures, statistical analysis of the tool's responsiveness would be instructive for verifying its ability to measure improvement.

The MELASQOL-BP was further used in a cross-sectional study examining the effects of melasma on the QOL of 85 Southern Brazilian women.[25] Patients were recruited from all clinics in a tertiary care teaching hospital to obtain a representative sample. The patients were scored using the MASI and completed a 55-item epidemiologic questionnaire and 10-item MELASQOL-BP. The original investigator of the MELASQOL-BP, T. Cestari, participated in its administration. Sample size calculation indicated that the study needed 85 patients to detect a moderate correlation between the MASI and MELASQOL-BP. However, the final sample size was 84 because of missing data in 1 patient. Most patients had a stable conjugal relationship and had attended at least 8 years of school. The mean age was 41.1 years and most had Fitzpatrick skin types III and IV. Malar melasma was present in 46.4% of patients, 20.2% had mandibular lesions, 11.9% had centrofacial pattern, and 21.4% had a combined pattern. Asymptomatic melasma was reported by 91.7% of the women, with a small number reporting pruritus or burning. More than half of the patients had a positive family history of melasma. The study found that approximately 26% of patients experienced a sudden onset of melasma a few days after significant sun exposure. Most women had previously used oral contraceptives or hormonal replacement therapy. Three-fourths of the women had been pregnant, and more than 50% of them reported the onset or worsening of melasma during pregnancy. Of the 25 women who had more than 1 pregnancy, 72% reported recurrence of melasma in subsequent pregnancies. A total of 15 patients perceived their menstrual cycle as influencing their melasma lesions. In addition, 26.3% of patients believed stress aggravated their melasma. Predictably, sun exposure was considered an important aggravating factor in 88.1% of patients.

The mean MELASQOL-BP score was 37.5, mean MASI was 10.6, and the mean duration of disease was 6 years. Although the significance of comparing the results of a MELASQOL study in one population with that of another completely different population is not clear, it is interesting to contrast these results to understand the populations studied and to develop hypotheses that could be tested in future studies. The mean MELASQOL-BP score in the Southern Brazilian study was very similar to the MELASQOL mean of 36 in Balkrishnan and colleagues' study and close to the Sp-MELASQOL mean of 43 in Dominguez and colleagues' study. The mean MASI of 10.6 was somewhat lower than the mean of 13 found in the previous Brazilian study by Cestari and colleagues, which may reflect the more fair-skinned population found in southern Brazil. The mean MASI was comparable to the mean MASI of 11 found in Dominguez and colleagues' Hispanic population in Texas. Unlike the MELASQOL and the Sp-MELASQOL scores, which were moderately correlated to MASI scores, Freitag and colleagues[25] found no correlation between MELASQOL-BP scores and disease severity as measured by MASI. The MELASQOL-BP had satisfactory internal consistency demonstrated by Cronbach α (Cronbach α = 0.9039), confirming the previous Brazilian study. The QOL domains

most affected by melasma were appearance, frustration, embarrassment, feeling depressed, relationships with others, and feeling unattractive. The magnified effect of melasma on emotional well-being is consistent with previous results published by Balkrishnan and colleagues and Dominguez and colleagues. Patients with a previous diagnosis of psychiatric disease had significantly higher MELASQOL-BP scores than those with no history, which is similar to Balkrishnan and colleagues' results. Similar to Dominguez and colleagues' study, patients with less than 8 years of schooling had significantly higher MELASQOL-BP scores than those with more education. About 37.6% of patients had already been treated by nonphysicians, suggesting there may be a need to improve access to dermatologic care in southern Brazil. Freitag and colleagues report that dermatologists in Brazil are in agreement that melasma may be more prevalent in the North region because of increased sun exposure and the predominance of darker skin types. Future studies could compare between treated and untreated groups as well as different socioeconomic statuses to determine correlation with QOL. This study provides evidence that the MELASQOL-BP is a culturally adapted, valid, and reliable Brazilian Portuguese-language QOL measure.

FRENCH MELASQOL

Misery and colleagues[26] constructed a French version of the MELASQOL (MELASQOL-F) following similar cross-cultural adaptation guidelines as Dominguez and colleagues. Independent French-language translations of the MELASQOL were reviewed by an expert committee that then composed one unique MELASQOL-F. Items that were changed included substituting "Melasma" for "Skin Condition," as Dominguez and colleagues did for the Sp-MELASQOL, using "Ressenti" to signify "To Feel" rather than other similar French words that translate as feeling in English, and substituting "Hyperpigmentation" for "Discoloration." A back-translation was performed along with pretesting using a probe technique with 30 female patients with melasma. The patients justified their answers and rewrote the meaning of each question in their own words. An item was deemed unreadable if more than 1 patient had difficulty understanding it. The questionnaire was also administered again 10 days later to assess reproducibility. The internal reliability of the MELASQOL-F was shown by a high Cronbach α with this pretesting group (Cronbach α = 0.95). Very good reproducibility was also achieved during this stage, which has not been demonstrated in the aforementioned MELASQOL studies. Validated French versions of the 12-Item Short Form Health Survey (SF-12) scale,[27] an abbreviated version of the generic health-related QOL questionnaire 36-Item Short Form Health Survey,[28] and the DLQI were also administered. During pretesting, the MELASQOL-F was found to correlate significantly with the DLQI scores on both days and also with the mental composite of the SF-12. As predicted, it did not correlate with the physical composite of the SF-12. After another revision, the final version of the MELASQOL-F was administered to 28 women recruited from an academic department of dermatology and a private clinical research center in France. Exclusion criteria were male sex, age less than 18 years, inability to read and understand French, and pregnancy in the last 6 months. In addition to the MELASQOL-F, patients completed the SF-12, DLQI, and Prévention Cardio-Vasculaire en Medecine du Travail[29] (PCV-Metra) to explore the various health-related QOL domains potentially affected by melasma.

About 60.7% of women in the study were younger than 45 years. Nearly half had melasma for 5 years or less, whereas 29.6% had it for 10 years or more. About 18.5% of the patients were being treated for melasma, of which 60% had melasma for more than 10 years. The mean MELASQOL-F score was 20.9, which is significantly lower than the scores found in the previously mentioned studies, possibly reflecting decreased severity of melasma in the French population. Misery and colleagues also found that women older than 45 years had a significantly higher score than those younger than 45 years (24.6 and 18.5, respectively), which contrasts with those in Balkrishnan and colleagues' study, in which the 20- to 30-year age group had significantly higher scores.[1] The mean MELASQOL-F score was 14.8 when the duration of melasma was less than 5 years, 28.7 for the duration of 6 to 10 years, and 23.6 for the duration of more than 10 years. Like the results of the Balkrishnan study, the treated group of patients had significantly higher scores than the untreated group, with a mean of 32.8 versus 17.7. These results suggest that negative effects of melasma on QOL do not decrease over time and may increase with the number of attempts to treat this frustrating chronic condition. High body mass index or an associated disease did not affect the MELASQOL-F score, which suggests that the new instrument may be specific for melasma. When the mental composite score of the SF-12 (MCS-12) was less than 50, the mean MELASQOL-F score was 23.0, whereas the MELASQOL-F score was 14.7 when the MCS-12 was greater than 50. Thus, patients who had poor functioning in the psychological life domain (MCS-12<50) also had poorer QOL as reflected by higher MELASQOL-F scores, and vice versa. MELASQOL-F scores were significantly correlated with the DLQI and the PCV-Metra. The investigators suggest these correlations to the DLQI, PCV-Metra, and MCS-12 sufficiently demonstrate the new MELASQOL-F scale's equivalent reliability to these instruments. The MELASQOL-F's specificity for melasma and reliability in comparison with other QOL measures establish its superior utility in French women affected by melasma compared with other measures. The MELASQOL-F and the validation questionnaires were again internally consistent by Cronbach α, although the values were not presented. Construct validity was demonstrated by a high correlation between the MELASQOL-F scale and the health-related QOL psychosocial domains previously shown to be affected by melasma. Patients identified many QOL domains as significantly affected by melasma, especially family relationships and social life. The study is limited by the low number of patients, but it did find that MELASQOL-F scores were higher in women older than 45 years, in women who had a longer duration of melasma, and in women who had been previously treated. Similar to the MELASQOL results, the MELASQOL-F scores suggest that melasma is not better accepted by patients with the passage of time. MASI data in this French study would allow these results to be better compared with those of previous MELASQOL studies and correlate severity with QOL. Misery and colleagues have developed a reliable, reproducible, and validated French-language adaptation of the MELASQOL useful in the melasma population found in France.

TURKISH MELASQOL

Dogramaci and colleagues[30] translated the MELASQOL to the Turkish language in 2009 following the established translation process of forward translation, an expert panel consensus translation, back-translation, and review by the original author R. Balkrishnan. Dogramaci and colleagues conducted pretesting on 20 female patients with melasma and corrected any problematic items. To validate the newly adapted Turkish version of the MELASQOL (MELASQOL-TR), the scale was administered to 114 patients with melasma recruited from the dermatology outpatient clinics of Mustafa Kemal University School of Medicine in Turkey. The validated Turkish version of the WHOQOL-BREF was also concurrently administered, and patients were evaluated by MASI.

Inclusion criteria included female sex, age of 18 years or more, and use of an effective nonhormonal contraceptive method. Exclusion criteria included pregnancy in the last 6 months, menopause, history of bilateral oophorectomy, use of photosensitizing drugs, estrogen or progesterone preparation in the last 6 months, and use of depigmenting agents in the last 30 days. The mean age was 31.8 years, and most patients were married. About 60.5% of patients completed primary school, 12.3% were uneducated, 19.3% were high school graduates, and 7.9% had attended a university. The mean MELASQOL-TR score was 29.9, which is somewhat lower than that in the studies by Balkrishnan and colleagues and Dominguez and colleagues; however, the mean age of this Turkish population was also significantly lower. Mean duration of melasma was not presented and would have been informative to compare the Turkish study with previous studies that reported older patients and those with long-standing melasma had worse MELASQOL scores. Unlike the American, Brazilian, and French studies, no statistical differences were found between education levels, age groups, and variations in other demographic factors, such as marital status and medical comorbidities. The Cronbach α value of the MELASQOL-TR was 0.88, which, although satisfactory, is slightly lower than the high internal consistency demonstrated by the other MELASQOL versions. The MELASQOL-TR found that patients were most affected by the appearance of the skin, frustration, feeling unattractive to others, and having a restricted sense of freedom. Like the validation study for the MELASQOL-BP, the MELASQOL-TR showed inverse significant correlation to the WHOQOL-BREF. The mean WHOQOL-BREF score in the Turkish study was much lower at 54.8 compared with the mean of 86.7 in the study by Cestari and colleagues.[23] Dogramaci and colleagues found that patients scored highest (better QOL) in the WHOQOL-BREF in the social relations domain, followed by the physical domain, then psychological domain, and lowest in the environment domain, nearly the opposite of the findings in the study by Cestari and colleagues. Importantly, the study showed the most significant correlation between the MELASQOL-TR and the psychological domain of the WHOQOL-BREF. In contrast to the lack of or moderate correlation found between the MASI and the MELASQOL scores in previous studies, Dogramaci and colleagues interestingly found the MELASQOL-TR and MASI to be significantly correlated. The group modified the Turkish translation to better adapt the MELASQOL to the Turkish culture but did not elaborate on the details of these changes. Further revision of the MELASQOL-TR involving repeated correction and back-translation may help to improve comprehension of this tool, since 20.2% of patients needed help answering items. Validation of the MELASQOL-TR to demonstrate equivalent or superior discriminatory power to the WHOQOL-BREF or to a dermatology-specific QOL instrument such as the DLQI would also be helpful, and health-related QOL domains previously shown to be most affected by melasma should also correlate to the most affected QOL domains identified by the MELASQOL-TR.

Box 4
Guide for adaptation of the MELASQOL

1. Forward translate the MELASQOL into the new language.

2. Consult an expert bilingual panel to assess understandability.

3. Back translate the new-language MELASQOL to make sure meaning is not lost.

4. Pretest the new-language MELASQOL by probe technique on at least 10 members of the target population (preferably 25 to achieve <4% difficulty comprehending any item) or by appraisal by bilingual members of the target population.

5. Revise according to the pretesting results by consulting the expert panel and back translating until the new-language MELASQOL is highly comprehensible and cross-culturally equivalent.

6. Validate the new-language MELASQOL in the target population by:

   a. Comparing it to a validated same-language dermatology-specific QOL measure (or generic health-related QOL measure if the former is unavailable)

   b. Conducting comparative analyses of demographics and melasma characteristics, including MASI

   c. Using statistical analyses to demonstrate internal reliability, construct validity, discriminatory power, and correlation with relevant psychosocial health-related QOL domains

Data from Guillemin F, Bombardier C, Beaton D. Cross-cultural adaptation of health-related quality of life measures: literature review and proposed guidelines. J Clin Epidemiol 1993;46(12):1417–32; and WHO. Process of Translation and Adaptation of Instruments. Available at: http://www.who.int/entity/substance_abuse/research_tools/translation/en/index.html.

SUMMARY

Melasma is an asymptomatic but disfiguring disorder; therefore, it is important to evaluate the patient's overall health status using a QOL questionnaire that emphasizes the psychosocial effects of melasma rather than its clinical effects. From the results summarized in this article, it is clear that melasma causes a significant effect on QOL in many aspects of daily life. Because melasma is common worldwide, particularly in individuals with skin of color, it is imperative that the MELASQOL is translated and cross-culturally adapted to multiple languages in a semantically equivalent manner. The tool has been successfully adapted and validated in Spanish, Brazilian Portuguese, and French, and much progress has been made in Turkish. These studies have demonstrated differing and interesting findings about the emotional and psychological effects of melasma in various affected populations. Translation following the guidelines outlined by Guillemin and colleagues[22] is a key step in this process. Translation issues should be rigorously discussed by investigators and by those who are fluent in the language being addressed. Back-translation is important to ensure the items stay true to the original meaning and for complete understanding of the questionnaire. A standard of less than 4% of participants needing assistance to answer questions should be a goal of future questionnaires to maximize comprehension (see Box 4). In addition, thorough validation of the new-language MELASQOL should include comparison with a validated dermatology-specific QOL questionnaire; comparison of affected QOL domains; comparative analyses between various demographic and melasma characteristics including MASI; and, most importantly, statistical analyses demonstrating internal reliability, construct validity, and superior discriminatory power. Furthermore, the validation study should survey patients with chronic melasma because these patients comprise the target population of the MELASQOL. Box 4 is a guide for future adaptations of the MELASQOL. Although much progress has been made to understand the effect of melasma on QOL in different populations, more work needs to be done. Many large populations of the world affected by melasma still do not have a validated MELASQOL instrument available, including individuals who speak Mandarin Chinese, Hindi, Arabic, Russian, and Japanese, to name a few. Development of these instruments and their administration will help to understand the impact of melasma worldwide and also determine the effect of treatment on this disorder.

REFERENCES

1. Balkrishnan R, McMichael AJ, Camacho FT, et al. Development and validation of a health-related quality of life instrument for women with melasma. Br J Dermatol 2003;149:572–7.
2. Dominguez AR, Balkrishnan R, Ellzey AR, et al. Melasma in Latina patients: cross-cultural adaptation and validation of a quality-of-life questionnaire in Spanish language. J Am Acad Dermatol 2006;55: 59–66.
3. Chren MM, Lasek RJ, Quinn LM, et al. Skindex, a quality-of-life measure for patients with skin disease: reliability, validity, and responsiveness. J Invest Dermatol 1996;107:707–13.
4. Finlay A, Khan G. Dermatology Life Quality Index (DLQI)—a simple practical measure for routine clinical use. Clin Exp Dermatol 1994;19:210–6.
5. Motley R, Finlay A. Practical use of a disability index in the routine management of acne. Clin Exp Dermatol 1992;17:1–3.
6. Finlay AY, Kelly SE. Psoriasis—an index of disability. Clin Exp Dermatol 1987;12:8–11.
7. Whalley D, Mckenna SP, Dewar AL, et al. A new instrument for assessing quality of life in atopic dermatitis: international development of the Quality of Life Index for Atopic Dermatitis (QOLIAD). Br J Dermatol 2004;150:274–83.
8. Baiardini I, Pasquali M, Braido F, et al. A new tool to evaluate the impact of chronic urticaria on quality of life: chronic urticaria quality of life questionnaire (CU-Q2oL). Allergy 2005;60:1073–8.
9. Werlinger KD, Guevara IL, Gonzalez CM, et al. Prevalence of self-diagnosed melasma among premenopausal Latino women in Dallas and Fort Worth, Tex. Arch Dermatol 2007;143:424–5.
10. Grimes PE. Management of hyperpigmentation in darker racial ethnic groups. Semin Cutan Med Surg 2009;28:77–85.
11. Sheth VM, Pandya AG. Melasma: a comprehensive update part I. J Am Acad Dermatol 2011;65(4): 689–97.
12. Pandya AG, Hynan LS, Bhore R, et al. Reliability assessment and validation of the Melasma Area and Severity Index (MASI) and a new modified MASI scoring method. J Am Acad Dermatol 2011; 64(1):78–83.e2.
13. Skevington SM, Sartorius N, Amir M, et al. Developing methods for assessing quality of life in different cultural settings. The history of the WHO-QOL instruments. Soc Psychiatry Psychiatr Epidemiol 2004;39(1):1–8.
14. Finlay AY, Khan GK, Luscombe DK, et al. Validation of Sickness Impact Profile and Psoriasis Disability index in psoriasis. Br J Dermatol 1990;123(6):751–6.
15. Beattie PE, Lewis-Jones MS. A comparative study of impairment of quality of life in children with skin

disease and children with other chronic childhood diseases. Br J Dermatol 2006;155(1):145–51.

16. Rapp SR, Feldman SR, Exum ML, et al. Psoriasis causes as much disability as other major medical diseases. J Am Acad Dermatol 1999; 41(3):401–7.

17. Chren MM, Lasek RJ, Sahay AP, et al. Measurement properties of Skindex-16: a brief quality-of-life measure for patients with skin diseases. J Cutan Med Surg 2001;5(2):105–10.

18. Bland JM. Medical statistics in obstetrics and gynaecology. Eur J Obstet Gynecol Reprod Biol 1997;75(1):99–102.

19. Balkrishnan R, Kelly AP, McMichael A, et al. Improved quality of life with effective treatment of facial melasma: the PIGMENT trial. J Drugs Dermatol 2004;3(4): 377–81.

20. Pichardo R, Vallejos Q, Feldman SR, et al. The prevalence of melasma and its association with quality of life in adult male Latino migrant workers. Int J Dermatol 2009;48(1):22–6.

21. Orwin RG. A fail-safe N for effect size in meta-analysis. J Educ Stat 1983;8(2):157–9.

22. Guillemin F, Bombardier C, Beaton D. Cross-cultural adaptation of health-related quality of life measures: literature review and proposed guidelines. J Clin Ep idemiol 1993;46(12):1417–32.

23. Cestari TF, Hexsel D, Viegas ML, et al. Validation of a melasma quality of life questionnaire for Brazilian Portuguese language: the MelasQol-BP study and improvement of QoL of melasma patients after

triple combination therapy. Br J Dermatol 2006; 156(Suppl 1):13–20.

24. WHO. Process of translation and adaptation of instruments. Available at: http://www.who.int/entity/ substance_abuse/research_tools/translation/en/index. html. Accessed October 3, 2011.

25. Freitag FM, Cestari TF, Leopoldo LR, et al. Effect of melasma on quality of life in a sample of women living in southern Brazil. J Eur Acad Dermatol Venereol 2008;22(6):655–62.

26. Misery L, Schmitt AM, Boussetta S, et al. Melasma: measure of the impact on quality of life using the French version of MELASQOL after cross-cultural adaptation. Acta Derm Venereol 2010; 90(3):331–2.

27. Gandek B, Ware JE, Aaronson NK, et al. Cross-validation of item selection and scoring for the SF-12 Health Survey in nine countries: results from the IQOLA project. J Clin Epidemiol 1998;51:1171–8.

28. Ware JE, Gandek B. Overview of the SF-36 Health Survey and the International Quality of Life Assessment (IQOLA) Project. J Clin Epidemiol 1998;51: 903–12.

29. Consoli SM, Taine P, Szabason F, et al. Elaboration et validation d'un questionnaire de stress perçu proposé comme indicateur de suivi en médicine du travail. Encephale 1997;23:184–93.

30. Dogramaci AC, Havlucu DY, Inandi T, et al. Validation of a melasma quality of life questionnaire for the Turkish language: the MelasQoL-TR study. J Dermatolog Treat 2009;20(2):95–9.

Quality-of-Life Instruments: Evaluation of the Impact of Psoriasis on Patients

Misha M. Heller, BA[a,b], Jillian W. Wong, BA[a,c],
Tien V. Nguyen, BA[a,d], Eric S. Lee, MD[a,e], Tina Bhutani, MD[a],
Alan Menter, MD[f,g], John Y.M. Koo, MD[a,*]

KEYWORDS

- Psoriasis • Quality-of-life instruments
- Psoriasis treatments • Biologics

Psoriasis is a chronic, inflammatory dermatologic disease that affects approximately 2% to 3% of the general population.[1] Psoriasis can be cosmetically disfiguring, with much attached social stigmata. Consequently, patients often suffer significant interpersonal and psychologic distress.

The negative impact of psoriasis on a patient's quality of life (QoL) is well described in the literature. Patients commonly feel embarrassed, self-conscious, or ashamed of their physical appearance. They experience many difficulties in social interactions, especially in meeting new individuals and forming romantic relationships. They frequently demonstrate psychologic problems, including poor self-esteem, frustration, anger, helplessness, anxiety, and depression. Sadly, some patients even develop suicidal ideation.[2–8]

Beyond its psychosocial effects, psoriasis can cause significant physical complaints, such as severe itching, irritation, and pain. For many patients, psoriasis can be a tremendous burden on their daily lives.[7] In a landmark study published in 1999, Rapp and colleagues[8] found that the negative impact of psoriasis on QoL is comparable with that of other major medical disorders, such as cancer, diabetes, heart disease, and major depressive disorder. Therefore, it has become increasingly clear that psoriasis can have detrimental effects on a patient's QoL. As such, evaluation of the extent to which the disease impacts a patient's

Conflicts of Interest Disclosure: JWW, TVN, MMH, ESL, and TB have no financial conflicts of interest to disclose. JYMK has the following conflicts of interest: Abbott, Amgen, Leo, Galderma, Glaxo-Smith-Klein, PhotoMedex, Pfizer, and Teikoku. AM has the following conflicts of interest: Abbott, Amgen, Astellas, Celgene, Centocor, Eli Lilly, Galderma, Genentech, Novartis, Novo Nordisk, Pfizer, Promius, Stiefel, Syntrix Biosystems, Warner Chilcott, and Wyeth. There were no funding sources for this manuscript.

[a] Department of Dermatology, Psoriasis and Skin Treatment Center, University of California San Francisco Medical Center, 515 Spruce Street, San Francisco, CA 94118, USA
[b] Keck School of Medicine, University of Southern California, 1975 Zonal Avenue, Los Angeles, CA 90089-9034, USA
[c] University of Utah School of Medicine, 30 North 1900 East, Room 1C029, Salt Lake City, UT 84132, USA
[d] University of Texas Health Science Center at San Antonio, School of Medicine, 7703 Floyd Curl Drive, San Antonio, TX 78229, USA
[e] University of Nebraska Medical Center, College of Medicine, 985527 Nebraska Medical Center, Omaha, NE 68198-5527, USA
[f] Department of Dermatology, Baylor University Medical Center, 3500 Gaston Avenue, Dallas, TX 75246, USA
[g] University of Texas Southwestern Medical Center, 5323 Harry Hines Boulevard, Dallas, TX 75390, USA
* Corresponding author.
E-mail address: john.koo@ucsfmedctr.org

Dermatol Clin 30 (2012) 281–291
doi:10.1016/j.det.2011.11.006

QoL should be a central aspect of the management and care of patients with psoriasis before initiating therapy and at subsequent visits.

DEFINITION OF QoL

QoL is a broad term used to evaluate the general well-being of an individual. It is meant to encompass all variables that may impact an individual's life, including physical, social, and psychologic factors. Some authors define QoL as an individual's perception of his or her position in life, in relation to his or her life goals and belief system.[9] Health-related QoL is a more limited concept used to describe the effects that a disease or its symptoms have on an individual's life. In terms of psoriasis, health-related QoL consists of physical disabilities (eg, itching, pain, insomnia, difficulty walking); psychologic effects (eg, embarrassment, frustration, anxiety, depression); social effects (eg, making new friends, going to social functions); occupation effects (eg, lost time from work, decreased work productivity); daily burdens (eg, wearing specific clothing to conceal psoriatic plaques, frequently vacuuming); and treatment impact (eg, time demands, cost of therapy, potential side effects).[10]

IMPORTANCE OF QoL EVALUATION

There are many reasons why it is especially important to measure the impact of psoriasis on a patient's QoL. Perhaps the most significant reason is in determining appropriate therapy for psoriasis. Presently, there are several highly effective, systemic therapies for psoriasis, such as cyclosporine, methotrexate. and the biologics including etanercept (Enbrel), adalimumab (Humira), infliximab (Remicade), and ustekinumab (Stelera). There are also many new systemic and biologic therapies currently in development. Unfortunately, all of these systemic therapies carry the potential risk of side effects, including nephrotoxicity, hepatotoxicity, tuberculosis, and malignancy. Thus, when a clinician makes the decision to go beyond topical therapies in the treatment of psoriasis, he or she considers whether the benefits of prescribing systemic therapies outweigh their possible side effects.

In evaluating this risk-to-benefit ratio, the clinician should consider whether the patient's clinical disease severity and the impact of the disease on the patient's QoL warrants more aggressive therapy. Generally speaking, a clinician can easily determine a near precise estimate of the clinical disease severity using such measures as the psoriasis area and severity index (PASI) or the psoriasis global assessment scores. However, a clinician may not be accurate in evaluating the impact of the disease on a patient's QoL. Here, the use of simple QoL instruments can assist the clinician in identifying those patients who would benefit most from systemic or biologic therapy. At the same time, it can provide the clinician with an added means of justifying to third-party payers and other interested parties the need to cover more aggressive, and often more expensive, therapies.

HEALTH-RELATED QoL INSTRUMENTS

Health-related QoL instruments are questionnaires designed to assess the impact of a disease on a patient's QoL. These QoL instruments can be generic, specialty-specific (ie, dermatology-specific), or disease-specific (ie, psoriasis-specific). Most have been developed for adult patients, but a few have been designed for children. To be a useful QoL instrument, it should demonstrate the following criteria: (1) validity (ie, the instrument evaluates well what it intends to measure); (2) reliability (ie, the instrument is reproducible over time); (3) capable of measuring health-related QoL regardless of the disease severity (ie, the instrument can be used for patients with either mild-to-moderate or moderate-to-severe psoriasis); (4) applicable to a wide variety of patients in different clinical settings; and (5) quick and easy for patients to fill out.

QoL INSTRUMENTS FOR PSORIASIS

Several useful generic, dermatology-specific, and disease-specific QoL instruments exist to evaluate the impact of psoriasis on patient's QoL.[9–12] Specifically, generic QoL instruments given to patients with psoriasis include the Short Form 36 (SF-36),[13,14] the Sickness Impact Profile (SIP),[15] the General Health Questionnaire (GHQ),[16] and the Psychological General Well-Being Index (PGWB).[17] The dermatology-specific QoL instruments commonly administered to patients with psoriasis include the Dermatology Life Quality Index (DLQI),[18,19] Dermatology Quality of Life Scales (DQoLS),[20] Dermatology Specific Quality of Life (DSQL),[21] and Skindex (Skindex-61, Skindex-29).[22] The dermatology-specific QoL instruments developed for children with psoriasis and other dermatologic disorders are the Children's Dermatology Life Quality Index (CDLQI) text version[23] and cartoon version.[24] Finally, the psoriasis-specific QoL instruments include Psoriasis Disability Index (PDI),[25,26] Psoriasis Life Stress Inventory (PLSI),[27] Psoriasis Specific Measure of

Quality of Life (PSORIQoL),[28] Salford Psoriasis Index (SPI),[29] and Koo-Menter Psoriasis Instrument (KMPI) (**Box 1**).[30] Although there may be overlap in the usage of these instruments, the generic instruments are most useful to compare psoriasis with other nonskin diseases, the skin-specific ones to compare psoriasis with other skin conditions, and the psoriasis-specific instrument to use in situations where small changes need to be measured or when psoriasis-specific QoL issues need to be elaborated.

GENERIC QoL INSTRUMENTS
Short Form 36

The SF-36 is a 36-question survey that measures eight broad health dimensions: (1) physical functioning, (2) social functioning, (3) role limitations caused by physical problems, (4) role limitations caused by emotional problems, (5) general mental health, (6) energy and fatigue, (7) bodily pain, and (8) general health perception.[13,14] In addition, there is a question regarding the change in general

---

Box 1
Useful QoL instruments for psoriasis

Generic QoL instruments
- Short Form 36
- Sickness Impact Profile
- General Health Questionnaire
- Psychological General Well-Being Index

Dermatology-specific QoL instruments
- Dermatology Life Quality Index
- Dermatology Quality of Life Scales
- Dermatology Specific Quality of Life
- Skindex (Skindex-61, Skindex-29)

Dermatology-specific QoL instruments: children
- Children's Dermatology Life Quality Index (text version)
- Children's Dermatology Life Quality Index (cartoon version)

Psoriasis-specific QoL instruments
- Psoriasis Disability Index
- Psoriasis Life Stress Inventory
- Psoriasis Index of Quality of Life
- Salford Psoriasis Index
- Psoriasis Quality of Life 12 items (a part of the Koo-Menter Psoriasis Instrument)

---

health in the past year. The SF-36 is scored from 0 (worst health state) to 100 (best health state).

The SF-36 meets stringent criteria of reliability and validity. It has been widely used in more than 200 clinical studies assessing QoL in various medical diseases, including those of the skin. It is considered to be most applicable for comparison of skin diseases with other systemic diseases. In evaluating the impact of psoriasis on QoL, the SF-36 demonstrates significant correlation with PASI scores (ie, worse SF-36 scores are associated with increased psoriasis severity).[31] The SF-36 is also a useful measure of mental health in skin conditions, such as palmoplantar psoriasis, where limited area of skin involvement can cause significant impairment of function.[32] A study of 100 patients with hand eczema recruited from an occupational dermatology clinic reported that the SF-36 was a more suitable measure of health-related QoL compared with the DLQI.[32] This was determined because the study had found that females had more impaired mental health using the SF-36 compared with males but that the DLQI was unable to differentiate the discrepancy in mental health impact between genders.

The SF-36 has been used to compare QoL of patients with psoriasis with the QoL of patients with other chronic health conditions. One study had 317 patients complete the SF-36, and responses were compared with patients who had other chronic conditions including depression, diabetes mellitus type 2, congestive heart failure, myocardial infarction, hypertension, cancer, arthritis, chronic lung disease, and dermatitis.[8] The impact of psoriasis on QoL was determined to be similar to other medical illnesses. The study supported the concept that psoriasis was not simply a cosmetic concern, but it had debilitating physical and emotional effects on patients.

Sickness Impact Profile

The SIP is a measure of health status based on assessment of an individual's performance on daily activities. The SIP has been used in a broad range of diseases in more than 2000 publications.[12] It has been shown to have high reliability and internal consistency.[15] In psoriasis, the overall SIP scores have been found to correlate well with PDI because both successfully measure the broad extent (in 12 different categories) to which psoriasis limits the patient's physical and psychosocial functions.[33] This measurement of disability is useful for those patients whose main issue with psoriasis is the functional and physical limitations rather than emotional.

General Health Questionnaire

The GHQ is a survey that identifies patients suffering from diagnosable psychiatric disorders. There are several versions of the GHQ, including the 60-, 30-, 28-, and 12-item versions.[12] The 28-item GHQ consists of four subscales (somatic symptoms, anxiety and insomnia, social dysfunction, and severe depression).[16] The 28-item GHQ is the version typically used on patients with psoriasis, and it has been shown to be highly correlated to psychologic distress specifically in a group of 22 patients with psoriasis undergoing psoralen-ultraviolet light A therapy.[34] In this study, patients were asked to complete a self-rating survey of disease severity, the PDI, and the GHQ. The GHQ, PDI, and patient-rated severity scores all correlated to each other. Overall, the results showed that psoriasis affects mental health through its impact on the daily life of the patient.[34]

Psychologic General Well-Being Index

The PGWB Index is a self-administered, validated psychometric instrument that measures an individual's emotional well-being. It is specifically designed to be suitable for assessing psychologic well-being of the general medical population as opposed to a psychiatric population. This 22-question instrument can be subdivided into six broad domains (anxiety, depressed mood, positive well-being, self-control, general health, and vitality). PGWB is graded on a five-point Likert-type scale, a psychometric scale commonly used in questionnaires in which answer choices range from "strongly disagree," "disagree," "neither agree nor disagree," "agree," to "strongly agree." The PGWB Index is a good tool for assessing the disability of psoriasis.[17] In a study of 32 patients with moderate-to-severe plaque psoriasis receiving adalimumab for 24 weeks, participants were asked to complete the PGWB.[35] Statistically significant improvement in the total PGWB score was documented by Week 4. By Week 24, all six PGWB domains showed statistically significant improvement from the pretreatment baseline. The authors then compared the PGWB scores of patients with psoriasis with those of patients with other chronic medical conditions. Based on PGWB scores, untreated patients with psoriasis have as much impairment in psychologic well-being as patients with other major medical diseases including breast cancer, coronary artery disease, congestive heart failure, and diabetes and that potent intervention improves psychologic well-being to where it is comparable with that of patients with asymptomatic hypertension. A prompt intervention with an effective dermatologic treatment is not only critical, but capable of restoring the physical and psychologic well-being of patients with psoriasis.

Each instrument has a different focus for the measurement of QoL in patients with psoriasis. The SF-36 inquires into the patient's perception of well-being and his or her attributions of limitations in daily life activities to psoriasis. SF-36 is thus a helpful tool for clinicians to deploy to monitor the effects of psoriasis treatment on the patient's overall QoL.[31] The SIP includes broad aspects of physical, emotional, and social behavior that suffer impairment as a result of their psoriasis, regardless of clinical symptom severity. SIP thus has a niche in measuring disability of patients with psoriasis and can be used complimentarily with other disability indices, such as the PDI.[33] Furthermore, such tools as the General Health Questionnaire and the Psychological General Well-Being Index are useful in assessing the psychiatric impact of psoriasis on a patient's QoL. They would not assist a physician who wishes to focus on physical constraints or social disability associated with psoriasis.

DERMATOLOGY-SPECIFIC QoL INSTRUMENTS

The dermatology-specific instruments allow for psoriasis to be compared with other skin conditions.

Dermatology Life Quality Index

Published by Finlay and Khan in 1994, the DLQI is the best known of all dermatologic questionnaires. The DLQI demonstrates high validity, reliability, and internal consistency. It has been widely used in numerous clinical studies in more than 17 countries and translated into more than 21 languages. It has been shown to be useful in psoriasis and 34 other dermatologic conditions.[12] It also offers the advantage of being short and easy for patients to complete. However, because of its brevity, some authors argue that the DLQI does not adequately address the emotional impact of dermatologic conditions.[11]

Dermatology Quality of Life Scales

DQoLS was initially based on the responses of 50 dermatologic outpatients in England. It was designed to complement the DLQI, with greater emphasis on the psychosocial issues. The DQoLS consists of a total of 41 items, divided into 17 items regarding psychosocial issues, 12 items concerning physical activity, and 12 items relating to disease severity. The psychosocial items are further divided into four subscales (embarrassment, despair, irritableness, distress), whereas the physical activity items are further divided into four subscales (everyday, summer, social, sexual). Each item is scored on a five-point scale, ranging from "very slightly or not at all," "a little," "moderately," "quite a bit," to "extremely."

In its development, the DQoLS was shown to have high internal consistency and test–retest reliability. Although the DQoLs was first tested on a wide variety of dermatologic conditions, further studies have focused mainly on acne and psoriasis. Recent clinical studies have also used the DQoLS to demonstrate that biologic therapy may help to improve QoL scores.[36] A multicenter, double-blinded study of 553 patients with plaque psoriasis was randomized to obtaining alefacept for two courses, alefacept in the first course and placebo in the second course, or placebo in the first course and alefacept in the second course. The DQOLS, DLQI, and SF-36 were administered. Scores for the DQOLS and DLQI were significantly reduced, and therefore improved, in the first course of treatment and during subsequent treatments.[35] The study found that patients who received a full two courses of the biologic treatment experienced additional increase in QoL measures during the second course. SF-36 also demonstrated that alefacept did not have a negative impact on the QoL of the patients.[35]

Dermatology Specific Quality of Life

The DSQL is a 52-item self-administered tool used to quantify the effects of dermatologic diseases on an individual's psychologic well-being.[12] Of the 52 items, 43 items are dermatology-specific falling into five scales (physical symptoms, daily activity, social function, work and school, and self-perception), and nine items are from two SF-36 scales (General Mental Health and Energy/Vitality).[21] To the authors' knowledge, no published studies have examined the use of the DSQL to psoriasis specifically.

Skindex

The Skindex was designed to measure the effects of dermatologic conditions on an individual's QoL. It is a 61-item self-administered survey composed of eight scales. Each scale addresses a component of QoL, including cognitive effects, physical limitations, embarrassment, anger, physical discomfort, social effects, depression, and fear.[22] Skindex is considered to be a useful tool to determine QoL in patients with many types of dermatologic diseases.[11] No published studies have examined the use of Skindex specifically for psoriasis.

DERMATOLOGY-SPECIFIC QoL INSTRUMENTS: CHILDREN
Children's Dermatology Life Quality Index

The CDLQI, published in 1995, is the children's version of the DLQI. It was standardized on 169 children (ages 3–16 years), who presented to a pediatric dermatologic clinic. The CDLQI was developed based on what these children, with the assistance of their parents, described to be all the ways in which their skin disease affected their lives. The CDLQI has a similar structure to the adult DQLI and has the same scoring system. Specifically, it is a 10-item text-only questionnaire (maximum score of 30).[23] The CDLQI is recommended for use in children ages 7 years or older.[11]

Children's Dermatology Life Quality Index (Cartoon version)

In 2003, a colored cartoon version of the CDLQI was developed. The cartoon version of the CDLQI is considered equivalent in assessing QoL measures as the written version of the CDLQI. However, it is easier and faster for children to complete. Children and parents prefer the cartoon version of the CDLQI.[12,24]

The CDLQI has been shown to produce consistent results in the pediatric population. In 1995, when the CDLQI was used to measure the quality-of-life impact of different dermatologic conditions in 233 pediatric dermatology outpatients compared with two different control groups, psoriasis had a mean score of 5.4, whereas those for scabies, eczema, and acne were 9.5, 7.7, and 5.7, respectively.[23] Patients with warts and moles scored the lowest (2.3 and 3.3, respectively).[23] Forty-six additional patients were recruited to complete the CDLQI on two separate occasions; their results indicated acceptable reliability of this questionnaire's test–retest capability.[23]

In 2010, 39 pediatric patients with psoriasis with almost equal gender distribution completed the CDLQI during outpatient dermatology clinic visits.[37] The mean CDLQI score for this study was 6,[37] which is not significantly different from that obtained from the aforementioned study. Moreover, the correlation coefficient calculated by the Spearman rho test between CDLQI and PASI was 0.47, whereas that between CLDQI and Physician Global's Assessment was 0.51.[37] Because perfect score for positive correlation is 1, a pediatric patient with psoriasis whose scores of clinical severity are high can be predicted with a moderate degree of confidence to have a relatively low QoL.

PSORIASIS-SPECIFIC QoL INSTRUMENTS

The psoriasis-specific instruments are the most sensitive and comprehensive to psoriasis. As such, they are best in two scenarios. The first is to detect small changes in psoriasis-specific QoL, which is relevant in both the clinical setting and in interventional trials. The second scenario is the need to elaborate what aspects of psoriasis is most important to the patient. The following instruments fit in these scenarios in differing ways.

Psoriasis Disability Index

Published by Finlay and Kelly in 1987, the PDI is one of the first questionnaires to specifically assess QoL in patients with psoriasis. The PDI consists of 15 questions divided into questions related to daily activities, work or school, personal relationships, leisure, and treatment. All questions are based on the patient's experiences over the last 4 weeks. There are two possible scoring systems (visual analog scale or tick box). On the visual analog scoring system, questions are answered on a scale of 1 to 7. On the tick box scoring system, questions are answered as either 0 ("not at all"), 1 ("a little"), 2 ("a lot"), or 3 ("very much").[25,26] The PDI has been used in numerous clinical studies over the past 20 years and has proved to be a valuable measure for psoriasis.[11] The niche for this questionnaire may be more appropriate to evaluate disability than to assess emotional impact.

Psoriasis Life Stress Inventory

The PLSI is a 15-item measure that evaluates the effect of daily stressors on patients with psoriasis. It aims to measure the social impact of psoriasis. It examines such questions as the following: do you feel self-conscious about your appearance among strangers, do you avoid public places like swimming pools or fitness centers, and do you wear clothing to cover affected areas? Each item is scored on a four-point scale, ranging from 0 ("not at all"), 1 ("slight degree"), 2 ("moderate degree"), and 3 ("a great deal"). The total score varies from 0 to 45, with higher scores indicating greater levels of daily stress.[27]

The PLSI has a high degree of internal consistency. It demonstrates comparability with PASI scores. Specifically, patients with PLSI score of 10 or greater have been found to have greater overall psoriasis severity. PLSI is also a useful measure to evaluate patients suffering from psoriatic arthritis.[38] Therefore, it can be used to identify stressors in psoriasis and psoriatic arthritis.

Psoriasis Index of Quality of Life

The PSORIQoL is a psoriasis-specific instrument that was developed from responses of 62 patients with psoriasis in the United Kingdom, Italy, and the Netherlands. It consists of a total of 25 items written as negative statements aimed at assessing the psychosocial impact of psoriasis. The PSORIQoL includes items related to fear of negative reactions from others, self-consciousness and poor self-confidence, problems with socialization, physical contact and intimacy, limitations on personal freedom and impaired relaxation, and sleep and emotional stability. For each item, patients receive one point for every negative statement with which they agree. The final scores range from 0 to 25, with higher scores indicating worse psychosocial impact.[28]

The PSORIQoL is a validated instrument, with high test–retest reliability and high internal consistency. Of note, the internal consistency of the PSORIQoL is higher than that of DLQI. The PSORIQoL is thought to be a useful tool for clinical trials in psoriasis.[12]

Salford Psoriasis Index

The SPI is made-up of three individually scored measures: (1) signs, (2) psychosocial disability, and (3) intervention. This three-measure model is meant to be a similar paradigm to the TNM (tumor, nodes, metastasis) classification system used for staging cancer. The signs measure converts the PASI score into a number ranging from 0 to 10. The psychosocial impact measure evaluates the effect of psoriasis on day-to-day life, using a visual analog scale of 0 ("not at all affected") to 10 ("completely affected"). The intervention measure reflects historical disease severity, where extra points are given for need of systemic treatment, admission to the hospital, and number of episodes of erythroderma.[29]

The SPI is a validated psoriasis-specific instrument with high reliability. The psychosocial impact measure is strongly associated with the PDI, but it is poorly correlated with PASI. Ultimately, the SPI instrument is considered to take a holistic approach to evaluating psoriasis by examining current clinical disease severity, psychosocial disability, and past disease severity based on treatment history.[29]

Psoriasis Quality of Life 12 Items and the Koo-Menter Psoriasis Instrument

The KMPI is a two-page questionnaire on a single sheet developed to assist dermatology providers in making the critical decision of whether it is necessary to go beyond topical therapies in treating psoriasis (**Fig. 1** illustrates the entire KMPI). The patient completes the front page of the KMPI and the physician completes the reverse side. The front page consists of three brief sections, including the psoriasis-specific QoL instrument (also known as, the Psoriasis Quality of Life 12-items [PQoL-12]); indication of the parts of the body currently affected by psoriasis; and symptoms of joint pain or history of psoriatic arthritis. On the reverse side, the

A

Koo-Menter Psoriasis Instrument

Patient Self-Assessment   Name: _____   Date: _____

Part 1: Quality of Life - Please answer each of the following questions as they pertain to your psoriasis <u>during the past month</u>. (Circle one number per question)

	Not at All				Somewhat					Very Much
1. How self-conscious do you feel with regard to your psoriasis?	0	1	2	3	4	5	6	7	8	9	10
2. How helpless do you feel with regard to your psoriasis?	0	1	2	3	4	5	6	7	8	9	10
3. How embarrassed do you feel with regard to your psoriasis?	0	1	2	3	4	5	6	7	8	9	10
4. How angry or frustrated do you feel with regard to your psoriasis?	0	1	2	3	4	5	6	7	8	9	10
5. To what extent does your psoriasis make your appearance unsightly?	0	1	2	3	4	5	6	7	8	9	10
6. How disfiguring is your psoriasis?	0	1	2	3	4	5	6	7	8	9	10
7. How much does your psoriasis impact your overall emotional well-being?	0	1	2	3	4	5	6	7	8	9	10
8. Overall, to what extent does your psoriasis interfere with your capacity to enjoy life?	0	1	2	3	4	5	6	7	8	9	10

How much have each of the following been affected by your psoriasis <u>during the past month</u>? (Circle one number per question)

	Not at All				Somewhat					Very Much
9. Itching?	0	1	2	3	4	5	6	7	8	9	10
10. Physical irritation?	0	1	2	3	4	5	6	7	8	9	10
11. Physical pain or soreness?	0	1	2	3	4	5	6	7	8	9	10
12. Choice of clothing to conceal psoriasis?	0	1	2	3	4	5	6	7	8	9	10

Total Quality-of-Life Score (0 - 120)
* (Medical staff to calculate) [ ][ ][ ]

12-item Psoriasis Quality of Life Questionnaire (PQOL-12), Copyright 2002, 2003, Allergan, Inc.

Part 2:

A. Using the figures below, place an "X" on the parts of your body that <u>currently</u> have psoriasis.

Front   Back

Part 3:

A. Have you ever been diagnosed with psoriatic arthritis?
Yes ☐   No ☐

B. Do you have swollen, tender, or stiff joints (e.g., hands, feet, hips, back)?
Yes ☐   No ☐

If yes, how many joints are affected? (Check one box)
1 ☐   2 ☐   3 ☐   4 ☐   More than 4 ☐

If yes, how much have your joint symptoms affected your daily activities?
Not at all ☐   A little ☐   A lot ☐   Very much ☐

STOP Once completed, please return to medical staff

Fig. 1. (*A, B*) Koo-Menter psoriasis instrument. (*Courtesy of* J.Y.M. Koo, MD, San Francisco, CA; and A.M. Menter, MD, Dallas, TX.)

B Koo-Menter Psoriasis Instrument

Physician Assessment Name:_____ Date:_____

Part 1: Total Quality-of-Life assessment score (from part 1 of previous page) ⟹	☐ ☐ ☐

Part 2: Area of total body involvement: % BSA (body surface area)

Head	☐ %	Head: up to 9% of total BSA	
Anterior Trunk	☐ %	Anterior Trunk: up to 18%	Note: Patient's open hand (from wrist to tips of fingers) with fingers tucked together and thumb tucked to the side equals approximately 1% body surface area
Posterior Trunk	☐ %	Posterior Trunk: up to 18%	
Right Leg	☐ %	Right Leg: up to 18% (includes buttock)	
Left Leg	☐ %	Left Leg: up to 18% (includes buttock)	
Both Arms	☐ %	Both Arms: up to 18%	
Genitalia	☐ %	Genitalia: 1%	
Total BSA	☐ ☐ %		

Part 3: In terms of psoriasis severity, does the patient have:	Check Answer	
Plaque, erythrodermic, or pustular psoriasis with >10% BSA involvement?	Yes	No
Persistent guttate psoriasis?	Yes	No
Localized (< 10% BSA) psoriasis but resistant to optimized attempts at topical therapy or physically disabling (e.g., palmar and/or plantar psoriasis)?	Yes	No
Localized (< 10% BSA) but serious subtype with possibility of progression (eg, pustular or pre-erythrodermic psoriasis)?	Yes	No
Psoriatic arthritis that affects daily activities (arthritis based on prior diagnosis or Part 3 of patient self-assessment and physician clinical assessment)?	Yes	No
Substantial psychosocial or quality-of-life impact documented by patient Quality-of-Life self-assessment score of ≥ 50?	Yes	No

Part 4: Is phototherapy an option?	Check Answer	
Is a suitable phototherapy unit readily accessible to the patient?	Yes	No
Does the anatomical location or form of psoriasis (e.g., scalp, inverse, erythrodermic) preclude phototherapy?	Yes	No
Does the patient have the dedication, time, stamina, or transportation for phototherapy?	Yes	No
Has phototherapy, as monotherapy, failed in the past?	Yes	No
Is phototherapy contraindicated (eg, photosensitive drugs, history of multiple skin cancers)?	Yes	No
In your clinical judgement, is phototherapy likely to yield substantial improvement to justify its use before systemic therapy?	Yes	No

Physician/Nurse comments: _____

_____

_____

If at least one of the shaded boxes in both Part 3 and Part 4 above are checked, then the patient is a candidate for systemic therapy.

CONCLUSION: The patient is a candidate for systemic therapy	Yes	No

Fig. 1. (*continued*)

physician sums the QoL score, calculates the body surface area involvement using the "rule of nines," and answers a series of "yes" or "no" questions that help characterize the patient's disease severity and treatment history. With this QoL score, the body surface area involvement, and the overall clinical assessment of the patient's disease, the dermatology provider is better able to determine the need for systemic therapy and thereby minimize the significant undertreatment of patients with moderate-to-severe psoriasis.[30,39–45]

The KMPI was initially drafted by the two authors, Dr Koo and Dr Menter. It has since been scrutinized, improved, and endorsed by the medical advisory board of the National Psoriasis Foundation. With this endorsement, the KMPI not only clarifies to dermatology providers when to go beyond to topical therapies, but also assists dermatology providers who are often put in the difficult position to defend the decision to use systemic and biologic therapies to third-party payers and other interested parties.[30,39–45] In the author's (JK) experience with general dermatology clinics and psoriasis centers across the United States, the assessment of QoL as part of the KMPI has been used to overturn denials of systemic and biologic therapies to patients with psoriasis by insurance companies with almost complete success.

The PQoL-12 is a subsection of the KMPI, consisting of 12 items completed by the patient while waiting to be evaluated by the physician. Compared with other QoL instruments (eg, DLQI, PDI, or Skindex), the PQoL-12 is unique in that it is a data-derived questionnaire. Initially, nearly 100 questions were developed based on a comprehensive literature review and focus group sessions in which patients discussed their experiences living with psoriasis. These questions were pilot tested on more than 500 patients with psoriasis, who were identified from a nationwide population-based, demographically balanced sample of 50,000 households in the United States. The questions were refined down to 41 of the most relevant questions according the input of patients with psoriasis, and this made up the original 41-item version of the PQoL instrument. Subsequently, a final multicenter study was performed, and the list of questions was further narrowed down to 12-items, which constitutes the current PQoL-12 instrument. The PQoL-12 instrument is valid and reliable, with statistically significant cut-off threshold separating those with significant QoL deficits from those with less significant QoL negative impact. The cut-off threshold was determined to be a QoL score of 50 or more from the possible range of 0 (best QoL score) to 120 points (worse QoL score). Furthermore, although other instruments including the DLQI and PDI, have variable correlations to improvement in physical disease parameters, such as PASI, the PQoL-12 was found to be predictive of PASI.[30,39–45]

SUMMARY

Psoriasis results in a significantly negative QoL impact for a large portion of the affected population. Although psoriasis may not be life-threatening, it is a potentially life-ruining disease with multiple comorbidities in addition to the psychosocial implications. Fortunately, there are many new systemic treatment options available, such as biologic agents, which more effectively treat psoriasis not just for the short-term, but also for the long-term maintenance of control. However, when making the decision to use these more powerful agents that carry potential side effects, as do traditional systemic agents, the dermatology provider should always incorporate the patient's negative QoL impact into the decision, and not solely base the decision on the physical disease severity. To do this, it is critical that dermatology providers are knowledgeable of reliable methods of measuring QoL impact in patients with psoriasis, most of which are not time consuming for the busy clinician.

REFERENCES

1. National Psoriasis Foundation. About psoriasis: statistics. Available at: http://www.psoriasis.org/netcommunity/learn/about-psoriasis/statistics. Accessed July 15, 2011.
2. de Korte J, Sprangers MA, Mombers FM, et al. Quality of life in patients with psoriasis: a systematic literature review. J Investig Dermatol Symp Proc 2004;9:140–7.
3. Gupta MA, Gupta AK, Kirkby S, et al. A psychocutaneous profile of psoriasis patients who are stress reactors. A study of 127 patients. Gen Hosp Psychiatry 1989;11: 166–73.
4. Gupta MA, Gupta AK. Quality of life of psoriasis patients. J Eur Acad Dermatol Venereol 2000;14: 241–2.
5. Gupta N. Comorbid disease in psoriasis. Don't forget mental illnesses. BMJ 2010;340:c781.
6. Russo PA, Ilchef R, Cooper AJ. Psychiatric morbidity in psoriasis: a review. Australas J Dermatol 2004;45: 155–9 [quiz: 60–1].
7. National Psoriasis Foundation. 2009 survey panel results. Available at: http://www.psoriasis.org/page. aspx?pid=668. Accessed July 15, 2011.
8. Rapp SR, Feldman SR, Exum ML, et al. Psoriasis causes as much disability as other major medical diseases. J Am Acad Dermatol 1999;41:401–7.
9. Walker C, Papadopoulos L. Psychodermatology. Cambridge (NY): Cambridge University Press; 2005.
10. Koo JY, Lee CS. Psychocutaneous medicine. New York: Marcel Dekker; 2003.
11. Harth W. Clinical management in psychodermatology. 1st edition. New York: Springer; 2008.
12. Lewis VJ, Finlay AY. A critical review of Quality-of-Life Scales for Psoriasis. Dermatol Clin 2005;23: 707–16.

13. Jenkinson C, Coulter A, Wright L. Short form 36 (SF36) health survey questionnaire: normative data for adults of working age. BMJ 1993;306:1437–40.

14. Garratt AM, Ruta DA, Abdalla MI, et al. The SF36 health survey questionnaire: an outcome measure suitable for routine use within the NHS? BMJ 1993; 306:1440–4.

15. Bergner M, Bobbitt RA, Carter WB, et al. The Sickness Impact Profile: development and final revision of a health status measure. Med Care 1981;19: 787–805.

16. Goldberg DP, Hillier VF. A scaled version of the General Health Questionnaire. Psychol Med 1979; 9:139–45.

17. Dupuy H. The Psychological General Well-Being (PGWB) Index. In: Wenger N, Mattson M, Furberg C, et al, editors. Assessment of quality of life in clinical trials of cardiovascular therapies. Washington: Le Jacq Publishing; 1984. p. 170–83.

18. Finlay AY, Khan GK. Dermatology Life Quality Index (DLQI): a simple practical measure for routine clinical use. Clin Exp Dermatol 1994;19:210–6.

19. Lewis V, Finlay AY. 10 years experience of the Dermatology Life Quality Index (DLQI). J Investig Dermatol Symp Proc 2004;9:169–80.

20. Morgan M, McCreedy R, Simpson J, et al. Dermatology quality of life scales: a measure of the impact of skin diseases. Br J Dermatol 1997;136: 202–6.

21. Anderson RT, Rajagopalan R. Development and validation of a quality of life instrument for cutaneous diseases. J Am Acad Dermatol 1997;37:41–50.

22. Chren MM, Lasek RJ, Quinn LM, et al. Skindex, a quality-of-life measure for patients with skin disease: reliability, validity, and responsiveness. J Invest Dermatol 1996;107:707–13.

23. Lewis-Jones MS, Finlay AY. The Children's Dermatology Life Quality Index (CDLQI): initial validation and practical use. Br J Dermatol 1995;132:942–9.

24. Holme SA, Man I, Sharpe JL, et al. The Children's Dermatology Life Quality Index: validation of the cartoon version. Br J Dermatol 2003;148:285–90.

25. Finlay AY, Kelly SE. Psoriasis: an index of disability. Clin Exp Dermatol 1987;12:8–11.

26. Finlay AY, Coles EC. The effect of severe psoriasis on the quality of life of 369 patients. Br J Dermatol 1995;132:236–44.

27. Gupta MA, Gupta AK. The Psoriasis Life Stress Inventory: a preliminary index of psoriasis-related stress. Acta Derm Venereol 1995;75:240–3.

28. McKenna SP, Cook SA, Whalley D, et al. Development of the PSORIQoL, a psoriasis-specific measure of quality of life designed for use in clinical practice and trials. Br J Dermatol 2003;149:323–31.

29. Kirby B, Fortune DG, Bhushan M, et al. The Salford Psoriasis Index: an holistic measure of psoriasis severity. Br J Dermatol 2000;142:728–32.

30. Koo JY. Moderate-to-severe psoriasis. 3rd edition. New York: Informa Healthcare; 2009.

31. Heydendael VM, de Borgie CA, Spuls PI, et al. The burden of psoriasis is not determined by disease severity only. J Investig Dermatol Symp Proc 2004; 9:131–5.

32. Wallenhammar LM, Nyfjall M, Lindberg M, et al. Health-related quality of life and hand eczema: a comparison of two instruments, including factor analysis. J Invest Dermatol 2004;122:1381–9.

33. Finlay AY, Khan GK, Luscombe DK, et al. Validation of sickness impact profile and psoriasis disability index in psoriasis. Br J Dermatol 1990;123:751–6.

34. Root S, Kent G, al-Abadie MS. The relationship between disease severity, disability and psychological distress in patients undergoing PUVA treatment for psoriasis. Dermatology 1994;189:234–7.

35. Bhutani T, Patel T, Koo B, et al. A prospective, interventional assessment of psoriasis quality of life utilizing a non-skin specific validated instrument that allows comparison with other major medical conditions. Accepted for Poster Presentation. American Academy of Dermatology's 70th Annual Meeting 2011. San Diego (CA), March 16–20, 2012.

36. Feldman SR, Menter A, Koo JY. Improved health-related quality of life following a randomized controlled trial of alefacept treatment in patients with chronic plaque psoriasis. Br J Dermatol 2004;150:317–26.

37. de Jager ME, van de Kerkhof PC, de Jong EM, et al. A cross-sectional study using the Children's Dermatology Life Quality Index (CDLQI) in childhood psoriasis: negative effect on quality of life and moderate correlation of CDLQI with severity scores. Br J Dermatol 2010;163:1099–101.

38. Zachariae H, Zachariae R, Blomqvist K, et al. Quality of life and prevalence of arthritis reported by 5,795 members of the Nordic Psoriasis Associations. Data from the Nordic Quality of Life Study. Acta Derm Venereol 2002;82:108–13.

39. Feldman SR, Koo JY, Menter A, et al. Decision points for the initiation of systemic treatment for psoriasis. J Am Acad Dermatol 2005;53:101–7.

40. Koo J, Kozma C, Reinke K. The development of a disease-specific questionnaire to assess the quality of life for psoriasis patients: an analysis of the reliability, validity, and responsiveness of the psoriasis quality of life questionnaire. Dermatol Psychosom 2002;3:171–9.

41. Koo J. Population-based epidemiologic study of psoriasis with emphasis on quality of life assessment. Dermatol Clin 1996;14:485–96.

42. Koo JY, Martin D. Investigator-masked comparison of tazarotene gel q.d. plus mometasone furoate cream q.d. vs. mometasone furoate cream b.i.d. in the treatment of plaque psoriasis. Int J Dermatol 2001;40:210–2.

43. Koo J, Menter A, Lebwohl M. The relationship between quality of life and disease severity: results from a large

cohort of mild, moderate, and severe psoriasis patients [abstract]. Br J Dermatol 2002;147:1078.

44. Koo J, Kozma C, Menter A. Development of a disease-specific quality of life questionnaire: the 12-item Psoriasis Quality of Life Questionnaire (PQOL-12). Presented at the 61st Annual Meeting of the American Academy of Dermatology. San Francisco (CA), March 21–26, 2003.

45. Ware J, Harris W, Gandeck B, et al. MAP-R for Windows: Multitrait/Multi-item Analysis Program-Revised User's Guide. Boston: Health Assessment Laboratory; 1997.

Quality of Life Measures for Acne Patients

Lauren E. Barnes, BS[a], Michelle M. Levender, MD[b,c],
Alan B. Fleischer Jr, MD[b], Steven R. Feldman, MD, PhD[b,d,e],*

KEYWORDS

- Psychosocial burden • Anxiety • Depression
- Psychometric

Acne vulgaris is a chronic condition affecting more than 85% of adolescents and two-thirds of adults aged 18 years and older.[1,2] Adolescents aged 15 to 17 years are the most represented of patients with acne; however, as the age of onset approaches as early as 8 or 9 years and a substantial portion of patients experience this condition in adulthood, addressing acne comorbidities and quality of life is gaining importance.[2,3] Although no correlation exists between acne severity and psychological burden, acne patients may experience psychological burdens. including depression, anxiety, and lower self-esteem.[4–8] Acne focus groups report social avoidance; feelings of anger, sadness, or frustration; and the development of negative attitudes.[9] Furthermore, acne episodes produce a financial burden on patients;

the cost of an acne episode averages $690 and ranges from $360 to $870, covering inpatient stays, outpatient services, emergency care, and pharmacy costs during the episode.[2]

Health-related quality of life (HRQOL) refers to the physical, psychological, and social well-being an the emotional, physical, and social functioning reported by patients.[10,11] Current acne therapy often involves the assessment of HRQOL from the negative impact acne can have on a patient's functioning. For example, facial blemishes in women are correlated with lower HRQOL and fear of negative perceptions; the simple presence of a facial blemish, and not just the type or size of blemishes, contributes to lower HRQOL in women.[12] Quality of life improves as acne clears with successful treatment.[13–17] Treatment may

Disclosure: The Center for Dermatology Research is supported by an unrestricted educational grant from Galderma Laboratories, L.P. Dr Feldman has received speaking, consulting and/or research support from Galderma Laboratories, L.P., Stiefel/GSK, Abbott Labs, Leo, Centocor, Amgen, Photomedex, Astellas, Coria, Novartis and Aventis, has received stock options from Photomedex and holds stock in www.DrScore.com. Dr Fleischer has received research, speaking and/or consulting support from Astellas, Amgen, Abbott Labs, Allergan, Best Doctors, Gerson Lehrman, Kikaku America International, Novan, Pfizer, Eisai, Upsher Smith, Galderma Laboratories, L.P., and Intendis, and is a member of the advisory board for Intendis, Neutrogena Dermatologics, and Merz. Ms Barnes and Dr Levender have no conflicts to disclose.

[a] Department of Dermatology, Center for Dermatology Research, Wake Forest School of Medicine, Box 2473, Medical Center Boulevard, Winston-Salem, NC 27157-1071, USA
[b] Department of Dermatology, Center for Dermatology Research, Wake Forest School of Medicine, Medical Center Boulevard, Winston-Salem, NC 27157-1071, USA
[c] Department of Dermatology, Columbia University Medical Center, 161 Fort Washington Avenue, New York, NY 10025, USA
[d] Department of Pathology, Center for Dermatology Research, Wake Forest School of Medicine, Medical Center Boulevard, Winston-Salem, NC 27157-1071, USA
[e] Department of Public Health Sciences, Center for Dermatology Research, Wake Forest School of Medicine, Medical Center Boulevard, Winston-Salem, NC 27157-1071, USA
* Corresponding author. Department of Dermatology, Center for Dermatology Research, Wake Forest School of Medicine, Medical Center Boulevard, Winston-Salem, NC 27157-1071.
E-mail address: sfeldman@wakehealth.edu

Dermatol Clin 30 (2012) 293–300
doi:10.1016/j.det.2011.11.001

have an even greater effect on improving HRQOL in patients with depressive symptoms at the outset of treatment.[18]

The use of HRQOL assessments in clinical practice provides physicians with valuable insight into the debilitating effects of acne that patients may not address themselves. One can determine the present psychosocial effects of acne on a patient and also track changes and improvements in HRQOL easily in the clinical setting. Several dermatology-specific and acne-specific HRQOL questionnaires have been developed and vary in both the number and content of items addressing quality of life. A longer questionnaire may better serve clinical trial visits, yet can also provide a more comprehensive profile of patients' HRQOL than a brief measure. This review explores several formal skin disease–specific and acne-specific HRQOL measures to determine the most beneficial use of these assessments. The review also briefly explores the psychological comorbidities in patients with acne; the risk factors for low quality-of-life scores; and recommendations for physician intervention to improve HRQOL.

METHODS

A MEDLINE literature search was performed using the key words *acne* and *quality of life*. The 246 resulting studies were limited to the English language and adolescents aged 13 to 18 years, which produced 115 studies. Adults older than 18 years can also have acne; however, adolescents are the most represented of patients and this review focuses on this age group. Nineteen reviews were eliminated, and the search was further narrowed using the keywords *depression*, *psychosocial*, and *anxiety*. Twenty-nine studies pertaining to acne quality-of-life indices and scales were reviewed (**Fig. 1**).

RESULTS
General Dermatology HRQOL Measures

Physicians and researchers use HRQOL measures to assess the emotional, psychological, and social effects of disease on patients' lives. General HRQOL measures provide a means of comparing effects of different conditions on patients' lives.[19] Skin disease–specific measures address the effects of multiple types of skin disease and offer a more sensitive HRQOL measure than a generic health questionnaire.

Finlay and Khan[19] developed the widely used Dermatology Life Quality Index (DLQI) for use in research studies and routine clinical practice. The details of the DLQI are discussed in the article by

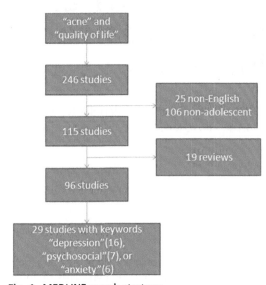

Fig. 1. MEDLINE search strategy.

Basra and colleagues[20] which is addressed elsewhere in this issue. The DLQI can be used in clinical practice to assess changes in HRQOL and is meant to provide a sensitive measure of patient HRQOL that streamlines its assessment for multiple dermatologic conditions. The DLQI has been modified for pediatric dermatology HRQOL (Children's DLQI) and to assess the secondary effects of a dermatologic condition on the patients' family (Family DLQI).[21] Application of the DLQI in acne shows that scores are lower in these patients than in those with atopic eczema, generalized pruritus, and psoriasis, yet were significantly higher than those for Finlay's control population.[19] The difference in scores can be attributed to the absence of items addressing depressive or anxious feelings; only 1 item of the 10 concerns the amount of embarrassment or self-consciousness experienced by the patient as a result of their skin condition. The DLQI item addressing the extent of the patient's itchiness, soreness, or pain is less applicable to patients with acne, which contributes to these patients' less-severe scores compared with patients with psoriasis or eczema.

The Skindex is another comprehensive dermatologic disease HRQOL measure developed by Chren and colleagues[22] and also discussed in detail in the article by Chren elsewhere in this issue. Skindex scores for patients with different dermatologic conditions varied; average scores for patients with inflammatory conditions such as acne, eczema, and psoriasis were higher than those for patients with isolated lesions. Patients with inflammatory conditions such as acne, eczema, or psoriasis had lower HRQOL scores than patients with isolated skin lesions. Acne patients' judgments of their acne severity correlated with both the physical limitation and embarrassment scales.[22] Nijsten and colleagues[23] used the Skindex-29 to categorize patient scores and examine whether scores differed among patients with acne, psoriasis, seborrheic dermatitis, alopecia areata, vitiligo, and nevi. Skindex-29 scores were categorized into emotions, symptoms, and functioning items. A higher percentage of acne patients ranked their emotions items as "moderate" or "severe" compared with psoriasis patients, yet a higher percentage of patients with psoriasis ranked their functioning and symptoms items as "moderate," "severe," or "extremely severe." Skindex supports a greater emotional and psychosocial burden of acne on patients compared with other inflammatory diseases like psoriasis.

Dermatology Quality of Life Scales (DQOLS) were developed by Morgan and colleagues[24] to complement the scores of Finlay's DLQI and focus on the psychosocial burden of dermatologic diseases. Morgan's DQOLS incorporates the impact of a dermatologic condition on patients' psychosocial burden and daily activities, with items generated by patients reporting on their psoriasis, acne, or eczema. Seventeen psychosocial items are categorized into four subscales (embarrassment, despair, irritableness, and distress); the 12 daily activities items fall into one of four subscales (everyday, summer, social, and sexual). The DQOLS offer a patient-generated measure of the impact of skin conditions such as psoriasis, eczema, and acne.[24] Patients with acne scored higher in the psychosocial categories than those with psoriasis or eczema, indicating that acne has a greater psychosocial impact than psoriasis. This finding was exemplified by 36% of patients with acne and 26% of those with psoriasis reporting their skin condition "extremely" affecting how they felt regarding the despair items (lack of hope, lack of understanding from others, isolated, worry about long-term effects, or ashamed).[24] A greater number of patients with acne (24%) than those with psoriasis (21%) also rated their skin condition as "extremely" affecting their feelings about the distress items (suicidal, anxious, depressed, or distressed).[24] Acne did not, however, have as great an effect on daily activities as psoriasis. The greater number of psychosocial items specifically addressed on the DQOLS lends to its usefulness in assessing the psychological impact of acne.

Niemeier and colleagues[25] evaluated the use of the Questionnaire of Chronic Skin Disorders (CSD) in patients with acne, which examines six aspects of coping behaviors in individuals with chronic skin diseases. The aspects include social anxiety and avoidance; cycle of itching and scratching; helplessness; anxious-depressive mood; impact on quality of life; and information seeking. Each of the six dimensions is a subscale of the CSD with a higher score, indicating lower HRQOL. Patients with acne had higher scores on every CSD subscale except the anxious-depressive mood subscale, and CSD scores were independent of the duration of patient symptoms. The CSD subscales correlated significantly with Beck's Depression Inventory (BDI) and indicated that, compared with patients with pain or depressive, patients with acne had depressive scores similar to healthy persons.[25,26] Although Niemeier and colleagues assessed the validity of the CSD in patients with acne, it can be used to compare different skin conditions, various presentations of acne, and methods of acne therapy.

Acne-Specific Health-Related Measures

Although skin disease quality-of-life indices and questionnaires serve the purpose of gauging the impact of dermatologic conditions on a patient's life and comparing the impacts of different skin diseases, an acne-specific HRQOL assessment can offer a focused examination of the negative effects of acne. An acne-focused HRQOL measure is the most sensitive way to determine the impact of acne and allows the dermatologist to assess the effects of acne on patients while excluding irrelevant symptoms.

The Acne Quality of Life Index (Acne-QOLI) is a 21-item measure covering three conceptual domains of HRQOL: social functioning, psychological functioning, and emotional functioning.[9] The scale has very good internal consistency and excellent test–retest reliability and validity. The Acne-QOLI is advantageous for use in clinical trials and everyday clinic operations, and offers a comprehensive yet concise analysis of the HRQOL of patients with acne. The 21 items cover a range of emotional and social effects of acne, including feeling uncomfortable, angry, unattractive to others, and wanting to avoid people, and 17 additional patient-reported feelings associated with acne.[9] The Acne-QOLI does not include acne severity or treatment items, and therefore avoids respondent confounding and provides a simple and effective measure of acne's negative effects on the patient. The length of the Acne-QOLI is not a major burden on respondents, and potentially could be incorporated into a routine clinic visit.

The Cardiff Acne Disability Index (CADI) was developed to quickly assess the level of disability caused by acne and to identify patients with increased disability and the need for additional intervention.[27] Health-related disability refers to any restriction or inability to perform an activity within the normal range of human ability.[28] The CADI is a condensed version of the Acne Disability Index (ADI), which consists of 48 items in eight HRQOL domains (psychological, physical, recreation, employment, self-awareness, social reaction, skin care, and financial).[29,30] The CADI consists of five questions, each with four graded responses, pertaining to disability caused by acne in the past month and addresses general psychological and social burdens of acne and the respondent's perception of the severity of their facial, chest, and back acne, if applicable.[27] Motley and Finlay[27] intended for the CADI to assess a patient's disability from acne and to identify patients who may benefit from psychological interventions in addition to acne therapy. Salek and colleagues[30] showed the validity of the CADI compared with ADI and a generic HRQOL measure, the United Kingdom Sickness Impact Profile (UKSIP), and determined that the CADI is more appropriate for routine clinical use and monitoring the HRQOL of patients with acne.[31] The CADI has been widely used and has been translated and adapted into French, Chinese, and Persian versions.[32–34]

The Acne-QoL is a 24-item questionnaire specific to facial acne in which the questions are organized into four domains: self-perception, role-emotional, role-social, and acne symptoms. Each question refers to the previous week of treatment for facial acne, thus allowing dermatologists to detect improvement over the course of therapy.[35] The Acne-QoL, which can be condensed into a 19-item questionnaire through eliminating five redundant items, is estimated to require 5 to 7 minutes to complete and offers a comprehensive score encompassing the psychosocial burden of facial acne.[35,36] Quality-of-life scores correlated strongly with patient-reported acne severity, more so than with physician-reported severity.[35] The Acne-QoL is a comprehensive assessment of patient-perceived acne severity; however, it addresses facial acne exclusively, and the extended time requirement to complete the questionnaire makes the Acne-QoL more useful in clinical trials than in the everyday clinic.

Tan and colleagues[37] condensed the 19-item Acne-QoL into a 4-item questionnaire (Acne-Q4), including the highest-ranked items from each of the four domains from the Acne-QoL. The four items include "Dissatisfied with appearance" (self-perception), "Feeling upset" (role-emotional), "Concern about meeting new people" (role-social),

and "Concern about scarring from facial acne" (acne symptoms). The Acne-Q4 was a good predictor of Acne-QoL score and also exhibited a relationship with physician-rated Investigators Global Assessment (IGA) scores of facial acne severity. The Acne-Q4 shares the Acne-QoL restriction to facial acne and is not applicable to patients with truncal acne or minimal facial acne. Although the Acne-Q4 is restricted to use with facial acne and does not offer the breadth of quality-of-life information, it is a practical substitution for the Acne-QoL in clinical practice.

An Acne Quality of Life scale (AQOL) was developed by Gupta and colleagues[38] to specifically address the social and occupational functioning aspects of quality of life. This 12-item scale can be divided into two subscales, social quality of life (9 items) and vocational quality of life (3 items), although the 9 social quality-of-life items constitute the final version of the AQOL. Social scores correlate significantly with Interpersonal Dependency Inventory (IDS), Carroll Rating Scale for Depression (CRSD), and other psychopathologic scales; thus, the AQOL serves as an accurate psychological measure for patients without serious psychopathology.[38–40] Respondents completed the AQOL in less than 5 minutes, indicating potential ease of use in the routine clinical setting.

For patients with signs of a psychological comorbidity such as depression, the Assessment of the Psychological and Social Effects of Acne (APSEA) is an effective 15-item psychological-specific measure. The APSEA was used in a study examining the psychological changes in patients with acne treated with oral isotretinoin.[41] APSEA scores in patients taking isotretinoin for acne correlated with Beck's Depression Inventory (BDI) scores, which address the cognitive, affective, and physical symptoms of depression.[41] APSEA scores and acne severity improved in patients after 8 weeks of treatment, suggesting that APSEA scores are responsive to clinical change. Hahm and colleagues[41] suggest that skin clearance from oral isotretinoin treatment can improve HRQOL, which in turn improves and reduces depressive symptoms. An acne-specific psychological assessment is an important tool to measure changes in HRQOL for patients with preexisting psychological symptoms, and APSEA provides an efficient clinical alternative to an in-depth psychological assessment.

DISCUSSION

Although acne-specific quality-of-life measures are important in addressing the associated physical and psychological symptoms of acne vulgaris, a combination of disease-specific and generic quality-of-life measures can be advantageous when evaluating patients with skin disease.[42] Klassen and colleagues[42] examined the use of a combined questionnaire, including the EuroQol (EQ-5D), Short Form 36 (SF-36), and DLQI to assess changes in quality of life after treatment of severe acne.[19,43–46] The EQ-5D is a five-question general health questionnaire that addresses mobility, self-care, daily activities, pain or discomfort, and anxiety or depression related to any health condition.[43] The SF-36 is a longer general HRQOL assessment from which two summary scores, the physical component and the mental component, are derived from HRQOL items in eight health domains (physical function, limitations caused by physical problems, limitations caused by emotional problems, social function, mental health, energy, pain, and health perception).[44–46] Klassen and colleagues[42] found the DLQI scores to be the most responsive to change in acne severity after treatment, although the generic assessments did detect health problems and changes in HRQOL after treatment in patients with acne. A combination of generic and acne-specific HRQOL measures can provide a comprehensive view of HRQOL for patients with multiple health conditions; however, such a combination may be best reserved for research use or when extended time can be allowed in the clinical setting.

Psychological comorbidities associated with acne include depression and anxiety, although whether acne precipitates depressive symptoms or if preexisting depressive symptoms are worsened by skin conditions such as acne is unknown. Depression is two to three times more prevalent in patients with acne than in the general population.[47] The smaller number of patients taking antidepressants while also being treated with acne therapy compared with those not undergoing acne therapy suggests that successful treatment of acne may contribute to improved mental health and consequently improved HRQOL. Depression in patients with acne can be assessed in the clinic using the Acne-QOLI, which addresses several emotional functioning items, or the APSEA, which correlated significantly with BDI scores.[9,41]

Niemeier and colleagues[25] discuss triggering factors in their use of the CSD to assess the HRQOL of patients with acne. The most common triggering factors reported by patients are pathogenically relevant and include "puberty," "hormonal influences," "bacteria," and "predisposition." Stress-related triggering factors, including professional or familial stress and professional or familial disputes, followed the pathogenic triggering factors in frequency. Quality-of-life measures that identify stress (DQOLS, Skindex-16) may be useful tools in the clinic for patients reporting elevated levels of stress.[24,48,49]

Certain psychological comorbidities in patients with acne relate to personality traits such as social sensitivity and trait anger. Social sensitivity is an individual's increased level of concern for others' reactions to and judgments of him or her. Higher social sensitivity is associated with poorer HRQOL and greater concerns in both casual and intimate social interactions.[1] Trait anger, the tendency to regularly experience anger, is weakly associated with acne severity and adherence to treatment; however, it may play an important role in patients' satisfaction with treatment and HRQOL scores.[50]

Patients with acne with psychological comorbidities place more confidence in medical therapy than in psychotherapy for treatment of their acne.[25] However, patients with depressive or other psychological symptoms may need adjunctive psychiatric treatment. To address psychological and HRQOL issues with patients, Rapp and colleagues[50] developed the acronym "I VOTE," as a guide:

Inquire about how acne affects patients' life, self-esteem, ability to fulfill their vocational duties, and leisure activities.

Validate and acknowledge the importance of how acne affects patients' quality of life.

Offer to find additional resources and suggestions for reducing the negative impacts. For example, women who used makeup to camouflage facial blemishes had improved HRQOL scores, appearance, and mental status.[51]

Tell patients you are committed to helping them manage the symptoms of acne and the negative effects.

Evaluate patients' HRQOL as acne severity, adherence, and treatment satisfaction are monitored.

The "I VOTE" acronym is a simple method for approaching how acne affects patients' HRQOL. Quality-of-life measures best suited for the "Evaluate" in a busy clinical setting are simple, short questionnaires that take minimal time for the respondent to complete. Physicians may rely on their physical examination of patients' affect and a very global quality-of-life evaluation ("How are you feeling today? Is the acne bothering you?") to assess psychological impact of the disease. To quickly evaluate acne-specific HRQOL in a more formal way, the four-item Acne-Q$_4$ (for

Table 1
Quality-of-life measures for patients with acne

Scale	Number of Items	Specific Features
Skin disease HRQOL measures		
DLQI	10	Addresses effects of acne treatment High test–retest reliability
Skindex	61	Responsive to clinical change
Skindex-29	29	Scores categorized to ease interpretation Translated into Spanish[53]
Skindex-16	16	Measures the amount of bother to patient rather than frequency of experiences Addresses depressive feelings
DQOLS	17	Explores the psychosocial burden and effects of skin disease on daily activities
CSD	51	Addresses coping behaviors of patients with skin disorders Correlates significantly with BDI scores
Acne-specific HRQOL measures		
Acne-QOLI	21	High test–retest reliability and excellent validity Addresses depressive feelings
CADI	5	Patient perception of acne severity Addresses depressive feelings Translated into French, Chinese, and Persian versions
Acne-QoL	24	Patient perception of acne severity Responsive to clinical change Addresses facial acne only
Acne-Q$_4$	4	Construct validity and correlation with IGA scores Addresses facial acne only
AQOL	9	Correlates significantly with psychopathologic scales
APSEA	15	Responsive to clinical change Correlates with BDI scores

Abbreviations: Acne-QOLI, Acne Quality of Life Index; APSEA, Assessment of the Psychological and Social Effects of Acne; AQOL, Acne Quality of Life scale; BDI, Beck's Depression Inventory; CADI, Cardiff Acne Disability Index; CSD, Questionnaire of Chronic Skin Disorders; DLQI, Dermatology Life Quality Index; DQOLS, dermatology quality of life scales; HRQOL, health-related quality of life; IGA, Investigators Global Assessment; QoL, quality of life.

facial acne only), five-question CADI, or nine-question AQOL is appropriate; however, a more comprehensive and in-depth view of the HRQOL of patients with acne can be assessed quickly with the Acne-QOLI.[9,27,37,38] When psychiatric co-morbidities are suspected, the psychological effects–focused APSEA can provide information to influence the pursuit of psychiatric assessments.[41] For patients with multiple dermatologic comorbidities, it may be most beneficial to assess dermatologic HRQOL. The DLQI and Skindex-16 are short dermatology questionnaires that can be easily incorporated into clinical practice.[19,48] The Skindex-29 and CSD are longer and more-involved dermatologic HRQOL measures that are better used in clinical trials.[25,52] Any HRQOL measure, whether dermatologic-specific or acne-specific, can help physicians determine the most successful therapy regimen for their patients and whether additional psychiatric resources will benefit their patients' well-being (**Table 1**).

SUMMARY

When selecting an HRQOL measure to assess changes in the HRQOL in a patient with acne, it is important to first identify the goals of assessment and the potential respondent burden of completing the questionnaire. Quality-of-life indices requiring only a few minutes for the respondent to complete are ideal for routine clinical use. Longer, more in-depth questionnaires are appropriate for clinical trial visits in which the goal is to obtain a sensitive measure of HRQOL response to treatment or when comparing effects of different acne therapies. Acne-specific measures provide the most sensitive assessment of patient HRQOL, although dermatologic HRQOL scales can provide a means to compare effects of different, comorbid dermatologic conditions. When clinical time permits, perhaps the most informative HRQOL measure is a combination of dermatologic-specific and acne-specific questionnaires. The clinician should choose an HRQOL measure based on the time necessary to respond, its applicable content, and its usefulness to clinicians in helping patients achieve a higher acne-related quality of life.

REFERENCES

1. Krejci-Manwaring J, Kerchner K, Feldman SR, et al. Social sensitivity and acne: the role of personality in negative social consequences and quality of life. Int J Psychiatry Med 2006;36(1):121–30.

2. Yentzer BA, Hick J, Reese EL, et al. Acne vulgaris in the United States: a descriptive epidemiology. Cutis 2010;86(2):94–9.

3. Friedlander SF, Eichenfield LF, Fowler JF Jr, et al. Acne epidemiology and pathophysiology. Semin Cutan Med Surg 2010;29(2 Suppl 1):2–4.

4. Jowett S, Ryan T. Skin disease and handicap: an analysis of the impact of skin conditions. Soc Sci Med 1985;20(4):425–9.

5. Koo J. The psychosocial impact of acne: patients' perceptions. J Am Acad Dermatol 1995;32(5 Pt 3): S26–30.

6. Koo JY, Smith LL. Psychologic aspects of acne. Pediatr Dermatol 1991;8(3):185–8.

7. Krowchuk DP, Stancin T, Keskinen R, et al. The psychosocial effects of acne on adolescents. Pediatr Dermatol 1991;8(4):332–8.

8. Smithard A, Glazebrook C, Williams HC. Acne prevalence, knowledge about acne and psychological morbidity in mid-adolescence: a community-based study. Br J Dermatol 2001;145(2):274–9.

9. Rapp SR, Feldman SR, Graham G, et al. The Acne Quality of Life Index (Acne-QOLI): development and validation of a brief instrument. Am J Clin Dermatol 2006;7(3):185–92.

10. Schipper H, Clinch JJ, Olweny CL. Quality of life studies: definitions and conceptual issues. In: Spilker B, editor. Quality of life and pharmacoeconomics in clinical trials. 2nd edition. Philadelphia: Lippincott-Raven; 1996. p. 11–23.

11. Shumaker SA, Wyman JF, Uebersax JS, et al. Health-related quality of life measures for women with urinary incontinence: the Incontinence Impact Questionnaire and the Urogenital Distress Inventory. Continence Program in Women (CPW) Research Group. Qual Life Res 1994;3(5):291–306.

12. Balkrishnan R, McMichael AJ, Hu JY, et al. Correlates of health-related quality of life in women with severe facial blemishes. Int J Dermatol 2006;45(2): 111–5.

13. Grosshans E, Marks R, Mascaro JM, et al. Evaluation of clinical efficacy and safety of adapalene 0.1% gel versus tretinoin 0.025% gel in the treatment of acne vulgaris, with particular reference to the onset of action and impact on quality of life. Br J Dermatol 1998;139(Suppl 52):26–33.

14. Jones-Caballero M, Chren MM, Soler B, et al. Quality of life in mild to moderate acne: relationship to clinical severity and factors influencing change with treatment. J Eur Acad Dermatol Venereol 2007; 21(2):219–26.

15. Kellett SC, Gawkrodger DJ. The psychological and emotional impact of acne and the effect of treatment with isotretinoin. Br J Dermatol 1999;140(2):273–82.

16. Layton AM, Seukeran D, Cunliffe WJ. Scarred for life? Dermatology 1997;195(Suppl 1):15–21 [discussion: 38–40].

17. Newton JN, Mallon E, Klassen A, et al. The effectiveness of acne treatment: an assessment by patients of the outcome of therapy. Br J Dermatol 1997; 137(4):563–7.

18. McGrath EJ, Lovell CR, Gillison F, et al. A prospective trial of the effects of isotretinoin on quality of life and depressive symptoms. Br J Dermatol 2010;163(6):1323–9.

19. Finlay AY, Khan GK. Dermatology Life Quality Index (DLQI)–a simple practical measure for routine clinical use. Clin Exp Dermatol 1994;19(3):210–6.

20. Basra MK, Sue-Ho R, Finlay AY. The family dermatology life quality index: measuring the secondary impact of skin disease. Br J Dermatol 2007;156(3): 528–38.

21. Lewis-Jones MS, Finlay AY. The Children's Dermatology Life Quality Index (CDLQI): initial validation and practical use. Br J Dermatol 1995;132(6):942–9.

22. Chren MM, Lasek RJ, Quinn LM, et al. Skindex, a quality-of-life measure for patients with skin disease: reliability, validity, and responsiveness. J Invest Dermatol 1996;107(5):707–13.

23. Nijsten T, Sampogna F, Abeni D. Categorization of Skindex-29 scores using mixture analysis. Dermatology 2009;218(2):151–4.

24. Morgan M, McCreedy R, Simpson J, et al. Dermatology quality of life scales–a measure of the impact of skin diseases. Br J Dermatol 1997;136(2):202–6.

25. Niemeier V, Kupfer J, Demmelbauer-Ebner M, et al. Coping with acne vulgaris. Evaluation of the chronic skin disorder questionnaire in patients with acne. Dermatology 1998;196(1):108–15.

26. Beck AT, Ward CH, Mendelson M, et al. An inventory for measuring depression. Arch Gen Psychiatry 1961;4:561–71.

27. Motley RJ, Finlay AY. Practical use of a disability index in the routine management of acne. Clin Exp Dermatol 1992;17(1):1–3.

28. World Health Organization. International classification of impairments, disabilities, and handicaps.

Geneva (Switzerland): World Health Organization; 1980.

29. Motley RJ, Finlay AY. How much disability is caused by acne? Clin Exp Dermatol 1989;14(3):194–8.

30. Salek MS, Khan GK, Finlay AY. Questionnaire techniques in assessing acne handicap: reliability and validity study. Qual Life Res 1996;5(1):131–8.

31. Finlay AY, Khan GK, Luscombe DK, et al. Validation of sickness impact profile and psoriasis disability index in psoriasis. Br J Dermatol 1990;123(6):751–6.

32. Aghaei S, Mazharinia N, Jafari P, et al. The Persian version of the Cardiff Acne Disability Index. Reliability and validity study. Saudi Med J 2006;27(1):80–2.

33. Dreno B, Finlay AY, Nocera T, et al. The Cardiff Acne Disability Index: cultural and linguistic validation in French. Dermatology 2004;208(2):104–8.

34. Law MP, Chuh AA, Lee A. Validation of a Chinese version of the Cardiff Acne Disability Index. Hong Kong Med J 2009;15(1):12–7.

35. Martin AR, Lookingbill DP, Botek A, et al. Health-related quality of life among patients with facial acne – assessment of a new acne-specific questionnaire. Clin Exp Dermatol 2001;26(5):380–5.

36. Girman CJ, Hartmaier S, Thiboutot D, et al. Evaluating health-related quality of life in patients with facial acne: development of a self-administered questionnaire for clinical trials. Qual Life Res 1996;5(5):481–90.

37. Tan J, Fung KY, Khan S. Condensation and validation of a 4-item index of the Acne-QoL. Qual Life Res 2006;15(7):1203–10.

38. Gupta MA, Johnson AM, Gupta AK. The development of an Acne Quality of Life scale: reliability, validity, and relation to subjective acne severity in mild to moderate acne vulgaris. Acta Derm Venereol 1998;78(6):451–6.

39. Carroll BJ, Feinberg M, Smouse PE, et al. The Carroll rating scale for depression. I. Development, reliability and validation. Br J Psychiatry 1981;138:194–200.

40. Hirschfeld RM, Klerman GL, Gough HG, et al. A measure of interpersonal dependency. J Pers Assess 1977;41(6):610–8.

41. Hahm BJ, Min SU, Yoon MY, et al. Changes of psychiatric parameters and their relationships by oral isotretinoin in acne patients. J Dermatol 2009; 36(5):255–61.

42. Klassen AF, Newton JN, Mallon E. Measuring quality of life in people referred for specialist care of acne: comparing generic and disease-specific measures. J Am Acad Dermatol 2000;43(2 Pt 1):229–33.

43. Kind P, Gudex C, Dolan P, et al. Practical and methodological issues in the development of the EuroQol: the York experience. Adv Med Sociol 1994;5:219–53.

44. Ware JE, Snow KK, Kosinski M, et al. SF-36 health manual and interpretation guide. Boston: The Health Institute, New England Medical Center; 1993.

45. Ware JE Jr, Sherbourne CD. The MOS 36-item short-form health survey (SF-36). I. Conceptual framework and item selection. Med Care 1992;30(6):473–83.

46. Ware JE Jr, Kosinski M, Bayliss MS, et al. Comparison of methods for the scoring and statistical analysis of SF-36 health profile and summary measures: summary of results from the Medical Outcomes Study. Med Care 1995;33(Suppl 4): AS264–79.

47. Uhlenhake E, Yentzer BA, Feldman SR. Acne vulgaris and depression: a retrospective examination. J Cosmet Dermatol 2010;9(1):59–63.

48. Chren MM, Lasek RJ, Sahay AP, et al. Measurement properties of Skindex-16: a brief quality-of-life measure for patients with skin diseases. J Cutan Med Surg 2001;5(2):105–10.

49. Nijsten TE, Sampogna F, Chren MM, et al. Testing and reducing skindex-29 using Rasch analysis: Skindex-17. J Invest Dermatol 2006;126(6):1244–50.

50. Rapp DA, Brenes GA, Feldman SR, et al. Anger and acne: implications for quality of life, patient satisfaction and clinical care. Br J Dermatol 2004;151(1):183–9.

51. Hayashi N, Imori M, Yanagisawa M, et al. Make-up improves the quality of life of acne patients without aggravating acne eruptions during treatments. Eur J Dermatol 2005;15(4):284–7.

52. Chren MM, Lasek RJ, Flocke SA, et al. Improved discriminative and evaluative capability of a refined version of Skindex, a quality-of-life instrument for patients with skin diseases. Arch Dermatol 1997;133(11):1433–40.

53. Jones-Caballero M, Penas PF, Garcia-Diez A, et al. The Spanish version of Skindex-29. Int J Dermatol 2000;39(12):907–12.

Quality-of-Life Measurement in Blistering Diseases

Deshan F. Sebaratnam, MBBS (Hons)[a,b,1],
John W. Frew, MBBS (Hons), MMed (Clin Epi)[a,b,1],
Fereydoun Davatchi, MD[c],
Dédée F. Murrell, MA, BMBCh, FAAD, MD, FACD[d,*]

KEYWORDS

- Quality of life • Vesiculobullous skin diseases
- Epidermolysis bullosa • Autoimmune blistering disease
- Pemphigus • Bullous pemphigoid

Quality of life (QOL) has been defined as "the individual's perception of their position in life, in the context of the cultural and value systems in which they live and in relation to their goals, expectations, standards and concerns."[1] It is an abstract multidimensional construct reflecting the physical, psychological, and social aspects of an individual's condition complementing the concept of health as "a state of complete physical, mental, and social well-being and not merely the absence of disease or infirmity."[2] Many dermatologic conditions pose minimal threat to patients in terms of mortality but have the capacity to significantly impinge upon a patient's QOL. This is often because of the disfiguring nature of skin disease with its adverse impact on body image and succeeding burden on social function, which may be independent of clinical severity. Physical symptoms such as pain and itch can strongly affect QOL, and auxiliary considerations such as functional limitations, financial burden, and side effects of treatment all exert a detrimental effect on QOL.

Accordingly, an assessment of QOL provides a suitable means to evaluate the impact of patients' dermatosis on their well-being, and quantifying this impact has stemmed from a desire to evaluate outcomes of medical intervention.[3] With the rise of QOL research and general qualitative inquiry in areas outside its traditional sociologic sphere, health care providers are increasingly looking toward semiqualitative measurement tools to assess and measure the impact of diseases within their patient population. Such measurements of QOL and burden of disease have multiple benefits, including

- An increased understanding of patient experiences in living with a disease
- Establishing serial measurements for longitudinal monitoring of a patient's condition
- Evaluating new innovations or interventions with regard to their impact of the patient as a whole rather than purely on biophysical measurements
- Eliciting areas of value in a patients' life that exert the greatest detrimental impact, facilitating the provision of personalized care
- Quantifying the burden of disease for patient advocacy relating to public perception of dermatologic conditions and the allocation of research support and clinical resources.

[a] Department of Dermatology, St George Hospital, Gray Street, Sydney, NSW 2217, Australia
[b] Faculty of Medicine, University of New South Wales, Sydney, NSW 2052, Australia
[c] Department of Rheumatology Research Center, Shariati Hospital, Tehran University for Medical Sciences, Tehran 1417613151, Iran
[d] Department of Dermatology, St George Hospital, University of New South Wales, Gray Street, Kogarah, Sydney, NSW 2217, Australia
[1] Dual first name authorship.
* Corresponding author.
E-mail address: d.murrell@unsw.edu.au

Dermatol Clin 30 (2012) 301–307
doi:10.1016/j.det.2011.11.008

A range of instruments has been used to assess QOL in the clinical setting, and these are classified as generic, dermatology specific, or disease specific. This paradigm has been discussed elsewhere in this edition in detail and thus is only highlighted here (see article by Kini and DeLong elsewhere in this issue for further exploration of this topic). Researchers often use a combination of specific and generic QOL instruments to obtain satisfactory responsiveness and comparability, and a recent systematic review suggested that the combination of a generic instrument (the Medical Outcome Study 36-item Short-Form Survey [SF-36][4]) and a dermatology-specific instrument (the Skindex-29[5]) may be the best selection of QOL instruments for use in dermatology.[6]

The use of such patient measurement tools is particularly useful in both congenital and acquired bullous diseases, which are chronic, burdensome, and painful afflictions.[7,8] Treatment modalities for these disorders vary in nature and efficacy, the mainstay of treatment in congenital blistering disorders being supportive care and immunosuppression in autoimmune bullous dermatoses.

Several qualitative and semiqualitative studies have emerged from the literature over the last 5 to 10 years addressing aspects of QOL in blistering disorders, and this article examines those findings with a view to understanding the impact blistering diseases have on their respective populations and assessing the utility of available measurement tools.

INHERITED BLISTERING DISEASES

The inherited blistering diseases consist of the variety of skin fragility syndromes classified under the general heading of epidermolysis bullosa (EB).[9] The main subtypes include EB simplex (EBS), junctional EB (JEB), and dystrophic EB (DEB), with other conditions such as Kindler syndrome, skin fragility–ectodermal dysplasia syndrome, and laryngoonychocutaneous syndrome recently reclassified as forms of EB on the basis of genetic and ultrastructural characteristics.[9]

The burden of disease in inherited blistering disorders is known to be high, although it does vary considerably between subtypes. A 2002 study by Horn and Tidman[10] of 116 Scottish patients with EB demonstrated that the QOL impairment in EBS and nongeneralized severe dystrophic subtypes (previously known as non–Hallopeau-Seimens syndrome) were comparable to moderate to severe psoriasis and atopic eczema as measured by the Dermatology Life Quality Index (DLQI)[11] questionnaire with an average DLQI score of 10.7/30 for adults and 15/30

for children. Generalized severe subtypes of EB had greater QOL impairment than any disease previously assessed, with average DLQI scores of 18/30 for adults and 22/30 for children.

Fine and colleagues[12] attempted to quantify the functional impairment and pain levels of an EB cohort using patient rating scales, demonstrating in their 2004 study that the subjective clinical severity of the disease did correlate with increased mobility and functional impairment and increased pain levels. Again, individuals with generalized severe recessive DEB (GS-RDEB) had the highest levels of pain and impairment across the EB cohort. This is demonstrated by 32% of all children with GS-RDEB rating their daily cutaneous pain greater than 5 out of 10 on a visual analog scale as opposed to 14% to 19% in all other subtypes of EB. More than 90% of the individuals with EBS surveyed by Fine and colleagues were rated as independent for activities of daily living (ADLs) in contrast to 73% of individuals with JEB or GS-RDEB who required full assistance with ADLs. The most problematic ADLs were identified as grooming and bathing across all EB subtypes, with toileting and feeding the most problematic in JEB and GS-RDEB subtypes.

These early studies were essential starting points to begin to assess the impact of EB on QOL; however, as subjective patient rating scales, they provided only semiqualitative data demonstrating a snapshot of QOL at one specific time point. These studies did give valuable insight into areas in patients' lives that were not previously thought to have a great impact on QOL.

These areas were then further explored in later studies, particularly with Fine and colleagues'[13] report on the impact of a child with EB on parental interpersonal relationships and the birth of subsequent children. This study described the significant impact of having a child with EB on parental relationships, including divorce rates of 31% in parents of a child with JEB[7] and the contribution a child with EB has on parental decisions to not have further children, with 26% and 64% of parents with a child with EBS or GS-RDEB, respectively, choosing not to have further children because of the potential risks of having a subsequently affected child. Fine's study demonstrated the wide impact of the disease, not just on the individual but also on family and caregivers alike.

A recent study by Tabolli and colleagues[14] has evaluated an Italian cohort of 125 patients with EB using several generic questionnaires, including the SF-36, Skindex-29, 12-item General Health Questionnaire (GHQ),[15] EuroQol 5-dimension questionnaire (EQ-5D) or EQ-5D child,[16] Family Strain Questionnaire,[17] and a 5-point Patient

Global Assessment scale.[14] The results mirror the results of earlier studies showing the significant burden on families and caregivers, as well as the variation in QOL and burden of disease, with those individuals with GS-RDEB and some forms of JEB having much lower QOL than milder forms of EBS. The investigators' results on the psychological impact of EB stated that mental health scores as measured by the SF-36 were only slightly lower than that in the general population.

A recent psychiatric study by Margari and colleagues[18] contradicts these findings, stating that 80% of all individuals within their EB cohort had psychiatric symptoms, the most common being anxiety/paranoia and depression. Such psychiatric symptoms were present but partially compensated for by well-developed psychological strategies and coping mechanisms. The investigators state that the role of family and caregiver support was instrumental in the facilitation of coping mechanisms to prevent exacerbations of psychiatric conditions in individuals with EB.[7] This highlights the importance of the holistic management of the patient, with attention being paid to not only the physical and functional but also the psychological and emotional aspects of the condition.

In the past 5 years, QOL research has moved from evaluation using preexisting generalized dermatologic and QOL questionnaires to a more qualitative approach through ascertaining areas of impact and burden from a grassroots level. The last decade has seen an increase in the use of qualitative methodologies in the medical field, and dermatology has been no exception. Although preexisting generalized dermatologic questionnaires have many uses in being able to compare quantitative scores between individuals and different diseases, the level of validity and reliability of such questionnaires can be brought into question when they are used for specific conditions such as EB. In severely affected individuals with GS-RDEB, lack of content validity and the presence of ceiling effects in general questionnaires such as the DLQI are significant in providing erroneous pictures and underestimates of disease burden, although these affect all EB subtypes to a greater or lesser degree.[7,19] Our research group based in Sydney, Australia, has demonstrated that DLQI scores in patients with EBS are highly similar to EB-specific QOL scores, whereas more burdensome subtypes such as GS-RDEB and JEB show definite ceiling effects, particularly with functional questions that hold preexisting assumptions regarding an individual's ability to go shopping, bathe oneself, or have an active sex life, which many individuals with severe EB subtypes are unable to perform.[19]

Another source of error in previous measurements of QOL in EB has been the way in which pediatric patients with EB have been approached. As with any inherited disorder, a large proportion of the patient cohort is understandably pediatric. The use of traditional pediatric dermatologic questionnaires has the same potential pitfalls as adult QOL questionnaires with poor content validity; ceiling effects; and, if inappropriately administered, increased potential for parental bias. The differences in understanding, vocabulary, and interpretation of questions geared toward QOL between adults and children have led to the use of more creative methodologies to assess burden of disease in pediatric populations. This is best demonstrated by van Scheppingen and colleagues'[20] recent qualitative study identifying specific issues that affect the QOL in children with EB, including itch, pain, the sense of feeling different, and difficulties in joining in other activities with children.[21] A second qualitative study by Dures and colleagues[21] in 2011 gave further focus to the psychosocial impact of EB with themes such as learning to live with EB, talking to others, and understanding EB contributing significantly to the degree of impact EB has on patients' psychosocial well-being. The investigators also touch on the coping strategies mentioned by Margari and colleagues,[18] which individuals with EB use, and how these can lessen the psychosocial impact of the disease, with the identification of social support and maintaining focus on abilities as opposed to disabilities being key components of these mechanisms.

The use of more qualitative approaches to overcome the downfalls of previous questionnaires has allowed the beginning of EB-specific QOL questionnaires and accurate quantification of burden of disease in this patient population. Our research group has designed and validated an EB-specific QOL questionnaire (the QOLEB questionnaire)[19] specifically for use with individuals with EB. The QOLEB was devised using an exhaustive item generation process with 26 patients with EB of various types and severities, their families, and experts in the field. A pilot questionnaire was devised and distributed to 130 patients with EB, and, from the data obtained, the instrument was revised using various methods, including factor analysis, to a 17-item questionnaire. The QOLEB has been shown to be a statistically valid and reliable means to evaluate QOL in EB, correlating well with existing QOL instruments and distinguishing EB subtypes by score. The QOLEB has been shown to have a high validity, specific enough to capture the QOL concerns particular to EB and broad enough to encompass the different subtypes of EB. Results from the QOLEB questionnaire conform with previous research regarding the varied impacts different EB subtypes have on QOL, with average QOLEB scores (with standard deviations in parentheses) of 13.7/51 (8.7) for EBS, 31.5 (17.6) for JEB, 18.1 (10.9) for dominant DEB, and 35.5 (12.7) for RDEB. The QOLEB has the potential to be a sensitive disease-specific tool to assess QOL in EB in future studies and has been used in a recent randomized control trial of cell therapy for recessive DEB.[22,23] At present, only an adult form of this questionnaire exists, although validation of the questionnaire in other languages, such as Spanish, Portuguese, Dutch, and French, are forthcoming. A pediatric form of this questionnaire is required to address the needs of the pediatric population, and further statistical validation is underway through anchor- and distribution-based banding methods to determine mild, moderate, severe, and extreme QOL impairment for ease of interpretation of this valid score and definition of a minimal clinically important difference in the QOLEB score. This would aid in use of the score as a longitudinal measurement tool and for use in evaluating new interventions in EB.

AUTOIMMUNE BLISTERING DISEASE

Studies exploring QOL in autoimmune bullous dermatoses have primarily focused on pemphigus (namely pemphigus vulgaris and pemphigus foliaceus) and bullous pemphigoid with a paucity of information regarding QOL in other forms of pemphigus as well as other acquired bullous diseases such as mucous membrane pemphigoid, EB acquisita, and linear IgA bullous dermatosis.

The earliest study exploring QOL in autoimmune blistering disease (AIBD) involved 380 patients with pemphigus in Japan.[24] Patients were stratified according to disease severity (with most patients [67.7%] having mild disease) and asked to complete a survey reviewing their ADLs and the financial impact of their condition. Patients were found to be independent in most ADLs; however, they experienced a considerable economic burden due to their disease. In the cohort, 41.9% described a decrease in income because of lost work time (60.0% in severe disease) and 41.3% described their financial status as being in poverty (57.9% in severe disease). However, only 2.2% of patients were in the active stage of disease, with the remainder in varying phases of remission, and, accordingly, the results illustrated that with appropriate treatment pemphigus does not significantly impinge upon the ADLs of patients. In

contrast, the financial impact of pemphigus may be burdensome even if the patient shows clinical improvement, probably because of extensive loss of time at work when the disease is in its visible state and takes weeks to months to come under control, and this should be remembered in the assessment of these patients.

Another study evaluating QOL in pemphigus was conducted using the SF-36[4] to compare QOL in patients with pemphigus with that in the wider population in Morocco.[25] The study cohort included 30 consecutive patients with pemphigus presenting to dermatology clinics or admitted to the hospital, and the control cohort consisted of 60 patients presenting with nondebilitating conditions such as verrucous warts. The SF-36 was translated into the Moroccan dialect, and, given the low literacy rate in Morocco, the questionnaires were administered by a single investigator rather than being patient administered. The investigators identified a significant difference between cohorts with the pemphigus group displaying decreased mean scores across all dimensions except for "Physical Pain" and "Change Compared to the Previous Year." Physical status and emotional status were the domains most affected by pemphigus, with facial involvement and the extent of lesions correlating well with overall scores. Within the group, 70% expressed enormous shame about their appearance, 60% were anxious about what others thought of their disease, and 63% reported a significant loss of confidence (N = 30). Repercussions for sexual function were also important, with 81% of patients reporting concerns in this domain. Cultural factors were noted to play an important role in the detrimental effect of pemphigus on QOL in these patients because of the misconceptions that existed within the community associating skin pathologies with poor hygiene or sexual practices that go against cultural mores. Auxiliary considerations include the disease's onerous and costly management and social issues such as the limitations placed on marriage prospects for young women. Using a generic QOL instrument, the investigators identified a significant impact of pemphigus on QOL and highlighted that beyond functional aspects of disease burden, the SF-36 also explores social domains and self-image issues, which are particularly relevant in pemphigus.

The QOL of patients with pemphigus vulgaris was also evaluated in one study of 27 German participants using a dermatology-specific instrument.[26] The DLQI score for the study cohort averaged 10.1 ± 6.6 compared with healthy individuals with a mean score of 0.5 ± 1.1, and the investigators concluded that a diagnosis of pemphigus conferred a large impairment in QOL. Patients with mucosal involvement were found to have a higher DLQI, averaging 10.4 ± 7.3, than those with mucosal sparing who averaged 9.3 ± 5.1, indicating a poorer QOL. Itching was also associated with decreased QOL as patients with itch scored 11.5 ± 7.5 compared with those without itch who scored 7.9 ± 4.8. Similarly, burning was found to impair QOL, with patients scoring 10.8 ± 6.6. This score was compared with that in those without burning, who scored almost half of that with an average DLQI of 5.5 ± 5.7. Possibly because of the small cohort size, none of the results achieved statistical significance, and, notably, 22.2% of patients felt that their QOL was not impaired by their illness at all. The mean DLQI for pemphigus was higher than the mean scores for similar blistering diseases such as bullous pemphigoid (6.92 ± 3.8) as well as other dermatologic pathologies such as basal cell carcinoma (2.0 ± 2.2) but lower than that of atopic eczema (12.5 ± 5.8), a comparison facilitated by the use of a skin-specific QOL instrument to compare severity.

A study reviewing the health status of 58 Italian inpatients undergoing treatment of pemphigus also demonstrated a significant decrease in QOL compared with the greater population.[27] Participants were issued the SF-36, Clinical Depression Questionnaire (CDQ),[28] and the Institute for Personality and Aptitude Testing Anxiety Scale Questionnaire (ASQ).[29] As expected, pemphigus had a larger impact on SF-36 scores than normative data.[30] Patients with disease duration of 5 years or more, recent-onset disease, disease that had worsened compared with the previous year, mucocutaneous involvement, higher anti-Dsg3 antibodies, and more severe disease subjectively had worse SF-36 scores (P<.05). The ASQ and CDQ values demonstrated a strong negative correlation with the SF-36 scores, indicating that poorer QOL scores were associated with higher levels of anxiety and depression.

Another study from Italy used generic and dermatology-specific QOL instruments in 126 inpatients with pemphigus.[31] Most patients had pemphigus vulgaris (N = 112), although the cohort included patients with pemphigus foliaceus (N = 10), paraneoplastic pemphigus (N = 2), and IgA pemphigus (N = 2). Patients completed the SF-36, the Skindex-29,[5] and the GHQ-12 to assess QOL with the Ikeda index[32] and Physician Global Assessment and autoantibody titers used to assess disease severity. The SF-36 and Skindex-29 scores of patients with pemphigus were adversely affected compared with normative scores for the general Italian population (P<.05). Disease severity was significantly associated with poorer QOL scores as was female sex, which had not been identified in previous QOL studies in pemphigus, although has been described in other dermatologic conditions.[33] No correlation was found between Dsg antibody titers, clinical severity, or QOL scores. GHQ positivity (suggesting probable minor nonpsychotic psychiatric conditions) was detected in 39.7% of participants compared with a general population prevalence of 10% to 12% and was significantly correlated with clinical severity. Patients with pemphigus foliaceus were found to have slightly poorer QOL than those with pemphigus vulgaris using the Skindex-29, with a significant difference in the symptom scale with 70% of patients with pemphigus foliaceus GHQ positive. However, there were only 10 patients with pemphigus foliaceus in this study compared with 112 patients with pemphigus vulgaris, and, as this study was completed in an inpatient setting, it is plausible that patients with pemphigus foliaceus were more severe at presentation. As no objective disease extent score, such as the Autoimmune Bullous Skin Disease Intensity Score[34] or Pemphigus Disease Activity Index,[35] was provided with this study, it is not known if this was the case.

Another cross-sectional study from Iran[36] compared the QOL in 76 patients with pemphigus for at least 3 months and 86 healthy controls who accompanied them to clinic appointments (ie, most likely relatives), so their environment and social status was similar using Farsi translations of the SF-36 and the Sweden Quality of Life instrument.[37] It is not reported whether the investigators used validated Farsi translations of the SF-36 and Swedish QOL instruments or the proficiency of patients in Farsi given the ethnic diversity in Iran. As expected, patients with pemphigus were found to have significantly lower QOL scores across all parameters, with a mean score of 69.38 compared with the control mean of 85.43 (P<.0001). Factors associated with poorer QOL scores included age greater than 50 years (P<.04), longer disease duration (P<.01), repeated hospitalization (P<.001), and treatment protocol (steroid and adjuvant, P<.001). Of note, better QOL scores were demonstrated amongst patients with a university education (P<.01) and with particular professions. Housekeepers had a higher number of poor QOL scores; however, this may have been because of confounding because all housekeepers within the study were women and, as mentioned previously and also found in this study, women had worse QOL scores.[33] No significant difference in QOL was identified between patients with higher and lower incomes, although the latter had slightly better scores. The reason may be the low number of patients in the study with high incomes.

The importance of QOL in the setting of AIBD is becoming increasingly appreciated, and many studies are now including this as an important outcome measure. For instance, a small study of Brazilian patients with pemphigus recently investigated the effects of physiotherapy with QOL, the only outcome of interest.[38] Seven patients received a 4-month course of 25 physiotherapy sessions with QOL assessed using the SF-36 at baseline and at the completion of the study. Patients who participated in the intervention showed a tendency for improvement in the symptom component of the SF-36 but not the social or psychological aspects. The only statistically significant improvement was in pain scores ($P<.005$); however, further studies are warranted with larger numbers before the effects of physiotherapy on QOL in pemphigus can be determined definitively. QOL is also appearing with increasing frequency as an outcome in clinical trials, and, accordingly, it is important that reliable validated instruments are available to evaluate this construct.

To our knowledge, no QOL instrument specific to AIBD has yet been developed, and our research group has been working on the development of such a measure: the Autoimmune Bullous Disease Quality of Life Questionnaire (ABQOL).[39] Following a comprehensive item-generation process, a pilot instrument was established that was administered to 73 patients with autoimmune bullous disease across Australia along with the DLQI. Results obtained from this pilot questionnaire were evaluated using factor analysis and review by experts in bullous disease to refine the measure to the final ABQOL questionnaire consisting of 17 questions. Psychometric evaluation of the ABQOL has shown it to be a valid and reliable instrument that may be used to monitor disease activity and serve as an end point in clinical trials. This measure has been presented at various conferences and is being submitted for publication.[40]

SUMMARY

Both congenital and acquired bullous dermatoses have the potential to impose a significant burden of disease, and the impact exerted on the QOL of patients is often multifaceted. As expected, the qualitative and quantitative studies reviewing QOL in patients with bullous have all reported a significant decrease in QOL scores compared with the greater population using a range of patient-based measures. Formal evaluation of QOL in this setting facilitates the assessment of disease severity and mapping of disease trajectory and can capture outcomes of therapeutic intervention relevant to the patient.

ACKNOWLEDGMENTS

We would like to thank the Independent Learning Program of the University of New South Wales, Sydney, for supporting the research years for D.F.S. and J.W.F. with D.F.M.; Dr James McMillan, University of Queensland, for assistance with the translation of the Japanese article; and Dr James Drummond for assistance with the translation of the French article.

REFERENCES

1. WHOQOL Group. The World Health Organization Quality of Life assessment (WHOQOL): position paper from the World Health Organization. Soc Sci Med 1995;41:1403–9.
2. World Health Organization. Constitution of the world health organization. In: Basic documents, 45th edition, Supplement, October 2006 from the Fifty-First World Health Assembly. Geneva (Switzerland): WHO; 2006. p. 1.
3. Chen S. Dermatology quality of life instruments: sorting out the quagmire. J Invest Dermatol 2007;127: 2726–39.
4. Ware J Jr, Sherbourne C. The MOS 36-item short form health survey (SF-36). Conceptual framework and item selection. Med Care 1992;30:472–83.
5. Chren MM, Lasek RJ, Floke SA, et al. Improved discriminative and evaluative capability of a refine version of Skindex, a quality-of-life instrument for patients with skin diseases. Arch Dermatol 1997; 133:1433–40.
6. Both H, Essink-Bot M, Bussschbach J, et al. Critical review of generic and dermatology-specific health-related quality of life instruments. J Invest Dermatol 2010;127:27726–39.
7. Frew JW, Murrell DF. Quality of life measurements in epidermolysis bullosa: tools for clinical research and patient care. Dermatol Clin 2010;28:185–90.
8. Sebaratnam DF, McMillan JR, Werth VP, et al. Quality of life in patients with bullous dermatoses. Clin Dermatol 2012;30:103–7.
9. Fine JD, Eady RA, Bauer EA, et al. The classification of inherited epidermolysis bullosa (EB): report of the Third International Consensus Meeting on Diagnosis and Classification of EB. J Am Acad Dermatol 2008; 58:931–50.
10. Horn HM, Tidman MJ. Quality of life in epidermolysis bullosa. Clin Exp Dermatol 2002;27:707–10.
11. Finlay A, Khan G. Dermatology Life Quality Index (DLQI)—a simple practical measure for routine clinical use. Clin Exp Dermatol 1994;19:210–6.

12. Fine JD, Johnson LB, Weiner M, et al. Assessment of mobility, activities and pain in different subtypes of epidermolysis bullosa. Clin Exp Dermatol 2004;29: 122-7.

13. Fine JD, Johnson LB, Weiner M, et al. Impact of inherited epidermolysis bullosa on parental interpersonal relationships, marital status and family size. Br J Dermatol 2005;152:1009-14.

14. Tabolli S, Sampogna F, Di Pietro C, et al. Quality of life in patients with epidermolysis bullosa. Br J Dermatol 2009;161:869-77.

15. Goldberg D, Williams P. A user's guide to the General Health Questionnaire. Windsor (United Kingdom): NFER-Nelson; 1988.

16. Brooks R, Rabin RE, de Charro F. The measurement and validation of health status using EQ-5D: a European perspective. Dordrecht (The Netherlands): Kluwer Academic; 2005.

17. Ferrario SR, Baiardi P, Zotti AM. Update on family strain questionnaire: a tool for the general screening of caregiving-related problems. Qual Life Res 2004; 13:1425-34.

18. Margari F, Leece PA, Santamato W, et al. Psychiatric symptoms and quality of life in patients affected by epidermolysis bullosa. J Clin Psychol Med Settings 2010;17:333-9.

19. Frew JW, Martin LK, Nijsten T, et al. Quality of life evaluation in epidermolysis bullosa (EB) through the development of the QOLEB questionnaire: an EB-specific quality of life instrument. Br J Dermatol 2009;161:1323-30.

20. van Scheppingen C, Lettinga AT, Duipmans JC, et al. Main problems experienced by children with epidermolysis bullosa: a qualitative study with semi-structured interviews. Acta Derm Venereol 2008;88:143-50.

21. Dures E, Morris M, Gleeson K, et al. The psychosocial impact of epidermolysis bullosa. Qual Health Res 2011;21:771-8.

22. Venugopal SS, Yan WF, Frew JW, et al. First double-blind randomized clinical trial of intradermal allogeneic fibroblast therapy for severe generalized recessive dystrophic epidermolysis bullosa randomized against placebo injections resulted in similar wound healing that is independent of collagen VII expression. J Invest Dermatol 2010;130:S67.

23. Frew JW, Venugopal SS, Murrell DF. Quality of life outcomes of cultured allogeneic fibroblast therapy recipients with epidermolysis bullosa. Aust J Dermatol 2011;52(Suppl 1):26.

24. Masahiro S, Shigaku I, Yutaka I, et al. An investigation of quality of life (QOL) of pemphigus patients in Japan (first report). J Dermatol 2000;110:283-8.

25. Terrab Z, Benchikhi H, Maaroufi A, et al. Quality of life and pemphigus. Ann Dermatol Venereol 2005;132:321-8.

26. Mayrshofer F, Hertl M, Sinkgraven R. Significant decrease in quality of life in patients with pemphigus vulgaris. Results from the German Bullous Skin Disease (BSD) Study Group. J Dtsch Dermatol Ges 2005;3:431-5 [in German].

27. Tabolli S, Mozzetta A, Antinone V, et al. The health impact of pemphigus vulgaris and pemphigus foliaceus assessed using the Medical Outcomes Study 36-item short form health survey questionnaire. Br J Dermatol 2008;158:1029-34.

28. Krug S, Laughlin J. Handbook for the IPAT depression scale. Champaign (IL): Institute for Personality and Ability Testing; 1976.

29. Krug S, Scheier I, Cattel R. Handbook for the IPAT anxiety scale. Champaign (IL): Institute for Personality and Ability Testing; 1976.

30. Sampogna F, Tabolli S, Soderfeldt B, et al. Measuring quality of life of patients with different clinical types of psoriasis using the SF-36. Br J Dermatol 2006;154:844-9.

31. Paradisi A, Sampogna F, Di Pietro C, et al. Quality-of-life assessment in patients with pemphigus using a minimum set of evaluation tools. J Am Acad Dermatol 2009;60:26-9.

32. Ikeda S, Imamura S, Hashimoto I, et al. History of the establishment and revision of diagnostic criteria, severity index and therapeutic guidelines for pemphigus in Japan. Arch Dermatol Res 2003; 295(Suppl 1):S12-6.

33. Sampogna F, Chren M, Melchi C, et al. Age, gender, quality of life and psychological distress in patients hospitalised with psoriasis. Br J Dermatol 2006; 154:325-31.

34. Pfütze M, Niedermeier A, Hertl M, et al. Introducing a novel Autoimmune Bullous Skin Disease Intensity Score (ABSIS) in pemphigus. Eur J Dermatol 2007; 17:4-11.

35. Rosenbach M, Murrell DF, Bystryn JC, et al. Reliability and convergent validity of two outcome instruments in pemphigus. J Invest Dermatol 2009;129:2404-10.

36. Darjani A, Ghanbari A, Sayadi Nejhad A. Comparison of the health-related quality of life of patients suffering from pemphigus with healthy people. Journal of Guilan University of Medical Sciences 2008;17:1-9.

37. Brorsson B, Ifyer J, Hays RD. The Swedish Health-Related Quality of Life Survey. Qual Life Res 1993; 2:33-45.

38. Timóteo P, Simões Marques L, Bertoncello D. Physiotherapy intervention promotes better quality of life for patients with pemphigus. Rev Soc Bras Med Trop 2010;43:580-3 [in Portuguese].

39. Hanna A, Sebaratnam D, Chee S, et al. A disease-specific quality of life instrument for autoimmune bullous diseases—the ABQOL. Aust J Dermatol 2010;52(Suppl 1):27.

40. Hanna A, Sebaratnam D, Chee S, et al. The development of a disease-specific quality of life instrument for autoimmune bullous dermatoses: the ABQOL. J Invest Dermatol 2011;131(Suppl 2):S33.

Pruritus

Suephy C. Chen, MD, MS[a,b,*]

KEYWORDS

• Pruritus • Quality of life • Itch

Pruritus is the Rodney Dangerfield of medicine, and perhaps even dermatology, because it commands very little respect relative to other symptoms. Why would this be the case? The definition of itch originated more than 340 years ago when Hafenreffer,[1] a German physician, characterized itch as an unpleasant sensation, provoking the desire to scratch. Since then, pruritus has been increasingly recognized as a common symptom. Population-based epidemiologic data are sparse; however, several recent studies have yielded data supporting this claim. Wolkenstein and colleagues[2] attempted to evaluate the prevalence and impact of main dermatologic disorders in France. From their data for skin conditions in which pruritus is commonly associated, the prevalence of pruritus can be extrapolated to be between 20% and 35%. Matterne and colleagues[3] performed a population-based cross-sectional study in the general German population with the specific aim of determining the prevalence of chronic pruritus. The investigators found a point prevalence of 13.5% (95% confidence interval [CI], 12.2%–14.9%), 12-month prevalence of 16.4% (95% CI, 15.0%–17.9%), and lifetime prevalence of 22.0% (95% CI, 20.4%–23.7%). Our preliminary data from nationally sampled US veterans suggest that 30% of veterans have suffered from chronic pruritus.

Data also suggest that diagnoses in which itch is often a primary symptom rank as the most common cutaneous diagnoses treated.[4] An example of a skin condition in which pruritus is common is psoriasis. Globe and colleagues[5] used physician interviews and patient focus groups to characterize the impact of itch symptoms when developing a disease model for psoriasis. Dermatologists most frequently mentioned pruritus as a major psoriasis symptom followed by arthralgia/arthritis, flaking, and pain. They also rated the importance of itch to patients highly (8–10 out of 10). In focus groups of patients with both severe and mild psoriasis, the overwhelming majority of the patients rated itch as the most important (31/39), most severe (31/39), and most troublesome (24/39) symptom and noted that itch negatively affected daily activities (eg, concentration, sleep, ability to attend work or school) as well as emotions (eg, anxiety and embarrassment).

However, the cause of chronic pruritus is not only from cutaneous disorders but also from systemic diseases such as uremia and liver failure or because of unknown origin. Weisshaar and colleagues[6] compared 2 populations with pruritus, one in Germany (132 patients) and one in Uganda (84 patients). Although 57% of the German patients had pruritus due to dermatoses, 36% had pruritus due to a systemic disease and 8% had pruritus of unknown origin. Affective reactions such as aggression and depression occurred more frequently in patients with dermatologic problems than those with systemic pruritus. The former group felt that pruritus had a greater impact on their lives. Almost all Ugandan patients had pruritus due to dermatoses, except for 3 with pruritus of unknown origin. Patients with pruritus in both populations showed an impaired quality of life (QoL).

Although pruritus has being recognized as a common symptom and although a core group of investigators have made progress in unraveling the pathophysiologic pathways of pruritus,[7–10] very few treatment options exist and exceedingly little research is being conducted to fill this void. One could argue that the study of pruritus is stunted and frustrating because it is not visible and is difficult to measure. However, other nonvisible symptoms such as pain and nausea are well

a Division of Dermatology, Atlanta Veterans Affairs Medical Center, Decatur, GA 30322, USA
b Department of Dermatology, Emory University, 101 Woodruff Circle, Atlanta, GA 30322, USA
* Department of Dermatology, Emory University, 101 Woodruff Circle, Atlanta, GA 30322.
E-mail address: Schen2@emory.edu

Dermatol Clin 30 (2012) 309–321
doi:10.1016/j.det.2011.11.012
0733-8635/12/$ – see front matter Published by Elsevier Inc.

studied and, as a result, have many treatment options. Historically, investigators used instruments that measured the physical sequela of itch, such as scratching or rubbing. However, not everybody who itches manifests scratching.

There is an increasing recognition in health care research of the value of patient-reported outcomes. The simplest patient-reported outcome is the visual analog scale, asking patients to rank their itch on a scale that ranges from "No Itch" to "Most Severe Itch Imaginable or Experienced." However, these scales are very limited in that they only address intensity and do not address health-related QoL issues.

Health-related QoL is a patient-reported outcome that describes the impact of the disease in question to all aspects of persons' life, including psychosocial, emotional, physical, and functional impact. As such, health-related QoL is particularly relevant in conditions that have no physical signs and need to rely on patient reports to know whether they are improving or not. Work is beginning in pruritus to develop instruments that can measure pruritus-related QoL. This article reviews the instruments that have been developed and used in pruritus and also reviews the literature regarding the impact of pruritus on QoL.

Health-related QoL instruments that detail the specifics of how a disease or condition affects QoL come in 3 main flavors: generic health, organ specific, and disease condition specific. Generic health QoL questionnaires contain items that are common to all health conditions. As such, they can be applied across diseases and populations. However, general health QoL measures may not be sensitive enough to detect issues specific to a particular disease/condition and thus may not be responsive to changes. Organ-specific, in our case skin-specific, QoL instruments can be applied to all diseases/conditions within the skin, and thus the impact on QoL can be compared across skin disorders. More specific than general health QoL measures, these measures may still not be sensitive enough to detect issues specific to a particular disease/condition. Disease/condition-specific QoL instruments are the most sensitive to issues at hand with the disease/condition in question but may not be compared with other populations. As discussed in detail elsewhere in this issue, one can distinguish health status instruments, which define the state of itching for the patient, from QoL instruments that address the impact of itch on the psychosocial as well as the physical aspects of the patients' lives. In this article, we attempt to identify health status instruments as such, recognizing that the labels of health status versus health-related QoL instruments are often blurred in the literature. There are preference-based health-related QoL measures that ask patients to quantify the amount of QoL impact in terms of a metric that they are willing to trade, such as risk, time, or money.

METHODS

To determine the published literature establishing the QoL impact of pruritus, we conducted a limited systematic review. We queried PubMed with the key words of "pruritus" and "quality of life" and obtained 528 articles. We eliminated those articles without at least an English abstract and those articles that did not have "pruritus" and a construct related to QoL in the title. This filtering left 25 articles, of which 8 related to instrument development or translation and 2 related to epidemiology, which are discussed previously.

RESULTS
Generic Health Instruments in Pruritus

One of the most commonly used generic health instruments was developed from the Medical Outcomes Study, called the Short Form 36 (SF-36). SF-36 is a measure of health status and consists of 8 scaled scores that are the weighted sums of the questions in each section. The 8 sections are vitality, physical functioning, body pain, general health perceptions, physical role functioning, emotional role functioning, social role functioning, and mental health. The SF-36 has been subsequently pared to a 12-item version, the SF-12, which consists of a physical health component and a mental health component. Specifically, the SF-12 addresses general health, daily and social activity limitations as a result of physical and/or mental health, impact of pain on normal work, as well as feelings of calm and peace, energy, and downheartedness/blue. Scores from both versions are compared with norms developed from a US general population.

Our search revealed 3 studies that used the Short Form instruments to investigate the impact of pruritus, one of which is discussed in this review because they also used a skin-specific QoL instrument. Paul and colleagues[11] examined itch in chronic venous disease. Their study was part of a larger investigation into the impact of intravenous drug use on the distribution and severity of chronic venous disorders. The 161-subgroup cohort evaluated for pruritus completed the SF-12 as well a visual analog scale for itch intensity. Using the clinical score of the Clinical-Etiology-Anatomy-Pathophysiology classification of the worst leg, the most common classification was Class 3, edema without skin changes (45.9%); 18.6% had severe venous disease (Classes 5 and 6). Eighty-eight participants (54.7%) reported itch somewhere on their body, with 74 of them (45.9%) reporting itch on the legs or feet. Persons with leg or feet itch had poorer scores on the physical component of the SF-12 than those without itch. The 2 groups did not differ significantly on the mental health component. One possible reason that there was no significant difference in the mental health scores is that the items in SF-12 are not sensitive enough to the emotional impact of pruritus. However, compared with the US norms, persons with itch were more than 1 SD below the mean for both their mental (57.45) and physical health (34.79) scores. The investigators concluded that legs or feet itch has lower QoL and is a clinically relevant problem that is related to the level of venous disease.

El-Baalbaki and colleagues[12] explored the association of pruritus with QoL and disability in 578 patients with systemic sclerosis after 1 or more years postenrollment in the Canadian Scleroderma Research Group Registry. Patients reported whether they experienced pruritus during the past month on most days and completed the SF-36. Disability was measured with the Health Assessment Questionnaire disability index. However, only the abstract was available, so scores for the assessments were not attainable. The investigators described that a total of 248 patients (43%) reported pruritus on most days. Patients with pruritus had significantly worse mental (Hedges g = −0.43; 95% CI, −0.59 to −0.26) and physical function (Hedges g = −0.51; 95% CI, −0.68 to −0.34) and greater disability (Hedges g = 0.46; 95% CI, 0.29 to 0.63) than those without pruritus. In multivariate analyses, controlling for age, sex, marital status, education, disease duration, skin score, number of tender joints, gastrointestinal symptoms, breathing problems, Raynaud phenomenon, and finger ulcers, pruritus was independently associated with mental ($P = .017$) and physical function ($P = .003$) but not disability ($P = .112$). The investigators concluded that pruritus is common and associated with QoL in systemic sclerosis.

Another general health instrument is the Symptom Checklist-90-R (SCL-90-R), which is designed to evaluate a broad range of psychological problems and symptoms of psychopathology. The 90 items yield 9 scores along primary symptom dimensions, including somatization, obsessive-compulsive disorder, interpersonal sensitivity, depression, anxiety, hostility, phobic anxiety, paranoid ideation, and psychoticism. van Os-Medendorp and colleagues[13] used the SCL-90-R to determine the predictors of psychosocial morbidity in patients with chronic pruritic skin diseases. They hypothesized that feelings of helplessness and lack of control can influence the perceived itch and psychosocial complaints. The investigators recruited 168 patients with pruritic skin diseases from 5 hospitals in the Netherlands. Skin-related psychosocial morbidity was measured with the Adjustment to Chronic Skin Diseases questionnaire (ACS); general psychosocial morbidity was measured with the Symptom Checklist-90 (SCL-90). The frequency and intensity of itching and scratching was recorded in diaries. Itch-related coping was measured with the Itching Cognitions Questionnaire. The investigators found that patients with pruritic skin diseases had higher SCL-90 scores than a healthy Dutch population. All patients had psychosocial complaints as measured with the ACS. About 39% of the variance in skin-related psychosocial morbidity was explained by catastrophizing and helpless coping; another 11% was explained by itching and scratching. Age and sex together explained another 10%. The frequency of itching and scratching (11%), catastrophizing and helpless coping (19%), and skin-related psychosocial morbidity (10%) explained the variance in general psychosocial morbidity. The investigators concluded that patients with a pruritic skin disease have a high level of psychosocial morbidity. Catastrophizing and helpless coping are the most important predictors of psychosocial morbidity, with itching, scratching, and demographic variables having a limited influence.

Skin-Specific QoL Instruments

Skin-specific QoL instruments have been developed and validated to measure the QoL impact for all skin disorders. The 2 most commonly used instruments, the Skindex and the Dermatology Life Quality Index (DLQI), have items that relate to pruritus. The DLQI, a frequency-based measure, has an item that asks, "Over the last week, how itchy, sore, painful or stinging has your skin been?" which should be noted to combine pruritus with 3 other symptoms. The Skindex-29, which describes the frequency of impairment to QoL, has 1 item that asks the frequency of "My Skin Itches," whereas the Skindex-16, which describes the level of bother for a QoL impairment, has an item that asks, "During the past week, how often have you been bothered by your skin condition itching?" Because both instruments ask items that relate to QoL impairment, one can ascertain the difference in QoL impairment when comparing those that itch more with those that do not. However, the way that the items are referred to "Your Skin Condition" can be problematic when trying to distinguish whether the QoL impact is purely because of the symptom of pruritus or some other aspect of the skin condition, such as appearance.

DLQI application in pruritus

The DLQI is the most commonly used skin-specific health status measure.[14] It consists of 10 questions querying how symptoms and feelings, daily activities, leisure, work, school, personal relationships, and treatment were affected by skin disease over the previous week. It has been reviewed in detail elsewhere in this issue but should be noted to primarily address disability rather than emotional impact of skin conditions. In addition, clinical meaning has been assigned to bands of DLQI scores: 0 to 1, no effect; 2 to 5, small effect; 6 to 10, moderate effect; 11 to 20, very large effect; and 21 to 30, extremely large effect on patient's QoL.[15] The DLQI was the instrument of choice in evaluating pruritus or skin diseases in which pruritus is a major symptom in 6 articles in our systematic review.

Chularojanamontri and colleagues[16] performed a cross-sectional study, administering a Thai version of the DLQI in patients with systemic sclerosis who attended the Department of Dermatology, Siriraj Hospital in Bangkok, Thailand, between August 2009 and April 2010. A total of 80 patients with systemic sclerosis were enrolled in this study. Twelve patients had limited disease, whereas 68 patients had diffuse sclerosis. DLQI scores were not reported or correlated to pruritus. However, the investigators note that pain/pruritus was the most significant problem in patients, whereas the salt-and-pepper appearance was the cutaneous finding that had association with high DLQI scores. The investigators concluded that the treatment of pain and pruritus and prominent cutaneous findings should be taken into account to improve the QoL of patients with systemic sclerosis.

Szepietowski and colleagues[17] surveyed 334 patients with end-stage renal disease with moderate to severe uremic xerosis for QoL assessment using the DLQI. Pruritus was self-assessed by patients, using a visual analog scale. Those subjects who reported pruritus had greater QoL impact than those who did not (5.99 ± 4.82 [moderate effect] vs 3.24 ± 3.99 [small effect], $P<.001$). Using a multiple linear regression model, the investigators found that age and pruritus intensity, but not xerosis intensity, were found to be independent contributors to DLQI deterioration ($P<.0005$). On the other hand, uremic xerosis without associated pruritus still resulted in DLQI alteration (3.24 ± 3.99). It was concluded that young age and intensity of uremic pruritus compromise QoL in patients with uremic xerosis. Some characteristics of uremic

xerosis other than xerosis intensity may also be involved in QoL alteration.

The DLQI was also used to determine the impact of pruritus on QoL in sulfur mustard–exposed Iranian veterans.[18] The rationale for this study is that one of the foremost negative effects of sulfur mustard, a chemical warfare agent, is chronic pruritus. The DLQI and a pruritus visual analog scale were administered to 125 consecutive chemically injured veterans suffering from pruritus. The distribution of subjects according to pruritus severity were as follows: 11%, mild; 35%, moderate; and 54%, severe itching with corresponding median DLQI scores of 16, 20, and 21, respectively ($P = .014$). Of note, the scores of 16 and 20 fall within the clinical band of "Very Large Effect on QoL," whereas 21 is the lower bound of "Extremely Large Effect on QoL." The DLQI subscores of symptoms and feelings ($P = .015$), personal relationships ($P = .002$), and daily activities ($P = .036$) were worst in patients with severe itching. The investigators concluded that chemically injured veterans suffering from severe itching have a significantly poorer QoL than patients with milder symptoms.

The DLQI was used in 2 studies for evaluation of pruritus in psoriasis. Zachariae and colleagues[19] explored the possible association between different dimensions of pruritus to psychological symptoms and QoL impact. The investigators also explored the role of sleep impairment as a possible mediator of the association between pruritus and psychological symptoms and QoL. A sample of 40 patients with psoriasis completed a scale with descriptors from the Structured Itch Questionnaire together with measures of depression, distress, sleep quality, and the DLQI. Of note, the investigators modified the DLQI by omitting irrelevant items and items relating directly to perceived itch, thus preventing the calculation of an overall DLQI score. The investigators also rephrased items to refer directly to difficulties due to itch. Psoriasis severity was assessed with the Psoriasis Area and Severity Index. Factor analysis of descriptors confirmed both an affective (eg, unbearable, bothersome) and a sensory (eg, pinching, tickling) pruritus severity dimension. Multivariate statistics, controlling for age, gender, disease duration, and severity, showed affective, but not sensory, pruritus severity to be a significant predictor of depressive symptoms, global distress, impairment of sleep, and QoL. Mediation analyses indicated that impaired sleep quality partly mediated the association between pruritus severity and psychological symptoms. The investigators concluded that pruritus is multidimensional and that the affective dimension may be the most important predictor of pruritus-related psychological morbidity and that the association may be mediated by its negative impact on sleep quality.

Reich and colleagues[20] used the DLQI to evaluate the relationship between pruritus and the well-being of patients with psoriasis. The mean DLQI score of the 91 patients who reported pruritus (of total 102 patients with psoriasis) was 12.2 ± 7.0. Patients with pruritus had significantly decreased QoL compared with those without report of pruritus (12.2 ± 7.0 vs 6.8 ± 7.1, $P = .02$ or very large vs moderate impact). The investigators also found that pruritus intensity correlated with feelings of stigmatization, stress, and depressive symptoms. They concluded that pruritus may have a significant negative influence of the psychosocial status of patients with psoriasis.

A pediatric version of the DLQI, the Children's Dermatology Life Quality Index (CDLQI), was administered to children with atopic dermatitis to evaluate improvement with pruritus after they and their families joined support groups.[21] The investigators based their study on preliminary evidence suggesting that support groups and educational programs are helpful in reducing stress, disease, and pruritus severity and improving QoL. Thirty-two patients and their relatives completed the questionnaires satisfactorily. The baseline overall QoL as measured by the CDLQI was 11.37 ± 7.26, which corresponds to "Very Large Effect" on the clinical interpretation of DLQI scores. The investigators noted significant change in CDLQI scores ($P<.01$) as well as specific domains, such as personal relationships ($P = .02$) and leisure ($P = .04$) with their intervention but did not report correlations with pruritus improvement. Thus, although the investigators concluded that support groups may be very effective accessory tools in the management of recalcitrant forms of atopic dermatitis, it is unclear regarding the relative impact of pruritus versus other aspects of atopic dermatitis improvement on the QoL benefits.

Skindex application

The Skindex instruments were designed to measure the effects of skin disease on health-related QoL across different populations and to aid in assessing change in this parameter in individual patients.[22,23] The Skindex-29 addresses frequency of items, whereas the Skindex-16 addresses level of bother. Similar to the DLQI, the Skindex has been extensively psychometrically tested. In addition, the Skindex has a broad emotional component that the DLQI lacks and can be reported as subscales of emotion, symptoms, and functional impact. The Skindex was used in 3 articles to measure QoL impact of itch.

Murota and colleagues[24] used the Skindex-16 to measure the impact of sedative and nonsedative antihistamines in patients with pruritic skin diseases in Japan. The investigators also examined work productivity and used a visual analog scale to measure itch intensity. They found that in 216 patients with pruritic skin diseases, there was a significant impairment of work, classroom, and daily productivity. All pruritic diseases in this study negatively affected daily activity to a similar degree. No scores and only correlations were reported for the Skindex results. The Skindex-16 change scores correlated well with changes in pruritus visual analog scale score (r = 0.58, $P<.001$) for the group that took the nonsedative antihistamines, whereas there was no significant correlation in the sedative antihistamine group. This may be explained by their finding that nonsedative antihistamines produced greater overall improvements in productivity than sedative antihistamines. However, this explanation also suggests that the Skindex might be measuring more than just pruritus-specific QoL impact.

Tessari and colleagues[25] examined the impact of pruritus on the QoL of 169 patients undergoing both hemodialysis (HD) and peritoneal dialysis (PD) using the Skindex-29. The investigators measured pruritus intensity on a visual analog scale and health status using the SF-36 and the General Health Questionnaire. Only the abstract was available to us, so we could not ascertain if SF-36 and Skindex scores were published. Pruritus was found in 52% of patients, with no differences between patients undergoing HD and PD. Prevalence of poor sleep in patients with pruritus was higher than in those without pruritus (59% vs 11%; $P<.001$). Neither physical nor mental scores of SF-36 correlated with the presence and the intensity of pruritus. Pruritus intensity was significantly related to poor scores in all 3 subscales of Skindex-29. This finding confirms the higher sensitivity of the skin-specific instrument as compared with the generic health instrument in measuring pruritus-specific impact on QoL. In the subscales of social function and emotions, worse scores were observed in patients undergoing HD and with minor psychiatric disorders. The investigators concluded that pruritus had a high level of impact on all aspects of QoL and was a predictor of poor sleep.

Duque and colleagues[26] explored the prevalence and QoL impact of itch, pain, and burning sensation in a convenience sample of 100 patients with mild to moderate chronic venous insufficiency. Patients who suffered from itch were assessed with a visual analog scale for itch intensity and a modified Skindex-16 questionnaire.

The investigators did not explicitly detail how the Skindex was modified. The prevalence of itch was 66%. Concomitant itch and burning sensation as well as itch and pain were noted in 47% and 44% of the patients, respectively. However, Skindex item and scale scores were not reported; only correlations with itch intensity were reported. The investigators reported a statistically ($P<.05$) significant negative relationship between itch intensity and bother by itch (r = 0.5), persistence (r = 0.2), being irritated (r = 0.2), feelings of frustration (r = 0.2), and depression (r = 0.4). Functionally, the itch intensity was correlated with the desire to be with other people (r = 0.3), with the desire to develop daily activities (r = 0.4), and with what they enjoy (r = 0.3). The investigators note that the intensity of itch was comparable to that of other populations that they have studied: uremic pruritus, urticaria, and psoriasis. In addition, despite the correlation analysis, the investigators conclude that patients did not attribute emotional distress to the sensation of itch, differing from their findings with patients with psoriasis and atopic dermatitis. Nevertheless, the investigators concluded that their study found that itch, pain, and burning sensation are common symptoms of mild to moderate chronic venous insufficiency with a significant impact on QoL.

Pruritus-specific instruments

Both pruritus health status instruments, which define the state of itching for the patient, and pruritus-specific QoL instruments, which address the impact of itch on the psychosocial as well as the physical aspects of the patients' lives, have been developed. One of the first pruritus-specific instruments to be developed is the Eppendorf Itch Questionnaire (EIQ)[27] that is based on the long form of the McGill Pain Questionnaire.[27] The instrument consists of 40 descriptive adjectives describing the itch sensation and 40 more descriptors of emotional aspects of itch. Investigators have critiqued the EIQ for not measuring QoL[28]; however, the instrument does address some emotional aspects of QoL, especially with items such as "Annoying," "Bothersome," and "Torturing."

Another pruritus-specific instrument is the Short-Form Itch Questionnaire by Yosipovitch and colleagues.[29] This questionnaire was based on the short-form McGill Pain Questionnaire,[30] which is a multidimensional instrument designed to measure the impact of chronic pain and has been translated into other languages such as Canadian French.[31] In addition to pruritus history, severity, and characteristics, there are questions that relate to QoL. The investigators define QoL items as those that ask about mood change, eating habits, as well

as sexual desire and function, but they also ask about the impact of sleep, which can be considered a functional impact of QoL. The investigators developed questions as to how daily activities affect pruritus but do not ask how pruritus affects daily activities. The questionnaire also contained several items that were termed affective dimensions and consisted of the itch being bothersome, annoying, unbearable, and worrisome. The questionnaire was tested in a cohort of patients with uremia and found to have reasonable test-retest reliability (r = 0.72, $P<.01$).

Our review of the literature revealed 5 articles that used the Yosipovitch Short Form Itch Questionnaire. Two involve the population with uremia on which the questionnaire was developed, and the others include patients with at least 30% body involvement of psoriasis,[32] chronic idiopathic urticaria,[33] and atopic dermatitis,[34] all populations from Singapore. All these patients had significant QoL impact because of their symptom of pruritus (**Table 1**).

The uremic population on which the Short Form Itch Questionnaire was developed included 264 patients receiving HD treatment in Israel. In this group, pruritus was a frequent cause of sleep difficulties in 33%. In 52%, pruritus did not have any effect on mood, but 36% reported nervousness and 8% reported depression related to pruritus. Two years later, Yosipovitch's group revisited the initial 264 patients with uremia, of which 219 were able to participate.[35] Pruritus-related QoL impact had not changed (see **Table 1**). The investigators concluded that pruritus is still a major problem for these patients with end-stage renal disease.

Amatya and colleagues[36] reported their findings from 109 Swedish patients with chronic plaque psoriasis regarding the pattern and characteristics of pruritus. The investigators had developed a questionnaire using focus groups of patients. Although they did not use the Short-Form Itch Questionnaire, the investigators modified the McGill Pain Questionnaire, similar to the work from Yosipovitch's group. We thus compare their data with those of Yosipovitch's group (see **Table 1**). Although both populations with psoriasis reported high prevalence of daily pruritus, the impact of the pruritus differed between the 2 populations. As compared with Amatya's Swedish population, Yosipovitch's Singaporean population with psoriasis reported less difficulty concentrating but more impact on sleep, eating, sexual function, and feelings of their pruritus being annoying and unbearable. These differences speak to the need to account for cultural and sampling differences.

The Itch Severity Scale (ISS, **Table 2**)[37] was developed in response to the fact that the Short

Table 1
Cohorts using Short Form Itch Questionnaire, QoL-related items only

Cohort (N)	Uremia (264)	FU Uremia	Psoriasis (108)[32]	Psoriasis (Amatya et al[36])	Chronic Idiopathic Urticaria (100)[33]	Atopic Dermatitis (100)[34]
Daily pruritus	46%	46%	77%	66%	68%	87%
Affects sleep	33%	61%	69%	35%	62%	84%
Nervousness or agitation	36%	36%	35%	NR	52%	55%
Depression	8%	8%	24%	NR	14%	37%
Difficulty concentrating	NR	—	30%	47%	43%	63%
Eating habits	NR	—	23%	11%	34%	54%
Decreased sexual desire	NR	—	40%	21%	33%	26%
Decreased sexual function	NR	—	35%	NR	27%	21%
Bothersome[a]	80%	—	53%	63%	76%	82%
Annoying[a]	68%	—	44%	20%	66%	83%
Unbearable[a]	33%	—	36%	13%	59%	70%
Worrisome[a]	NR	—	18%	NR	44%	51%

Abbreviation: NR, not reported.
[a] Affective items with moderate to great extent.

Form Itch Questionnaire was designed to be administered by a trained interviewer. Investigators modified the Short Form so that it could be self-administered by the patient. In their study, subjects with psoriasis-associated pruritus were asked to answer the modified survey along with the RAND-36 Health Status Inventory and DLQI. The investigators found that 7 of the initial 11 components of the modified Short Form were included in the ISS. The different component responses to each of the 7 questions are summed separately and divided by the highest possible total score for the respective question. The 7 values are then added together and multiplied by 3 to get a total out of 21. Total ISS scores can range from 0 (no pruritus) to 21 (most severe pruritus). ISS scores correlated moderately with physical ($r = -0.483$) and mental ($r = -0.492$) health composite scores of the RAND-36 and strongly with DLQI scores ($r = 0.628$), evidence of construct validity. It had an internal consistency reliability of 0.80 and a test-retest reliability of 0.95. The principal component analysis identified 2 meaningful factors: pruritus severity, which explained 50.8% of the total variance, and temporal aspects, which explained 12.3% of the total variance. The investigators also found a clinically

important difference in ISS scores to be approximately 2 points. They concluded that the new 7-item ISS may be useful in comparing pruritus severity among different disease populations or in assessing pruritus treatment effectiveness. The ISS has subsequently been translated into Spanish using patients with atopic dermatitis[38] and Danish using patients with atopic dermatitis, psoriasis, urticaria, genital pruritus, and nephrogenic pruritus.[39]

The ISS has been used in assessing external auditory canal pruritus by Acar and colleagues.[40] The investigators modified the ISS to use 5 of the 7 parameters (daytime incidence, itch type, itch severity, effect on sleep, and effect on general psychological state) because 2 were unsuitable for assessment of the external auditory canal pruritus. They summed together the scores for the 5 parameters and multiplied by 3 to obtain the total score. The investigators did not psychometrically test their modified version but concluded that it was a useful tool to measure outcomes in external auditory canal pruritus because it did show significant difference between baseline and follow-up after topical treatments.

Another health status measure of pruritus, the 5-D itch scale, was developed as a brief but

Table 2
Pruritus-specific instruments, QoL items only

ISS	ItchyQoL (Frequency Version: 1 = Never to 5 = All the Time; S, Symptom; F, Function; E, emotions)	AGP (QoL Items Only) (1 = Not at All to 4 = Quite a Lot)	Patient Benefit Index[44] (Therapeutic Needs: 0 = Not at All to 4 = Very Important) Listed in Decreasing Order of Relevance to Respondents
Mood change (none, depressed, agitated, difficult concentration, anxious; can pick more than one)	Bleeds (S)	Sleep disturbance	No longer experience itching
How has itch affected sexual desire or function (no change vs decrease)	Hurts (S)	Impact on relationships	Find a clear diagnosis and therapy
How often does this happen (never, sometimes, almost always) in falling asleep, awakening to itch, and use of sleep medications	Burns/stings (S)	Impact on leisure activities	Have confidence in the therapy
	Scars (S)	Impact on quality of life	Be less dependent on doctor and clinic visits
	Scratch (S)	Drowsiness and lack of drive	Be healed of all skin alterations
	Temperature aggravation (S)	Detriment impact on mood	Be able to sleep better
	Spend money (F)	Less joy and fun in life	Have no fear that disease will progress
	Hard to work (F)	Reduced optimism	No longer have a burning sensation on the skin
	Interaction with others (F)		Be able to lead a normal life
	Sleep (F)		Have fewer side effects
	Concentrate (F)		Gain in joy of living

Soaps, detergents, and lotions (F)	Have lower out-of-pocket treatment costs
Types of clothes (F)	Need less time for daily treatments
Frustrated (E)	Be less nervous
Embarrassed (E)	Be less of a burden to relatives and friends
	Be able to concentrate better
Crazy (E)	Be able to bathe and shower normally
Personality change (E)	Be free of pain
Angry (E)	Be more productive in everyday life
Worry what others think (E)	Be able to engage in normal leisure activities
Worry last forever (E)	Be less burdened in partnership
Self-conscious (E)	Be less depressed
Sad (E)	Be able to wear all types of clothing
	Be able to have more contact with other people
	Dare to show oneself more
	Be able to have a normal sex life
	Be able to lead a normal working life

multidimensional questionnaire to be used as an outcome measure in clinical trials.[41] The 5 dimensions of the instrument are degree, duration, direction, disability, and distribution. The instrument was tested for validity, reliability, and response to change by administering it at baseline and 6 weeks later to 234 individuals with chronic pruritus due to liver disease (N = 63), kidney disease (N = 36), dermatologic disorders (N = 56), AIDS (N = 28), and burn injuries (N = 51). A subset of 50 untreated patients was retested after 3 days to assess test-retest reliability. The 5-D score correlated strongly with a visual analog score at all time points (r = 0.7–0.9). The 5-D demonstrated responsiveness with significant changes in pruritus over the 6-week follow-up period (P<.0001) and a lack of change in mean score between days 1 and 3 in untreated individuals (intraclass correlation coefficient = 0.96, P<.0001).

It should be recognized that these instruments provide a way for patients to characterize the status of their itch, which can be quite textured and nuanced. The 5-D allows for quantifying the status across time, useful for monitoring changes with an intervention. The Short Form additionally incorporates questions that relate to pruritus history, which is often valuable in documenting the severity of the condition. However, although several of these instruments contain QoL items, none of these instruments were developed with QoL as their target.

In 2008, our group introduced the ItchyQoL,[42] which is a validated pruritus-specific instrument that addresses the symptom and emotional and functional impact of pruritus. There is an overall score as well as subscale scores to address the 3 types of impact. The instrument was developed using the Skindex as a model, so there is some overlap in the items, but the items refer to the pruritus rather than to skin condition. Items were developed from in-depth interviews with 21 consecutive patients without regard for etiology of pruritus until no more new items were elicited. In this manner, we were able to comprehensively capture all items relevant to the way pruritus affects QoL and ensure content validity for our instrument. The instrument was developed with 2 versions, one that assesses for frequency of items and the other for level of bother. A total of 89 individuals with pruritus participated in the psychometric testing. Both ItchyQoL versions were demonstrated to be reliable with internal consistency (Cronbach α: frequency, 0.72–0.93; bother, 0.78–0.81) and reproducibility (intraclass correlation coefficient: frequency, 0.91; bother, 0.84–0.87). We demonstrated responsiveness using paired t tests. The ItchyQoL scores were statistically significantly improved for the group that reported improvement in pruritus. The scores did not demonstrate significant difference in those who reported no change. The instrument also demonstrated construct and discriminant validity. The ItchyQoL is being developed into a variety of languages, including Spanish, German, Mandarin Chinese, and French.

The ItchyQoL has been used to assess pruritus in a small cohort (N = 30) of patients with cutaneous T-cell lymphoma (CTCL).[43] There was representation for each of the stage categories (13 IA-IIA, 7 IIB, 7 III, 3 IV). Overall, 77% reported pruritus and 100% reported itching over greater than 24% of their body surface area (BSA). The BSA scores correlated significantly with the total ItchyQoL score (r = 0.5, P<.01), as well as with the 3 subscale scores (r = 0.4–0.5, P<.05). The ItchyQoL total score correspond to moderate impact (mean, 2.4; standard deviation, 0.8) overall. There was a trend in overall ItchyQoL scores, with stage IV patients reporting greater overall impact (3.4 [0.6]) as compared with the other stages (P = .09). The functional subscale demonstrated a similar trend (2.8 [0.6]) with the stage IV patients as compared with other stages (P = .07). The symptom and emotional subscales did not demonstrate such trends (2.4 [0.9] and 2.3 [0.9], respectively) as mean subscale scores for all subjects. The investigators concluded that pruritus seems to be a significant component of patients with CTCL, particularly in those whose disease is not well controlled.

In 2009, Blome and colleagues[44] introduced the Patient Benefit Index (PBI) for pruritus (PBI-P), which was based on the standardized PBI (PBI-S), a validated instrument to assess patients' treatment needs and benefits in skin diseases. The idea of the PBI instruments is for the patient to rate the importance of predefined treatment goals; after therapy, the patient rates the extent to which these goals have been achieved. Items for the PBI-P were generated by open-ended questionnaire to 50 patients with pruritus regarding impairments due to pruritus and treatment needs. A panel of dermatologists, psychologists, and persons with pruritus reduced the more than 300 mentioned items into 27 nonredundant and relevant items. Of note, only 4 treatment objectives were not already covered by the PBI-S. The investigators then tested the PBI-P for feasibility by 36 patients with pruritus and validated it in a sample of 100 patients with pruritus.

The instrument was feasible in clinical practice, requiring only 11 minutes to complete both the before- and after-therapy questions. There were less than 2% missing values. Reliability was demonstrated with a Cronbach α of 0.93. Convergent validity was demonstrated with a high correlation with change in pruritus intensity (r = 0.57, P<.001) and change in QoL score as measured by the DLQI (r = 0.41, P = .001). The investigators also asked patients to identify items with "Does Not Apply to Me" and compared consistency in answering the same question in this manner both before and after therapy. They found that depending on the item, 4% to 36% of patients answered inconsistently; only 14% of patients answered all the items consistently. The investigators concluded that the lack of consistency should be addressed in further studies by relating the idea of "Apply to Me" to disease characteristics or item content.

In 2011, Weisshaar and colleagues[45] developed a German language questionnaire for assessing chronic pruritus (Arbeitsgemeinschaft Pruritusfor-schung der Deutschen Dermatologischen Gesell-schaft DLQI [AGP questionnaire]) with the goal of usage in epidemiologic studies. It comprises questions on course, intensity and quality of pruritus, general health status, sociodemographic data, QoL, and pruritus cognition. The questions were developed from published literature and experts. Patients were asked after item develop-ment for comprehension, but there was an evalua-tion sheet at the end of the questionnaire inviting participants to comment on the missing aspects. The QoL portion inquired about impairment and effect of itch on affect (see **Table 2**). A total of 100 patients with chronic pruritus from the univer-sity hospitals of Giessen, Heidelberg, Munich, and Muenster participated in the study. There was satisfactory internal consistency on the impair-ment (Cronbach α = 0.8). The Cronbach α was not available for the affect subscale but was re-ported as sufficiently high. The investigators plan further testing of validity and sensitivity.

There have been studies in which validated QoL instruments for particular diseases have been used to investigate the impact of pruritus. Thus, rather than a pruritus-specific instrument, a disease-specific instrument has been used to correlate with itch intensity. One such study is the German Atopic Dermatitis Intervention Study that included 823 children and adolescents, investigating age-related educational programs in long-term man-agement of atopic dermatitis.[46] The investigators also investigated whether the itch severity ob-tained in the scoring of atopic dermatitis correlated with QoL using a validated German questionnaire, Quality of Life in Parents of Children with Atopic Dermatitis, which comprises 26 items that can be divided by factor analysis into 5 clearly interpret-able subscales: psychosomatic well-being, effects on social life, confidence in medical treatment, emotional coping, and acceptance of the disease.

Significant correlations were found between itch severity and QoL (r = 33–0.42, P<.001), but low correlations were found between the severity of atopic dermatitis and the itch intensity. Itch and sleeplessness were significantly correlated too. The investigators concluded that QoL, itch inten-sity, and coping strategies should be considered when treating patients with atopic dermatitis. From their results, we also point out that itch inten-sity should be explicitly queried when assessing atopic dermatitis because the physical attributes of atopic dermatitis have low correlation with itch intensity.

Preference-based measures

A complementary approach to measuring health-related QoL is using preference-based measures. The topic has been reviewed extensively elsewhere in this issue by Seidler and colleagues, but, essen-tially, the burden of disease can be measured by asking patients what they prefer: their current health state or a different health state by giving up some currency of value. This currency may be money, time, or risk. This method is rooted in health economic theory and has the advantage of allowing QoL to be incorporated into health economic analyses.

Our group used the time trade-off utility method to assess the burden pruritus and to compare it with pain.[47] Our rationale to compare with pain is based on the fact that although the 2 symptoms are very similar (both subjective and causes QoL impairment), pain is better appreciated than pruritus. We recruited 138 patients with chronic pain and 73 patients with chronic pruritus. Partici-pants reported their symptom severity on a visual analog scale and participated in an interview to elicit their utility value for their current health state. We used a computerized utility instrument to pro-vide subjects with a hypothetical decision: living the rest of their life in their current health state or living for a shorter period of time in perfect health. These data were used to generate utility scores, which quantified the burden of the health state on a scale of 0 (death) to 1 (perfect health). Demo-graphically the groups were similar, although patients with pain were more likely to describe this symptom as severe (36% vs 28% with pruritus). Participants with pruritus had a mean utility score of 0.87, whereas participants with pain had a mean utility score of 0.77. Using a multi-variate regression model, we analyzed the rela-tionship of symptom type to utility values, adjusting for symptom severity, symptom dura-tion, age, sex, race, marital status, as well as educational and income levels. We found that only marital status and severity of symptom, and not symptom type, were the only predictors of utility score. These data indicate that chronic pruritus has a significant burden of disease, with subjects willing to hypothetically trade 13% of their life expectancy to not have pruritus. Also, our results from this small study indicate that chronic pruritus may have a QoL impact comparable to that of chronic pain, especially because it was severity and not symptom type that best predicted the QoL impact.

SUMMARY

This review has demonstrated that pruritus should be a symptom to be respected. Preference-based QoL measures indicate that patients with pruritus are willing to give up 13% of their life expectancy to not have pruritus. Generic health QoL instruments indicate that pruritus secondary to chronic venous disorders had clinically significant QoL impact as compared with United States norms.[12] Significant correlations were also seen with pruritus and QoL as measured by skin-specific QoL measures. This review also demonstrates that patient-reported tools are indeed available to assist future researchers in studying pruritus. Generic health instruments and preference-based measures are available to perform studies to compare the QoL impact in other populations and diseases. The preference-based QoL measures can also be used in pharmacoeconomic studies to determine whether new interventions are cost effective relative to currently available therapies. Skin-specific instruments allow researchers to compare QoL impact with other skin conditions. Pruritus-specific health status and health QoL measures are available to measure changes in pruritus, particularly relevant to those researchers who wish to test new interventions. With this armamentarium of tools, clinicians can better appreciate the impact of pruritus and researchers are better armed to develop therapies for patient sufferers.

REFERENCES

1. Samuel Hafenreffer. Available at: http://en.wikipedia.org/wiki/Samuel_Hafenreffer. Accessed November 24, 2011.
2. Wolkenstein P, Grob J, Bastuji-Garin S, et al. French people and skin diseases: results of a survey using a representative sample. Arch Dermatol 2003; 139(12):1614–9.
3. Matterne U, Apfelbacher C, Loerbroks A, et al. Prevalence, correlates and characteristics of chronic pruritus: a population-based cross-sectional study. Acta Derm Venereol 2011;91(6):674–9.
4. Fleischer AJ, Herbert C, Feldman S, et al. Diagnosis of skin disease by nondermatologists. Am J Manag Care 2000;6(10):1149–56.
5. Globe D, Bayliss M, Harrison D. The impact of itch symptoms in psoriasis: results from physician interviews and patient focus groups. Health Qual Life Outcomes 2009;7:62.
6. Weisshaar E, Apfelbacher C, Jäger G, et al. Pruritus as a leading symptom: clinical characteristics and quality of life in German and Ugandan patients. Br J Dermatol 2006;155(5):957–64.
7. Reddy V, Shimada S, Sikand P, et al. Cathepsin S elicits itch and signals via protease-activated receptors. J Invest Dermatol 2010;130(5):1468–70.
8. Reddy V, Iuga A, Shimada S, et al. Cowhage-evoked itch is mediated by a novel cysteine protease: a ligand of protease-activated receptors. J Neurosci 2008;28(17):4331–5.
9. Maddison B, Parsons A, Sangueza O, et al. Retrospective study of intraepidermal nerve fiber distribution in biopsies of patients with nummular eczema. Am J Dermatopathol 2011;33(6):621–3.
10. Papoiu A, Tey H, Coghill R, et al. Cowhage-induced itch as an experimental model for pruritus. A comparative study with histamine-induced itch. PLoS One 2011;6(3):e17786.
11. Paul J, Pieper B, Templin T. Itch: association with chronic venous disease, pain, and quality of life. J Wound Ostomy Continence Nurs 2011;38(1):46–54.
12. El-Baalbaki G, Razykov I, Hudson M, et al. Association of pruritus with quality of life and disability in systemic sclerosis. Arthritis Care Res 2010;62(10):1489–95.
13. van Os-Medendorp H, Eland-de Kok P, Grypdonck M, et al. Prevalence and predictors of psychosocial morbidity in patients with chronic pruritic skin diseases. J Eur Acad Dermatol Venereol 2006;20(7):810–7.
14. Finlay A, Kahn G. Dermatology Life Quality Index (DLQI): a simple practical measure for routine clinical use. Clin Exp Dermatol 1994;19:210–6.
15. Hongbo Y, Thomas C, Harrison M, et al. Translating the science of quality of life into practice: what do dermatology life quality index scores mean? J Invest Dermatol 2005;125(4):659–64.
16. Chularojanamontri L, Sethabutra P, Kulthanan K, et al. Dermatology life quality index in Thai patients with systemic sclerosis: a cross-sectional study. Indian J Dermatol Venereol Leprol 2011;77(6):683–7.
17. Szepietowski J, Balaskas E, Taube K, et al. Quality of life in patients with uraemic xerosis and pruritus. Acta Derm Venereol 2011;91(3):313–7.
18. Panahi Y, Davoudi S, Sadr S, et al. Impact of pruritus on quality of life in sulfur mustard-exposed Iranian veterans. Int J Dermatol 2008;47(6):557–61.
19. Zachariae R, Zachariae C, Lei U, et al. Affective and sensory dimensions of pruritus severity:

associations with psychological symptoms and quality of life in psoriasis patients. Acta Derm Venereol 2008;88(2):121–7.

20. Reich A, Hrehorow E, Szepietowski J. Pruritus is an important factor negatively influencing the well-being of psoriatic patients. Acta Derm Venereol 2010;90: 257–63.

21. Weber M, Fontes Neto Pde T, Prati C, et al. Improvement of pruritus and quality of life of children with atopic dermatitis and their families after joining support groups. J Eur Acad Dermatol Venereol 2008;22(8):992–7.

22. Chren M, Lasek R, Flocke S, et al. Improved discriminative and evaluative capability of a refined version of Skindex, a quality-of-life instrument for patients with skin diseases. Arch Dermatol 1997;133:1433–40.

23. Chren M, Lasek R, Sahay A, et al. Measurement of properties of Skindex-16, a brief quality-of-life measure for patients with skin diseases. J Cutan Med Surg 2001;5(2):105–10.

24. Murota H, Kitaba S, Tani M, et al. Impact of sedative and non-sedative antihistamines on the impaired productivity and quality of life in patients with pruritic skin diseases. Allergol Int 2010;59(4):345–54.

25. Tessari G, Dalle Vedove C, Loschiavo C, et al. The impact of pruritus on the quality of life of patients undergoing dialysis: a single centre cohort study. J Nephrol 2009;22(2):241–8.

26. Duque M, Yosipovitch G, Chan Y, et al. Itch, pain, and burning sensation are common symptoms in mild to moderate chronic venous insufficiency with an impact on quality of life. J Am Acad Dermatol 2005;53(3):504–8.

27. Darsow U, Mautner V, Scharein E, et al. Der Eppendorfer Juckreizfragebogen. Hautarzt 1997;48: 730–3.

28. Yosipovitch G. Itch questionnaires as tools for itch evaluation. In: Yosipovitch G, Greaves M, Fleischer A, et al, editors. Itch. New York: Marcel Dekker, Inc; 2004. p. 169–82.

29. Yosipovitch G, Zucker I, Boner G, et al. A questionnaire for the assessment of pruritus: validation in uremic patients. Acta Derm Venereol 2001;81:108–11.

30. Melzack R. The short-form McGill Pain Questionnaire. Pain 1987;30:191–7.

31. Parent-Vachon M, Parnell L, Rachelska G, et al. Cross-cultural adaptation and validation of the Questionnaire for Pruritus Assessment for use in the French Canadian burn survivor population. Burns 2008; 34(1):71–92.

32. Yosipovitch G, Goon A, Wee J, et al. The prevalence and clinical characteristics of pruritus among patients with extensive psoriasis. Br J Dermatol 2000;143: 969–73.

33. Yosipovitch G, Ansari N, Goon A, et al. Clinical characteristics of pruritus in chronic idiopathic urticaria. Br J Dermatol 2002;147:32–6.

34. Yosipovitch G, Goon A, Wee J, et al. Itch characteristics in Chinese patients with atopic dermatitis using a new questionnaire for the assessment of pruritus. Int J Dermatol 2002;41:212–6.

35. Zucker I, Yosipovitch G, David M, et al. Prevalence and characterization of uremic pruritus in patients undergoing hemodialysis: uremic pruritus is still a major problem for patients with end-stage renal disease. J Am Acad Dermatol 2003;49:842–6.

36. Amatya B, Wennersten G, Nordlind K. Patients' perspective of pruritus in chronic plaque psoriasis: a questionnaire-based study. J Eur Acad Dermatol Venereol 2008;22(7):822–6.

37. Majeski C, Johnson J, Davison S, et al. Itch Severity Scale: a self-report instrument for the measurement of pruritus severity. Br J Dermatol 2007;156(4):667–73.

38. Daudén E, Sánchez-Perez J, Prieto M, et al. Validation of the Spanish Version of the Itch Severity Scale: the PSEDA study. Actas Dermosifiliogr 2011;102(7): 527–36.

39. Zachariae R, Lei U, Hædersdal M, et al. Itch severity and quality of life in patients with pruritus: preliminary validity of a Danish adaptation of the Itch Severity Scale. Acta Derm Venereol 2011. [Epub ahead of print].

40. Acar B, Karabulut H, Sahin Y, et al. New treatment strategy and assessment questionnaire for external auditory canal pruritus: topical pimecrolimus therapy and Modified Itch Severity Scale. J Laryngol Otol 2009;124:147–51.

41. Elman S, Hynan L, Gabriel V, et al. The 5-D itch scale: a new measure of pruritus. Br J Dermatol 2010;162(3):587–93.

42. Desai N, Poindexter G, Monthrope Y, et al. A pilot quality-of-life instrument for pruritus. J Am Acad Dermatol 2008;59(2):234–44.

43. Chen S, Nguyen L, Pugliese S, et al. Pruritus in CTCL patients: prevalence and quality of life impact. First World Congress of Cutaneous Lymphomas. Chicago, September 25, 2010. p. 101.

44. Blome C, Augustin M, Siepmann D, et al. Measuring patient-relevant benefits in pruritus treatment: development and validation of a specific outcomes tool. Br J Dermatol 2009;161(5):1143–8.

45. Weisshaar E, Ständer S, Gieler U, et al. Development of a German language questionnaire for assessing chronic pruritus (AGP-questionnaire): background and first results. Hautarzt 2011;62(12): 914–27.

46. Weisshaar E, Diepgen T, Bruckner T, et al. Itch intensity evaluated in the German Atopic Dermatitis Intervention Study (GADIS): correlations with quality of life, coping behaviour and SCORAD severity in 823 children. Acta Derm Venereol 2008;88(3):234–9.

47. Kini S, DeLong L, Veledar E, et al. The impact of pruritus on quality of life: the skin equivalent of pain. Arch Dermatol 2011;147(10):1153–6.

Health-Related Quality-of-Life Assessment in Dermatologic Practice: Relevance and Application

O.D. van Cranenburgh, MSc[a,1], C.A.C. Prinsen, MSc[a,1],
M.A.G. Sprangers, MA, PhD[b], Ph.I. Spuls, MD, PhD[c],
J. de Korte, MA, PhD[a,*]

KEYWORDS

- HRQoL assessment • Dermatology • Clinical practice
- Chronic skin disease

The following is a brief summary of important points and objectives for recall:

- Health-related quality-of-life (HRQoL) data of patients may be used for various purposes: (1) to increase a patient's self-awareness and empowerment, (2) to increase patient-centeredness in health care, (3) to make an optimal choice for treatment, (4) to monitor treatment over time and determine treatment effectiveness, and (5) to improve treatment outcome.

- HRQoL assessment is particularly relevant for patients with chronic skin diseases that are known to have substantial and enduring adverse effects on HRQoL.

- Many HRQoL questionnaires are currently available. The selection of a HRQoL questionnaire will depend on several factors, such as the functions it has to fulfill in clinical practice, the specific patient population, the psychometric characteristics of a specific questionnaire, and the local policy and conditions.

- We have chosen the Skindex-29 as the questionnaire of first choice to be used in dermatology.

- An electronic assessment may facilitate the application of HRQoL in dermatologic practice.

- To use HRQoL data in clinical practice, scores should be interpreted promptly and accurately. Information on the interpretation of Skindex-29 scores is currently available.

- In discussing HRQoL scores, it is important not to focus on the overall score of the Skindex-29, but on the 3 domain scores.

Conflict of interest: The authors state no relationship with a commercial company that has direct financial interest in the subject matter or materials described in the article or with a company making a competing product.

[a] Department of Dermatology, Aquamarine Foundation, Academic Medical Center, University of Amsterdam, Meibergdreef 9, 1105 AZ Amsterdam, The Netherlands

[b] Department of Medical Psychology, Academic Medical Center, University of Amsterdam, Meibergdreef 9, 1105 AZ Amsterdam, The Netherlands

[c] Department of Dermatology, Academic Medical Center, University of Amsterdam, Meibergdreef 9, 1105 AZ Amsterdam, The Netherlands

[1] In alphabetical order; both authors contributed equally to this paper.

* Corresponding author.
E-mail address: j.dekorte@amc.uva.nl

Dermatol Clin 30 (2012) 323–332
doi:10.1016/j.det.2011.11.004
0733-8635/12/$ – see front matter © 2012 Elsevier Inc. All rights reserved.

derm.theclinics.com

Patient-reported outcomes (PROs) are reports or assessments of any aspect of a patient's health status or impact of treatment that come directly from the patient, without the interpretation of the responses by anyone else. Regulatory agencies in many countries take patient-relevant criteria into consideration in decisions on reimbursement of new therapies, resulting in an increased importance of PROs in clinical trials.[1] The application of PROs in clinical practice is growing as well. Assessment of PROs, such as patients' experienced disease severity, health-related quality of life (HRQoL), treatment adherence, and treatment satisfaction, appears to have added value for daily clinical practice.[2]

In a systematic review of studies on the impact of PRO assessment in clinical practice, Valderas and colleagues[3] stated that (1) PRO assessment can be time consuming, (2) both patients and physicians may perceive PRO questionnaires as burdensome, (3) the interpretation of PRO scores in a clinically meaningful manner requires additional resources, and (4) the implications for treatment are not apparent. On the other hand, PRO assessment can also have a positive impact on clinical practice, specifically by improving the diagnosis and recognition of problems, and in patient–physician communication.[3] The investigators also pointed out that studies included in their review were heterogeneous and of an inferior methodological quality and that, as a result, no evident conclusion could be drawn with regard to the effect of PRO assessment in clinical practice.

An important PRO in health care is HRQoL. HRQoL reflects patients' evaluation of the impact of disease and treatment on their physical, psychological, and social functioning and well-being. Chronic skin diseases, such as acne, eczema, hidradenitis suppurativa, psoriasis, and vitiligo, have been found to adversely affect patients' HRQoL. In many patients, this impact is profound.[4]

In such chronic skin diseases, dermatologic treatment can offer a temporary suppression and/or remission of severity and symptoms. As a result, many patients have to cope with the burden of their skin disease for years, or even throughout their entire lives. Patients often consider improvement of HRQoL as an important treatment goal[5,6]; hence, dermatologic treatment should aim to decrease disease severity and to increase patients' HRQoL.

HRQoL is gradually becoming a standard outcome parameter in clinical studies and health care management.[7] Because the major goal of therapeutic interventions is to make patients feel better, HRQoL assessment is likely to become even more important in the future.[8] Because of this development, the quality of HRQoL assessment itself, correct management and interpretation of HRQoL data, and the communication of such data with the patient, deserve attention.

HRQoL is generally measured with reliable and valid self-reported instruments (ie, questionnaires). The application of such questionnaires in daily clinical practice may improve evidence-based practice, facilitate communication with the patient, and, herewith, the process of shared decision making between patients and physicians. In a randomized controlled trial (RCT) in the field of oncology,[9] HRQoL assessment resulted in a significant increase of relevant information on and discussion of chronic symptoms; moreover, the explicit use of HRQoL information during patients' consultations was associated with a significant improvement in patients' well-being. Another RCT indicated that HRQoL assessment in daily clinical oncology practice facilitates the discussion of HRQoL issues and heightens physicians' awareness of their patients' HRQoL.[10]

Nevertheless, the application of HRQoL assessment is not customary in dermatologic practice and there are several practical and attitudinal barriers. A deeper understanding of the benefits of HRQoL assessment for both dermatologists and patients may improve its application. Hence, members of a Dutch expertise center on HRQoL in dermatology took the initiative to start a working group, consisting of 10 dermatologists, a psychologist, and a clinical epidemiologist, on HRQoL assessment in clinical practice. This working group produced a guideline to support the application of HRQoL assessment in routine dermatologic practice.[11] In this article, and following this guideline, we attempt to provide answers to the following 3 questions: (1) What is the relevance of HRQoL assessment to dermatologic practice? (2) Which patients would benefit most from routine HRQoL assessment? (3) How can HRQoL assessment be applied in clinical practice? In answering these questions, we aim to contribute to the discussion on and the implementation of HRQoL assessment in routine dermatologic practice.

HRQoL ASSESSMENT IN DERMATOLOGY: WHY?
Patients' Self-Awareness and Empowerment

By filling out an HRQoL questionnaire and communicating about the answers to the questions, patients may gain more insight into the impact of the skin disease on their own physical, psychological, and social functioning and well-being. Most likely, this insight will increase patients' self-awareness; for instance, awareness of specific psychological problems and of specific health care needs. Such awareness, and the acknowledgment of needs by the dermatologist, may further empower patients to share and discuss their problems with significant others, such as a partner, relatives, and friends.[12–14]

Patient-Centered Health Care

Clinical evaluations of the severity of a skin disease are not highly correlated with patients' perceptions of HRQoL.[15,16] Consequently, HRQoL assessment is of particular importance to enable the dermatologist to grasp the impact of the skin disease and/or its treatment on an individual patient.[17] In addition, such data may highlight specific aspects of HRQoL that are affected the most, for instance shame or depression. In patients with a chronic skin disease, this information might be of relevance, particularly because of a relatively high prevalence of psychosocial problems, often hidden "under the skin."[7,16,18]

Furthermore, insight into these problems creates an opportunity to communicate in an empathic and responsive way, thereby supporting patients in coping with their problems more effectively. Communication about HRQoL may also be helpful in engaging patients in a discussion on treatment preferences to allow mutual or shared decision making.

An Optimal Choice of Treatment

HRQoL data, in addition to clinical information, contribute to a more comprehensive insight into a patient's situation after diagnosis and before the choice for a specific treatment. By including HRQoL data into the decision-making process, the dermatologist and the patient can make an optimal, shared choice for a specific treatment in terms of its setting (eg, inpatient, outpatient, day care, specialty care), intensity or invasiveness, position in the conceivable order of treatments over time, and/or combinations with other treatments. For instance, if a patient experiences a high level of symptomatic burden, a more intensive or invasive treatment can be considered. A better-tailored treatment is expected to be better tolerated and adhered to by the patient. Additionally, feasible aims of a specific treatment can be discussed using HRQoL data; for instance, a reduction of itch, a decrease in or clearance of visible lesions, or a reduction in the degree of disease severity within a specific time frame.

Furthermore, patients' needs for additional care, as a supplement to regular dermatologic care, can be identified and addressed. Some patients may experience low levels of HRQoL that cannot be explained by disease severity only. Other patients may have serious problems with respect to specific domains or aspects of HRQoL, such as suffering from depression, feeling socially isolated, or encountering problems at work. In such instances, referral to a social worker, a psychologist, or a psychiatrist might be indicated, and can result in a valuable adjuvant therapy.

Monitor Treatment over Time and Determine Treatment Effectiveness

HRQoL scores of a patient before treatment may be compared with scores at follow-up visits. In this way, the treatment process can be monitored over time. HRQoL data obtained at follow-up visits may also be helpful in checking negative consequences or side effects of treatments; for instance, an increase of itch, pain, irritation, tiredness, sleep, or depression. Such HRQoL data alert the dermatologist to adjust the treatment whenever necessary (eg, dose, switch treatment, combination with other treatment); moreover, this tailored treatment is expected to be better tolerated and adhered to by the patient.

In the end, after completion of treatment, HRQoL scores of a patient can be compared with scores before treatment. An improvement in HRQoL, which is a main treatment goal for many patients,[5,6] can be monitored, and may indicate treatment effectiveness.

Improvement of Treatment Outcome

Although the aforementioned functions suggest that application of HRQoL primarily has a positive effect on the *process* of health care, a positive effect on the *outcomes* of dermatologic treatment itself is expected as well. Empowerment of the patient, patient-centered health care, an optimal choice for treatment, monitoring treatment over time, and the explicit attention to HRQoL and/or the patient's point of view is likely to have a positive impact on the patient's HRQoL, treatment satisfaction, and disease severity. As evidence suggests that clinical and psychological outcomes, such as adherence to treatment advice, are optimized when patients' emotional concerns are addressed, it is critical to recognize and manage the psychological needs of patients.[19]

Because of lack of evidence in dermatology concerning the aforementioned functions, a randomized controlled trial (Dutch Trial Register, NTR1364) was started to assess the efficacy of HRQoL assessment and HRQoL communication in dermatologic practice. The study is ongoing and we expect to publish the results in 2012.

HRQoL ASSESSMENT IN DERMATOLOGY: WHO?

HRQoL assessment is particularly relevant for patients with chronic skin diseases that exert a large, negative impact on HRQoL. Psoriasis and eczema have been found to induce substantial decreases in patients' HRQoL.[4,20–22] These skin diseases also have high incidence rates, a high degree of chronicity, and may require long-term treatment; however, many more skin diseases affect HRQoL adversely, including acne, alopecia areata, hand/foot eczema, hidradenitis suppurativa, lichen planus, lichen sclerosus, pruritus/prurigo, seborrhoeic eczema, ulcers, urticaria, and vitiligo.

In addition to a specific diagnosis, the degree of disease severity, social visibility of the condition, age, personal circumstances, and the presence or absence of social support may influence patients' HRQoL. So, a patient with severe psoriasis may experience a relatively good HRQoL, whereas another patient with only a mild degree of eczema may experience a relatively poor HRQoL. Assessments are thus relevant whenever a negative impact on HRQoL is suspected and whenever treatment does not meet the patient's expectations.

The treatment setting itself may also play a role in selecting patients for HRQoL assessment. The inclusion of patients may be influenced by local policy, local conditions, presence or absence of facilities, and availability of staff. For instance, some dermatologists prefer to integrate HRQoL assessment in inpatient care or in a day care center rather than in outpatient settings. This preference may arise from the availability of sufficient room, accommodation, and staff; longer duration of treatment; and/or feasibility of counseling. Others prefer integration in specific outpatient consultation hours, for instance a biologic therapy consultation hour in a psoriasis treatment center.

Although HRQoL assessment can be applicable to all aforementioned patients and settings, we do not recommend assessments in all attending patients. In patients with a skin disease that hardly affects their HRQoL, such as in most patients with actinic keratoses, naevi, warts, and onychomycosis, or in skin diseases where a single consultation or short-term treatment is sufficient, it does not appear to be of relevance. Last, HRQoL assessment should not induce aversion or resistance, for instance in patients who consider questions on psychosocial functioning as unnecessary, intrusive, or inappropriate.

HRQoL ASSESSMENT IN DERMATOLOGY: HOW?
HRQoL Questionnaires

There are simple ways to ask patients about their HRQoL, for instance by asking "How does your skin disease affect your daily life?" In fact, many dermatologists do ask patients how they are doing, and many patients do inform their dermatologists spontaneously about the impact of their skin disease on aspects of HRQoL, for instance on their mood, work, or family life. To collect data in a more objective and systematic way, however, reliable and validated HRQoL questionnaires may be required.

HRQoL questionnaires consist of a number of items or questions, most often to be answered by ticking off a multiple-choice answer. Multiple-choice responses may refer to intensity (eg, from "mild" to "severe") or frequency (eg, from "never" to "all the time") or may invite an opinion with respect to given statements (eg, from "strong disagreement" to "strong agreement"). Because HRQoL is a multidimensional construct (eg, consisting of a physical, psychological, and social functioning domain), responses may result in domain scores, as well as an overall score.

Currently, many questionnaires are available. In general, these can be distinguished into *generic* and *specific* HRQoL questionnaires. Generic questionnaires can be used for the measurement of HRQoL in all kinds of diseases and in the general population, whereas specific questionnaires are designed for the measurement of HRQoL in a specific disease, subgroup of disease, group of diseases, or patient population. Within dermatology, we distinguish *dermatology-specific* questionnaires designed for all kinds of skin diseases, and *disease-specific* questionnaires designed for a specific skin disease, for instance eczema or rosacea. The selection of an HRQoL questionnaire will depend on many factors, such as the functions it has to fulfill in clinical practice, the specific populations of patients, local policy and local conditions, and the psychometric characteristics of a specific questionnaire.

One could start using a simple, practical question to screen HRQoL, for instance a "questionnaire" consisting of only one question with multiple-choice responses: "To what extent does your skin disease affect your quality of life?" A more comprehensive questionnaire is the Dermatology Life Quality Index (DLQI), originally developed for routine dermatologic practice.[23] The DLQI consists of only 10 questions and mainly focuses on limitations, for instance limitations in daily and social activities.

De Korte and colleagues[24] and Both and colleagues[25] systematically reviewed the quality of generic and dermatology-specific HRQoL questionnaires that are used in dermatology. For research, they recommended the use of a generic questionnaire in combination with a dermatology-specific questionnaire. A dermatology-specific questionnaire was explicitly recommended, as it encompasses all relevant dermatologic aspects and domains that a generic questionnaire may not include. For dermatology, the dermatology-specific questionnaire Skindex-29 was recommended.[24,25]

Based on these reviews, we have chosen the Skindex-29 as the questionnaire of first choice for dermatologic practice in the Netherlands. Therefore, in this article we illustrate application of HRQoL assessment with the Skindex-29; however, there could be many reasons for making a different choice in different situations.

The Skindex-29 is a multidimensional questionnaire, assessing HRQoL during the past week, and consisting of 29 items that form 3 domains: symptoms, emotions, and functioning.[15,26] **Box 1** provides an overview of all Skindex-29 items, categorized per domain. Items are answered on a 5-point scale: Never = 0, Rarely = 25, Sometimes = 50, Often = 75, and All the Time = 100. The overall and domain scores are expressed on a 100-point scale, where higher scores indicate lower levels of quality of life. One item (item 18) about possible side effects of medication and/or treatment has been added to the questionnaire, but is not included in one of the domains, nor in the calculation of the overall score and domain scores. Research on the psychometric characteristics of the Skindex-29 indicated its reliability and validity.[15,24–26] The Skindex-29 is currently available and psychometrically tested in many languages, including English, Dutch, French, German, Italian, and Spanish.[27–31]

Electronic HRQoL Assessment

Assessment of HRQoL with a paper questionnaire has the advantage of simplicity. Nevertheless, it has several disadvantages. Apart from all the paperwork, and the integration of data into the medical record, it also implies the calculation of domain and overall scores by hand. Previous

---

Box 1
An overview of Skindex-29 items categorized per domain

Symptoms
1. My skin hurts
7. My skin condition burns or stings
10. My skin itches
16. Water bothers my skin condition (bathing, washing hands)
19. My skin is irritated
24. My skin is sensitive
27. My skin condition bleeds

Emotions
3. I worry that my skin condition may be serious
6. My skin condition makes me feel depressed
9. I worry about getting scars from my skin condition
12. I am ashamed of my skin condition
13. I worry that my skin condition may get worse
15. I am angry about my skin condition
21. I am embarrassed by my skin condition
23. I am frustrated by my skin condition
26. I am humiliated by my skin condition
28. I am annoyed by my skin condition

Functioning
2. My skin condition affects how well I sleep
4. My skin condition makes it hard to work or do hobbies
5. My skin condition affects my social life
8. I tend to stay at home because of my skin condition
11. My skin condition affects how close I can be with those I love
14. I tend to do things by myself because of my skin condition
17. My skin condition makes showing affection difficult
20. My skin condition affects my interactions with others
22. My skin condition is a problem for the people I love
25. My skin condition affects my desire to be with people
29. My skin condition interferes with my sex life
30. My skin condition makes me tired

Side effects
18. I worry about side effects from skin medications/treatments

research showed that pen-and-paper HRQoL questionnaires that have to be scored by hand take too much time and are costly in the long term.[32] Electronic assessment, on the other hand, may lower the resource burden and thereby encourage a more widespread use in clinical practice.[8]

To facilitate the application of HRQoL assessment in dermatologic clinical practice in the Netherlands, an electronic version of the Skindex-29 was developed. This enables patients to complete the questionnaire on a computer by touching the answers of choice on the screen. To our knowledge, this is the only dermatology-specific HRQoL questionnaire that is currently available as an electronic application. Completion of the electronic Skindex-29 takes no longer than 5 minutes and, immediately after answering all questions, all data are available: an overview of questions and answers arranged per domain, and an overview of scores visualized in a bar chart. Both can be printed, and answers that are bothersome, that is, marked with "often" or "all the time," are displayed in bold on the screen as well as in the printout.

International research indicates that electronic HRQoL assessment is increasingly applied within other specialties (eg, oncology and hepatology) and has many advantages for clinical practice.[33–38] Of course, a main advantage of this electronic version, compared with the paper version, is that answers and scores are immediately available and, thereby, facilitate "real-time" discussion with the patient, directly after the assessment (Fig. 1). For this discussion, answers are displayed on screen, but it is preferable that both the dermatologist and the patient have a printed overview of the results as well. Answers in bold can serve as guidance during the patient's consultation with the dermatologist, and the patient may take home the printout, enabling him or her to discuss the results with significant others. The dermatologist may easily include the printed overview of HRQoL results in the patient medical record or may link the results to an electronic patient record.

Another advantage of the electronic version, compared with the paper version, is that the patient's answers and scores are saved in a Skindex file and are automatically transferred to an MS Excel file. Saved scores can be used to analyze data on a group level and to follow the course of HRQoL of an individual patient over time: repeated assessments are graphically presented in a single bar chart (Fig. 2). In this way, the treatment process of a specific patient can be monitored and the effect of a treatment can be determined. Anonymous scores on a group level can be used for scientific research as well.

Interpretation of Scores

To use HRQoL data in clinical practice, scores should be interpreted promptly and accurately; however, the interpretation of scores of any HRQoL questionnaire is not straightforward and has little or no direct meaning. A score of 18 or 63 on a scale running from 0 to 100 cannot be interpreted without additional resources. Two types of methods to establish a clinically meaningful interpretation of HRQoL scores exist: distribution-based and anchor-based methods.[7] For interpretation of scores on the aforementioned DLQI we refer to Hongbo and colleagues.[39]

In the case of the Skindex-29, a first psychometric study on the distribution of Skindex-29 scores among 454 Italian patients with various skin diseases resulted in a categorization of levels of severity,[40] namely "very little," "mild," "moderate," "severe," and "extremely severe." This study, using a distribution-based method, was a first attempt to interpret Skindex-29 scores. In a study performed in the Netherlands

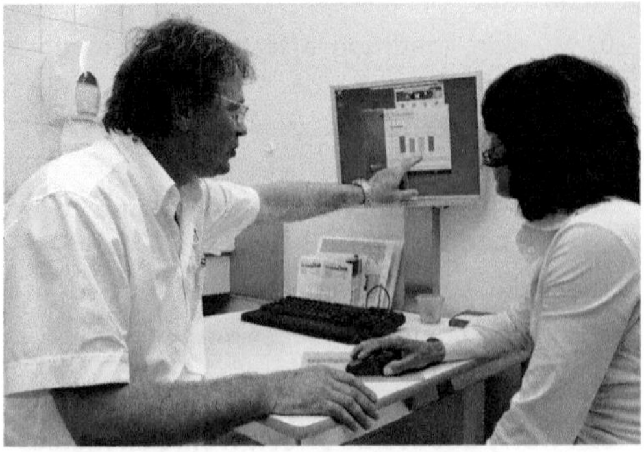

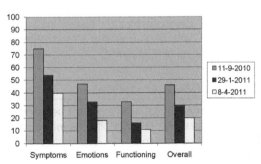

Fig. 1. Discussion of domain scores with the patient, directly after the self-assessment on a computer.

Fig. 2. Repeated assessments of Skindex-29 over time: an overview of domain scores.

Table 1
Identification of patients with mild, moderate, and severe impairment of HRQoL according to Prinsen and colleagues

Level of Severity	Skindex-29 Domains			
	Symptoms	Emotions	Functioning	Overall
Mild	≥39	≥24	≥21	≥25
Moderate	≥42	≥35	≥32	≥32
Severe	≥52	≥39	≥37	≥44

Data from Prinsen CA, Lindeboom R, Sprangers MA, et al. Health-related quality of life assessment in dermatology: interpretation of Skindex-29 scores using patient-based anchors. J Invest Dermatol 2010;130:1318–22; and Prinsen CA, Lindeboom R, Korte JD. Interpretation of Skindex-29 scores: cutoffs for mild, moderate, and severe impairment of health-related quality of life. J Invest Dermatol 2011;131:1945–7.

among 339 patients at 9 general dermatologic outpatient clinics, Prinsen and colleagues[7,41] used an anchor-based method to identify patients with mild, moderate, and severe impairment of HRQoL. The resulting cutoff scores for the Skindex-29 are presented in **Table 1**. To illustrate this: a patient with a score of 39 or higher on the emotions domain is likely to have a severe impairment, and a patient with a score of 32 or higher on the functioning domain is likely to have moderate impairment of HRQoL.

At first glance, these cutoff scores are not easy to apply in clinical practice; however, by using different colors in the bar chart (green for mild, yellow for moderate, and red for severe impairment), one is able to make prompt interpretations at a glance. To facilitate the application of the cutoff scores, one may also, as a rule of thumb or memory aid, round off the cutoff scores for mild, moderate, and severe impairment of HRQoL to 20 or higher, 30 or higher, and 40 or higher, respectively, with the exception of the symptoms domain.[41]

Patients with scores equal to or above the presented cutoff scores for "severe" (see **Table 1**) in at least 1 of the 3 domains are significantly affected by their skin disease. Prinsen and colleagues[7] indicated that these scores may signal a need for (adjustment of current) treatment or for additional care or support, but that scores do not automatically indicate what kind of treatment, care, or support is appropriate, and therefore the specific needs of an individual patient should be explored in direct contact with the patient.

Although the preceding paragraphs provide some guidance in the interpretation of scores and answers, it may be clear that discussion with the patient may yield important additional information and promote a patient-specific interpretation.

Discussion of HRQoL Data

Once a patient has completed the questionnaire, the summation of the domain scores provides a specific profile of a patient's HRQoL. This profile may indicate which domain of HRQoL was influenced most during the preceding week. Because large differences may exist among the 3 domain scores of a patient, it is important not to discuss the overall score solely, but to focus on the domain scores separately. In fact, 2 patients may have about the same overall score, but when taking the domain scores into account, it might appear that the impact of the skin disease focuses on different domains of HRQoL. This is illustrated in **Fig. 3**.

To focus on HRQoL in greater detail, answers to single questions might also be of relevance. In fact, we recommended this, as single questions often provide relevant, additional information that

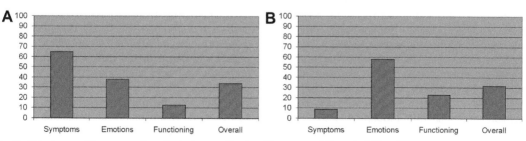

Fig. 3. Skindex profiles: examples of random patients with eczema (*A*) and vitiligo (*B*).

Box 2
A case to illustrate the relevance of HRQoL assessment in dermatologic practice as measured with the Skindex-29

Female, 26 years, psoriasis since the age of 7. Until the age of 20, psoriasis was under control with topical agents and phototherapy. Since then, the patient had extensive psoriasis, active without treatment. Only during pregnancies did the patient have a relatively stable disease. The patient had been on sickness leave regularly.

During the past 6 years, the patient used several systemic agents and underwent several intensive outpatient treatments, resulting in a temporary effect. After the last systemic treatment, her psoriasis aggravated. At that moment, her Psoriasis Area and Severity Index (PASI) was 25.

The patient acted relatively introverted, gave the impression of being very tired, and provided a more favorable picture of herself and her burden of disease than warranted. Skindex-29 assessment resulted in the following domain scores: Symptoms 96, Emotions 78, and Functioning 75.

During the consultation, Skindex-29 scores were discussed with the patient. The patient indicated that she had avoided social contacts and public places on several occasions because of her skin condition, and that there were some problems in handling psychic stress. The possibility of referral to a primary care psychologist for additional treatment with cognitive behavioral therapy was discussed. Also, support from a psoriasis patients' organization was mentioned.

By discussing HRQoL data, the patient became more aware of the consequences of her skin condition and the need to address her problems. At that moment, the patient preferred to wait with additional treatment by a psychologist, but did decide to join the psoriasis patients' organization. During a shared decision-making process concerning the patient's treatment, it was decided to start treatment with a biologic.

Treatment with the biologic agent exerted a rapid improvement. After 4 weeks, Skindex-29 assessment was repeated, showing reduced domain scores: Symptoms 57, Emotions 60, and Functioning 46.

It became evident that the patient did understand the cause of her fatigue more clearly and, thereby, was able to change her coping behavior. Because of contacts with the psoriasis patients' organization, the patient became more outgoing, showed a more open attitude, and talked about her problems more easily with others. Additional therapy was waived.

---

can be used in clinical practice. For instance, a patient may have a low symptoms score but could have indicated "often" or "all the time" to the question about itch, or a low functioning score but with answers "often" or "all the time" to questions about tiredness or sleep. This may signal patients' specific needs. In **Box 2**, a case is described to illustrate the relevance of HRQoL assessment in dermatologic practice, using the Skindex-29 as an example.

SUMMARY

The aim of this article was to contribute to the discussion on and the implementation of HRQoL assessment in routine dermatologic practice. With respect to the relevance of HRQoL assessment, we focused on self-awareness and empowerment, patient-centered health care, and optimal dermatologic treatment. With respect to patients, we focused on patients with a chronic skin disease in which substantial and enduring adverse effects on HRQoL are suspected. With respect to implementation in routine practice, we described

the application of the electronic version of the Skindex-29 in the Netherlands.

We realize we have presented an optimistic view on HRQoL assessment in clinical practice. We would like to stress that a clinically meaningful interpretation of scores and the implications for dermatologic treatment and care are not self-evident. We already referred to a systematic review in which no unambiguous conclusion could be drawn with regard to the effect of PRO assessment in clinical practice[3]; and even in our local, Dutch situation, there are some drawbacks to report. For instance, installation of the Skindex-29 software was sometimes complicated by technical limitations, such as information technology system requirements or safety boundaries that differ from organization to organization. Another problem in some of the clinics was lack of accommodation and staff, and budget problems with respect to computers, laptops, or pocket computers for the patients. Meanwhile, to overcome some of the technical limitations, a Web-based version of the Dutch Skindex-29 has been developed. This Web-based version enables patients to gain access to the Skindex-29 from any computer with an Internet connection. In the Netherlands, a considerable percentage of the citizens have a personal computer with an Internet connection at home. As Skindex data are saved on an external, protected server, potential technical problems during installation of software or constraints owing to safety requirements in a clinic are avoided. In the future, other HRQoL and PRO questionnaires can be added, thus resulting in a "Web portal" for PROs in dermatology. For instance, questionnaires measuring disease severity from a patient's perspective, adherence, or treatment satisfaction.

Although the available evidence on the added value of HRQoL assessment for clinical practice, especially the application of PRO assessment in general, is ambiguous, we believe that initiatives to integrate HRQoL data into the management of patients are most welcome, and will help create a more solid body of evidence. If HRQoL is considered to be an important outcome of routine dermatologic treatment, would it not be a bit "careless" not to measure this patient-reported outcome?

ACKNOWLEDGMENTS

The authors thank the members of the Dutch Working Group "Quality of Life Assessment in Dermatologic Practice" (in alphabetical order): M.T.W. Gaastra, MD; D.B. de Geer, MD; A.Y. Goedkoop, MD, PhD; C.L.M. van Hees, MD; W.J.A. de Kort, MD; C.M. Legierse, MD; T.E.C. Nijsten, MD, PhD; M.C.G. van Praag, MD, PhD; M.L.A. Schuttelaar, MD; A.M.E. Visser–van Andel, MD.

REFERENCES

1. Krenzer S, Radtke M, Schmitt-Rau K, et al. Characterization of patient-reported outcomes in moderate to severe psoriasis. Dermatology 2011;223:80–6.

2. Valderas JM, Alonso J, Guyatt GH. Measuring patient-reported outcomes: moving from clinical trials into clinical practice. Med J Aust 2008;189: 93–4.

3. Valderas JM, Kotzeva A, Espallargues M, et al. The impact of measuring patient-reported outcomes in clinical practice: a systematic review of the literature. Qual Life Res 2008;17:179–93.

4. Rapp SR, Feldman SR, Exum ML, et al. Psoriasis causes as much disability as other major medical diseases. J Am Acad Dermatol 1999;41:401–7.

5. Chren MM. Interpretation of quality-of-life scores. J Invest Dermatol 2010;130:1207–9.

6. Holm EA, Wulf HC, Stegmann H, et al. Life quality assessment among patients with atopic eczema. Br J Dermatol 2006;154:719–25.

7. Prinsen CA, Lindeboom R, Sprangers MA, et al. Health-related quality of life assessment in dermatology: interpretation of Skindex-29 scores using patient-based anchors. J Invest Dermatol 2010; 130:1318–22.

8. Guyatt GH, Ferrans CE, Halyard MY, et al. Exploration of the value of health-related quality-of-life information from clinical research and into clinical practice. Mayo Clin Proc 2007;82:1229–39.

9. Velikova G, Booth L, Smith AB, et al. Measuring quality of life in routine oncology practice improves communication and patient well-being: a randomized controlled trial. J Clin Oncol 2004;22:714–24.

10. Detmar SB, Muller MJ, Schornagel JH, et al. Health-related quality-of-life assessments and patient-physician communication: a randomized controlled trial. JAMA 2002;288:3027–34.

11. Working Group Quality of Life Assessment in Dermatological Practice. Kwaliteit van leven assessment in de dermatologische praktijk: een praktische leidraad. Amsterdam: Stichting Aquamarijn; 2008.

12. Bozcuk H, Erdogan V, Eken C, et al. Does awareness of diagnosis make any difference to quality of life? Determinants of emotional functioning in a group of cancer patients in Turkey. Support Care Cancer 2002;10:51–7.

13. Forlani G, Zannoni C, Tarrini G, et al. An empowerment-based educational program improves psychological well-being and health-related quality of life in Type 1 diabetes. J Endocrinol Invest 2006;29:405–12.

14. Tu YC, Wang RH, Yeh SH. Relationship between perceived empowerment care and quality of life among elderly residents within nursing homes in Taiwan: a questionnaire survey. Int J Nurs Stud 2006; 43:673–80.

15. Chren MM, Lasek RJ, Flocke SA, et al. Improved discriminative and evaluative capability of a refined version of Skindex, a quality-of-life instrument for patients with skin diseases. Arch Dermatol 1997; 133:1433–40.

16. Picardi A, Abeni D, Melchi CF, et al. Psychiatric morbidity in dermatological outpatients: an issue to be recognized. Br J Dermatol 2000;143:983–91.

17. Renzi C, Abeni D, Picardi A, et al. Factors associated with patient satisfaction with care among dermatological outpatients. Br J Dermatol 2001; 145:617–23.

18. Sampogna F, Picardi A, Chren MM, et al. Association between poorer quality of life and psychiatric morbidity in patients with different dermatological conditions. Psychosom Med 2004;66:620–4.

19. Richards HL, Fortune DG, Griffiths CE. Adherence to treatment in patients with psoriasis. J Eur Acad Dermatol Venereol 2006;20:370–9.

20. Carroll CL, Balkrishnan R, Feldman SR, et al. The burden of atopic dermatitis: impact on the patient, family, and society. Pediatr Dermatol 2005;22:192–9.

21. Chamlin SL, Frieden IJ, Williams ML, et al. Effects of atopic dermatitis on young American children and their families. Pediatrics 2004;114:607–11.

22. Finlay AY, Coles EC. The effect of severe psoriasis on the quality of life of 369 patients. Br J Dermatol 1995;132:236–44.

23. Finlay AY, Khan GK. Dermatology Life Quality Index (DLQI)—a simple practical measure for routine clinical use. Clin Exp Dermatol 1994;19:210–6.

24. de Korte J, Mombers FM, Sprangers MA, et al. The suitability of quality-of-life questionnaires for psoriasis research: a systematic literature review. Arch Dermatol 2002;138:1221–7.

25. Both H, Essink-Bot ML, Busschbach J, et al. Critical review of generic and dermatology-specific health-related quality of life instruments. J Invest Dermatol 2007;127:2726–39.

26. Chren MM, Lasek RJ, Quinn LM, et al. Convergent and discriminant validity of a generic and a disease-specific instrument to measure quality of life in patients with skin disease. J Invest Dermatol 1997; 108:103–7.

27. Abeni D, Picardi A, Pasquini P, et al. Further evidence of the validity and reliability of the Skindex-29: an Italian study on 2,242 dermatological outpatients. Dermatology 2002;204:43–9.

28. Aksu AE, Urer MS, Sabuncu I, et al. Turkish version of Skindex-29. Int J Dermatol 2007;46:350–5.

29. Augustin M, Wenninger K, Amon U, et al. German adaptation of the Skindex-29 questionnaire on quality of life in dermatology: validation and clinical results. Dermatology 2004;209:14–20.

30. Jones-Caballero M, Penas PF, Garcia-Diez A, et al. The Spanish version of Skindex-29. An instrument for measuring quality of life in patients with cutaneous diseases. Med Clin (Barc) 2002;118:5–9 [in Spanish].

31. Leplege A, Ecosse E, Zeller J, et al. The French version of Skindex (Skindex-France). Adaptation and assessment of psychometric properties. Ann Dermatol Venereol 2003;130:177–83 [in French].

32. Lofland JH, Schaffer M, Goldfarb N. Evaluating health-related quality of life: cost comparison of computerized touch-screen technology and traditional paper systems. Pharmacotherapy 2000;20: 1390–5.

33. Goodhart IM, Ibbotson V, Doane A, et al. Hypopituitary patients prefer a touch-screen to paper quality of life questionnaire. Growth Horm IGF Res 2005;15: 384–7.

34. Gutteling JJ, Busschbach JJ, de Man RA, et al. Logistic feasibility of health related quality of life measurement in clinical practice: results of a prospective study in a large population of chronic liver patients. Health Qual Life Outcomes 2008;6:97.

35. Kleinman L, Leidy NK, Crawley J, et al. A comparative trial of paper-and-pencil versus computer administration of the Quality of Life in Reflux and Dyspepsia (QOLRAD) questionnaire. Med Care 2001;39:181–9.

36. Larsson BW. Touch-screen versus paper-and-pen questionnaires: effects on patients' evaluations of quality of care. Int J Health Care Qual Assur Inc Leadersh Health Serv 2006;19:328–38.

37. Velikova G, Wright EP, Smith AB, et al. Automated collection of quality-of-life data: a comparison of paper and computer touch-screen questionnaires. J Clin Oncol 1999;17:998–1007.

38. Wright EP, Selby PJ, Crawford M, et al. Feasibility and compliance of automated measurement of quality of life in oncology practice. J Clin Oncol 2003;21:374–82.

39. Hongbo Y, Thomas CL, Harrison MA, et al. Translating the science of quality of life into practice: What do dermatology life quality index scores mean? J Invest Dermatol 2005;125:659–64.

40. Nijsten T, Sampogna F, Abeni D. Categorization of Skindex-29 scores using mixture analysis. Dermatology 2009;218:151–4.

41. Prinsen CA, Lindeboom R, Korte JD. Interpretation of Skindex-29 scores: cutoffs for mild, moderate, and severe impairment of health-related quality of life. J Invest Dermatol 2011;131:1945–7.

Clinical Meaning in Skin-specific Quality of Life Instruments: A Comparison of the Dermatology Life Quality Index and Skindex Banding Systems

Anna Rogers, BS[a], Laura K. DeLong, MD, MPH[b,c], Suephy C. Chen, MD, MS[c,d],*

KEYWORDS

• Quality of life • Clinical meaning • Dermatology

Skin disease is ubiquitous and can affect patients' lives in various ways. The World Health Organization defines quality of life (QOL) as "the individuals' perception of their position in life, in the context of the cultural and value system in which they live and in relation to their goals, expectations, standards and concerns."[1] Health-related QOL (HRQOL) includes the aspects of overall QOL that affect health: physical, psychological, and social. On an individual level, this includes health risks and conditions, functional status, social support, and socioeconomic status.

Several tools have been developed to assess the ways that skin disease is a burden to patients. This assessment is important because measuring HRQOL can help determine the burden of preventable disease and disability, help identify subgroups with poor perceived health, and help guide interventions to avoid more serious complications or burden. The functions of HRQOL assessment are numerous and include describing patients' overall state; screening for early disease or disability; monitoring disease status, progression, and response to treatment; developing treatment plans; justifying the use of drugs that are expensive or have associated risk; improving patient-physician communication; and assisting in the allotment of limited resources.

HRQOL assessment is also important because physicians' judgments of disease severity have been shown to not consistently correlate with patient-reported scores.[2] Additionally, measurements that focus on the clinical severity of disease may not accurately reflect its effects on patients' lives.[3,4] For example, in a study of patients with psoriasis, HRQOL, rather than clinical severity of

The authors have nothing to disclose.

[a] Department of Dermatology, Emory University School of Medicine, 1648 Pierce Drive, NE, Atlanta, GA 30322, USA

[b] Department of Dermatology, Emory University School of Medicine, Emory Clinic, Building A, 1365 Clifton Road Northeast Suite 1100, Atlanta, GA 30322, USA

[c] Division of Dermatology, Atlanta Veterans Affairs Medical Center, Decatur, GA 30322, USA

[d] Department of Dermatology, Emory University, 101 Woodruff Circle, Atlanta, GA 30322, USA

* Corresponding author. Department of Dermatology, Emory University, 101 Woodruff Circle, Atlanta, GA 30322.

E-mail address: schen2@emory.edu

Dermatol Clin 30 (2012) 333–342

doi:10.1016/j.det.2011.11.010

0733-8635/12/$ – see front matter © 2012 Published by Elsevier Inc.

disease, was an independent predictor of work productivity. In these same patients, indirect costs of loss of productivity have been shown to clearly exceed the total direct cost; thus, savings from regaining work productivity might counterbalance the high costs of biologic agents.[5]

Many skin-specific and skin disease–specific QOL instruments have been developed and validated to address the previously discussed needs. However, exceedingly few have explored the assignment of clinical meaning to the scores or changes in scores of the instrument. Currently, studies use statistical definitions (eg, $P<.05$) to claim a significant change in QOL after interventions. However, it is conceivable that a statistically significant change does not translate into a clinically significant change or a patient-oriented significant change. The most commonly used skin disease–specific instrument is the Dermatology Life Quality Index (DLQI), and it is the first to explore the issue of assigning a clinical meaning to DLQI scores. The other commonly used skin-specific instrument is the Skindex, for which investigators have also explored the assignment of clinical meaning. This article reviews the banding system, methods to assign clinical meaning to QOL measures, and specifically reviews methods behind the DLQI and Skindex scores. This article also includes pilot data that compare the DLQI and Skindex using these previously validated banding systems.

DERMATOLOGY LIFE QUALITY INDEX

The DLQI was the first dermatology-specific QOL assessment tool. Finlay and Kahn developed the DLQI in 1994 as a simple, practical questionnaire for routine clinical use.[6] The DLQI is comprised of 10 questions that focus on disability in the following domains: symptoms and feelings, daily activities, leisure, work and school, personal relationships, and the effects of treatment on daily life. The questionnaire states that the aim is to measure the QOL impact over the previous 1 week. It has tick-box answers scored from 0 to 3, and the response options include the following: very much (score 3), a lot (score 2), a little (score 1), or not at all (score 0). Individual scores are added to yield a total score with a maximum of 30; a higher score indicates greater disability. The DLQI has been used in at least 36 skin conditions in 32 countries, is available in 55 languages, and has been described in more than 270 full articles. The most commonly assessed skin conditions using the DLQI are psoriasis, atopic dermatitis, acne, and vitiligo. The questionnaire usually takes less than 5 minutes to complete, with average completion time reported at 2 minutes.[7]

Other than the original text-only version of the DLQI, there is also an illustrated version, which has a quicker average completion time of 88 seconds and has been shown to correlate strongly with the text-only version.[7] Variants of the original DLQI include the Family Dermatology Life Quality Index[8] and the Children's Dermatology Life Quality Index.[9]

The DLQI has been used widely for multiple purposes, including monitoring the effect of different therapeutic interventions, assessing the effectiveness of clinical practices and health services on patients' QOL, and monitoring the efficacy of topical and systemic drugs. The DLQI has also been used in at least 2 national registers of psoriasis in the United Kingdom and Sweden. Additionally, the National Institute for Health and Clinical Excellence in the United Kingdom has incorporated a requirement of a DLQI score of greater than 10 to be eligible to start certain systemic therapies for psoriasis.[10]

Multiple studies have proven that the DLQI has excellent psychometric properties, including validity, factor structure and dimensionality, internal consistency, sensitivity to change, and test-retest reliability.[6,11] However, several weaknesses of the DLQI include the lack of incorporation of the aspect of worry or concerns regarding future health and the lack of assessment of itch-scratch problems and perceived stigmatization.[12,13] There has also been some concern about item bias of the DLQI questions across variables, including gender, age, cultural background, diagnosis, and disease severity.[14] The lack of incorporation of emotional or mental health aspects has led some to recommend the combination of the DLQI with assessments more geared at these emotional aspects, such as the Short Form-36 (SF-36), which contains a mental health summary measure[10,15]; in their review of QOL questionnaires for psoriasis, although the DLQI is not included, de Korte and colleagues[16] also recommend the combination of the generic SF-36 with a dermatology-specific instrument to fully assess the QOL impact for dermatology patients.

SKINDEX

Skindex-29, developed in 1997 by Chren and colleagues,[17] is a refined version with decreased respondent burden and improved discriminative and evaluative capability. It includes 3 domains: symptoms (10 items), emotions (7 items), and functions (12 items); and it has an average completion time of 5 minutes. Skindex-16 was developed in 2001 to improve the sensitivity of some of the items to better distinguish among patients with different QOL effects.[18] The Skindex-16 is more concise, the questions are phrased to answer the level of bother, whereas the Skindex-29 is phrased to ask the frequency of a QOL aspect. Skindex-17 is a Rasch-reduced version of Skindex-29 in which the scores that are collapsed into a 3-point scoring system and the 3 subscales with an overall score have been replaced by 2 subscales, psychosocial and symptoms, with 2 independent scores.[19]

CLINICAL MEANING ASSIGNED TO SCORE

There are several ways to assign clinical meaning to scores of health status measures, which can be divided into anchor-based or distribution-based methods. The anchor-based approach involves determining the difference on a QOL scale that corresponds to a self-reported small but important change on a global scale given concomitantly, which serves as an independent standard or anchor. This approach can be further divided into population-focused and individual-focused approaches. In population-focused methods, multiple anchors, such as diagnosis, symptoms, disease severity, and so forth, are used to present population differences based on the status of anchors. In individual-focused methods, a single anchor is used to establish a minimum important difference (MID) or "the smallest difference in score in the domain of interest which patients perceive as beneficial and which would mandate, in the absence of troublesome side effects and excessive cost, a change in the patient's management,"[20] and then examine the proportion who achieved the MID.

Distribution-based approaches use statistical characteristics of the results, such as standard deviation or standard error of measurement, to express the magnitude of effect in terms of the distribution of results.[21,22] Each approach has its advantages and disadvantages, and best interpretations of meaningful change in QOL scores are achieved when combining anchor-based and distribution-based approaches. Despite these many approaches, the authors focus on the anchor-based banding approach given that the previous work used this technique.

DLQI

Hongbo and colleagues[12] used an anchor-based approach by pairing the DLQI with a Global Question (GQ) concerning patients' views of their overall impairment of their QOL caused by their skin disease to identify bands of DLQI scores that corresponded with each GQ descriptor. They selected patients from the dermatology outpatient wait lists or from patients seen in the previous 2

months at UK hospital dermatology departments. The most frequent diagnoses were nonmelanoma skin cancers and premalignant lesions (22.7%); benign skin and vascular tumors (21.1%); benign pigmented lesions and nevi (10.1%); eczematous conditions (9.7%); acne and other disorders of sebaceous, apocrine, and eccrine glands (8.9%); viral skin lesions (6.1%); and hair and scalp disorders (2.6%). Other less-common diagnoses included keloid scars, genital skin disorders, pigmentary disorders, urticarial disorders, nail disorders, superficial fungal infections, pruritus, reactive skin disorders and drug reactions, and infections.

To devise banding of DLQI scores, the mean, mode, and median of the GQ scores for each DLQI score were used. The kappa coefficient, which is a measure of the level of agreement beyond that which could be expected by chance, for each proposed banding set was calculated. Based on the kappa coefficients as well as other factors, such as improved sensitivity and ease of remembering the scale, the proposed banding system is the following: DLQI scores 0 to 1 indicate no effect on patients' QOL; DLQI scores 2 to 5 indicate a small effect on patients' QOL; DLQI scores 6 to 10 indicate a moderate effect on patients' QOL; DLQI scores 11 to 20 indicate a very large effect on patients' QOL; and DLQI scores 21 to 30 indicate an extremely large effect on patients' QOL ($\kappa = 0.489$) (**Table 1**). This study did not show any significant gender difference among overall responses, so the same banding system can be used for both genders.

Based on this banding system, a DLQI score greater than 10 indicates a very large impairment in QOL caused by skin disease, perhaps meriting intervention. This finding has led to the development of the rule of tens for severe psoriasis: "Current severe psoriasis equals >10% body surface area involved, or Psoriasis Area and Severity Index score >10, or Dermatology Life Quality Index score >10."[23] The application of this rule is for a clinical setting to serve as an adjunct for deciding when active intervention is likely to be required. Several other studies have

Table 1
Proposed banding system for the DLQI

DLQI Band	Scores	QOL Effect
Band 0	0–1	None
Band 1	2–5	Small
Band 2	6–10	Moderate
Band 3	11–20	Very large
Band 4	21–30	Extremely large

also used this banding system as a grading system for the impact of skin disease, specifically psoriasis[24-26] and hidradenitis suppurativa.[27] Other studies have also used this banding system to compare preintervention and postintervention mean DLQI scores. Woods and colleagues[28] found that a novel formulation of fluocinonide cream improved QOL in 25 patients with atopic dermatitis that had a moderate effect to having a mean of a small effect after only 2 weeks of treatment. In total, the Hongbo and colleagues banding article has been cited in more than 85 articles, some of which are reviews about QOL assessment instruments, whereas others use the banding to categorize patients according to QOL impact at different intervention time points[29-32] or to simply apply a clinical meaning to DLQI scores that were reported from their study population.[33-37]

Skindex

Three studies have explored methods to assign clinical meaning to scores from the Skindex-29 questionnaire. Nijsten and colleagues[38] (2009) used mixture analysis, a distribution-based approach, to categorize both the total and the subscale scores. As they describe, "mixture analysis assesses whether a distribution of a variable consists of different overlapping but independent 'subdistributions.'" They recruited patients from outpatient clinics at a large Italian dermatologic hospital, and the most common listed diagnoses were acne (33%), nevi (22%), psoriasis (17%), seborrheic dermatitis (12%), alopecia areata (12%), and vitiligo (6%). This method resulted in 4 levels of impairment for the composite Skindex-29 score: very little for scores less than 5, mild for scores 6 to 15, moderate for scores 18 to 36, and severe for scores greater than 37; it also divided the functioning and emotions subscales into 4 levels of impairment and the symptoms subscale into 5 levels of impairment.

Prinsen and colleagues (2010 and 2011) used an anchor-based approach with 4 global questions along with Skindex-29 to identify clinically meaningful cutoffs to develop a banding system. Patients were recruited from 9 outpatient dermatology clinics in the Netherlands, and the most common diagnoses were psoriasis (42.0%); eczematous lesions (23.6%); acne or other disorders of sebaceous, apocrine, or eccrine glands (5.9%); and nonmelanoma skin cancers and premalignant lesions (5.3%). Other less-common diagnoses (each <3%) included autoimmune disorders, genetic disorders, pigmentary disorders, pruritus, urticarial disorders, viral skin lesions, lichen sclerosis, ulcers, reactive skin disorders and drug reactions, and skin malignancies

not otherwise specified. Receiver operating characteristic–curve analysis was used to determine the optimal cutoff scores, and the Youden index was used to determine the optimal balance between sensitivity and specificity for these scores. This method also resulted in 4 levels of impairment for the composite Skindex-29 score: none for scores 0 to 25, mild for scores 26 to 32, moderate for scores 33 to 44, and severe for scores 45 to 100.[39,40] They also reported cutoffs for 4 levels of impairment for the 3 subscales of symptoms, emotions, and functioning.

Our group (Chen and colleagues) also used an anchor-based approach with a single GQ along with Skindex-29 to develop their banding system.[41] The patient population represented a good variety of general dermatology diagnoses, with the most frequently listed diagnoses being eczematous dermatoses (21%); benign skin lesions, such as seborrheic keratoses, keloids, cysts, and nevi (16%); and infectious processes, such as condyloma, folliculitis, and various types of tinea (13%). Other diagnoses included papulosquamous dermatoses (9%); acneiform dermatoses (8%); malignant lesions, such as nonmelanoma skin cancers, melanoma, and cutaneous lymphomas (6%); and premalignant lesions, such as actinic keratosis and dysplastic nevi (5%). The remaining diagnoses were reported by 12 or fewer patients and included alopecia, connective tissue disorders, acantholytic dermatoses, lichenoid dermatoses, primary pruritus, sarcoidosis, urticaria, vitiligo, and the panniculitides.[42] The mean, median, and mode of the GQ scores for each 5-point interval of Skindex scores were used to create a series of bands. The series with the highest kappa coefficient was deemed the most appropriate, resulting in a 5-band scoring system for the clinical impact of the composite Skindex scores: none for scores 0 to 10, mild for scores 11 to 25, moderate for scores 26 to 50, severe for scores 51 to 70, and very severe for scores 71 to 100. Analysis to generate a banding system for the 3 subscales is pending.

SKINDEX VERSUS DLQI

The Skindex and the DLQI have rarely been compared in a head-to-head manner using the same patient population, perhaps because of the different scoring systems, as previously detailed. Now that there are methods to assign clinical meaning to scores, a comparison can be attempted. Moreover, a comparison between the different Skindex clinical meaning systems can be explored.

In an Institutional Review Board–approved study conducted at Emory University from 2006 to 2008, consecutive available adult subjects were recruited prospectively from The Emory Clinic and the outpatient dermatology clinic at Grady Memorial Hospital. After informed consent was obtained and before their appointment time, subjects were asked to complete demographic questions, the Skindex-29, and the DLQI. A total of 382 subjects were enrolled, but only 374 completed both QOL surveys (Emory [n = 108] and Grady [n = 274]). The diagnoses are the same as previously listed with the Chen and colleagues article because the same data were used.

Composite scores for Skindex-29 and overall scores for DLQI were calculated. These scores were then assigned to bands using the different clinical meaning-assignment systems described above and listed in **Table 2**. Because the Njisten and Prinsen systems have 4 bands, for comparison purposes, the Hongbo banding system for DLQI and the Chen banding system for Skindex were collapsed into 4 bands too. The authors explored two approaches to determine which method provided better concordance: first by combining the lower 2 bands and second by combining the 2 higher bands (**Table 3**). Each Skindex banding system was then compared to the DLQI banding system to measure the agreement between the scales; the individual Skindex banding systems were also compared with each other to see how well they agreed.

Results

When comparing the DLQI system with the Skindex systems by merging the lower 2 bands of the Hongbo system, the Hongbo banding system placed patients in the same band as the Prinsen system 52.1% of the time and the Nijsten system 17.9% of the time (**Tables 4** and **5**). When the 2 higher bands, rather than the lower bands, of the Hongbo system were combined for comparison purposes, the Hongbo system placed patients in the same band as the Prinsen system 52.7% of

the time and the Nijsten system 46.0% of the time. Because the Hongbo and Chen systems both use 5 bands, only 1 direct comparison between the 5 bands of these two was performed; the Hongbo system placed patients in the same band as the Chen system 50% of the time.

All 3 systems trended toward placing patients in higher bands (ie, assigning more QOL impact, see **Table 4**) than the Hongbo system when the lower bands of the Hongbo DLQI system were combined, with the Nijsten system placing 82%, the Prinsen system placing 42%, and the Chen system placing 32% in higher-impact categories. With the higher 2 bands of the Hongbo DLQI system combined, the Prinsen system placed patients with higher impact 15% of the time, whereas Nijsten did so 48% of the time.

The Hongbo and Nijsten systems were in least agreement, with all patients being placed in higher bands by the Nijsten system with the exception of 1 patient when the lower bands of the Hongbo system were combined. This outcome improved somewhat when the higher bands of the Hongbo system were merged, but the Nijsten system still placed most patients in higher bands.

Subanalysis Without Most Emotionally Impacted: Comparison of Hongbo versus Prinsen

To better compare the DLQI and Skindex banding, a subanalysis excluding patients who had a severe emotional effect was performed (**Table 6**). These patients were chosen because the DLQI has been criticized for lacking an emotional element. The Prinsen banding system was used because it best agreed with the Hongbo scoring system; also, Prinsen and colleagues included banding systems for the subscales in addition to the banding for the composite Skindex scores. The cutoff of greater than or equal to 39 was found to correlate with severely impaired HRQOL on the emotions domain, so patients that fell into that category

Table 2
Banding systems for DLQI and Skindex

Band	Effect	DLQI Hongbo	Skindex Versions		
			Chen	Nijsten	Prinsen
0	None/very little	0–1	0–10	0–5	0–25
1	Mild	2–5	11–25	6–17	26–32
2	Moderate	6–10	26–50	18–36	33–44
3	Severe	11–20	51–70	>37	>44
4	Very severe	21–30	71–100	—	—

Table 3
Banding systems for DLQI and Skindex with lower and higher bands combined

		Combining Bands 0&1		Combining Bands 3&4	
Band	Effect	Hongbo	Chen	Hongbo	Chen
0	None/very little	0–5	0–25	0–1	0–10
1	Mild	6–10	26–50	2–5	11–25
2	Moderate	11–20	51–70	6–10	26–50
3	Severe	21–30	71–100	11–30	51–100

were not included in this comparison. After excluding those patients, 187 patients remained for comparison.

When the lower bands of the Hongbo system were merged, the Hongbo and Prinsen systems placed patients in the same band 78.6% of the time (as compared with only 52% when all patients were compared). The Prinsen system placed patients in higher bands 12% of the time. When the higher bands of the Hongbo system were merged, the Hongbo and Prinsen systems placed patients in the same band 47.1% of the time (vs 53.0%). The Prinsen system placed patients in higher bands 3% of the time and in lower bands 50% of the time.

Skindex Systems

When comparing within the Skindex systems, Chen and Prinsen agree 66.3% of the time, Prinsen and Nijsten agree 42.0% of the time, and Chen and Nijsten agree 18.2% of the time when the lower 2

bands of the Chen system were merged into 1. The Nijsten system tended to place patients in higher bands (82% more compared with Chen and 58% compared with Prinsen), whereas the Prinsen placed patients in higher bands compared with Chen 34% of the time.

When the higher 2 bands of the Chen system were merged, Chen and Nijsten agree 60% of the time and Chen and Prinsen agree 54% of the time. This time, the Nijsten system placed patients in higher bands 40% of the time, whereas the Prinsen tended to place patients in lower bands (40%).

Discussion

Although until now studies have not directly compared the DLQI with Skindex, others have graded the different available dermatology-specific life quality indices. In a review of generic and dermatology-specific HRQOL instruments, Both and colleagues[14] recommend Skindex-29 as the dermatology-specific instrument of choice.

Table 4
Comparisons between DLQI and Skindex and between different Skindex banding systems (lower bands combined)

	DLQI vs Skindex			Skindex Versions		
Difference	Hongbo-Prinsen	Hongbo-Chen	Hongbo-Nijsten	Chen-Prinsen	Prinsen-Nijsten	Chen-Nijsten
−4	...	1 (0.27)	...	...	...	...
−3	9 (2.4)	0	20 (5.3)	0	0	0
−2	42 (11.2)	15 (4.0)	126 (33.7)	22 (5.8)	61 (16.3)	120 (32.1)
−1	107 (28.6)	104 (27.8)	160 (42.8)	104 (27.8)	156 (41.7)	186 (49.8)
0	195 (52.1)	187 (50.0)	67 (17.9)	248 (66.3)	157 (42.0)	68 (18.2)
1	17 (4.5)	60 (16.0)	1 (0.27)	0	0	0
2	4 (1.1)	6 (1.6)	0	0	0	0
3	0	1 (0.27)	0	0	0	0
4	...	0	...	...	...	...

Note: Differences in the banding of the first system minus the second system. Results are listed as total number of patients with given difference (%).

Table 5
Comparisons between DLQI and Skindex and between different Skindex banding systems (higher bands combined)

	DLQI vs Skindex		Skindex Versions	
Difference	Hongbo-Prinsen	Hongbo-Nijsten	Chen-Nijsten	Chen-Prinsen
−3	2 (0.53)	4 (1.1)	0	0
−2	11 (2.9)	34 (9.1)	0	0
−1	42 (11.2)	143 (38.2)	150 (40.1)	22 (5.9)
0	197 (52.7)	172 (46.0)	224 (59.9)	202 (54.0)
1	101 (27.0)	20 (5.3)	0	150 (40.1)
2	17 (4.5)	0	0	0
3	4 (1.1)	0	0	0

They note the major limitations of the DLQI to be focus on disability, response distribution, and dimensionality and item bias. Because of the focus on disability or functioning in daily activities, they think the DLQI does not fully encompass the emotional and mental health aspects that might be affected. They claim that this suggests that the DLQI may lack conceptual validity in patients with minor dermatologic conditions or in diseases primarily affecting mental health, such as vitiligo and alopecia. The authors' pilot data provide evidence that the DLQI and the Skindex (at least with the Prinsen system) agree much better when the severely emotionally impaired patients are removed from analysis. Thus, given the excellent psychometric properties of the DLQI and its translation into so many languages, the DLQI should remain a favored QOL instrument when disability is a primary focus. However, in situations or diseases whereby the emotional aspect is important to measure or with diagnoses that potentially carry a large emotional burden, such as vitiligo and alopecia areata, investigators should consider the Skindex. Also, conditions that carry an aspect of worry, such as a concern that a spot is a skin cancer, might not be best assessed with the DLQI.

Aside from the comparison between the DLQI and the Skindex, the authors have highlighted the variability in the different clinical-assignment systems for the Skindex. The Nijsten system tended to place patients in higher bands when comparing with the other 2 systems, indicating higher QOL impact, whereas the Prinsen and Chen systems were more closely aligned. This finding is not a surprising result because the Nijsten's highest band encompasses more than half the Skindex scale (37–100). Indeed, when the higher 2 bands of the Chen system were merged, the agreement was higher between it and the Nijsten system (18.2% vs 60.0%). Thus, one could argue that for the more severely affected populations, the Chen or Prinsen system may be better in discerning differences in QOL impact.

The utility of HRQOL assessment tools lies in the ability to assign a clinical significance to the score generated by the tool. The results provided earlier illustrate that the implication of a score on either the DLQI or Skindex questionnaire can be significantly altered depending on which scoring system is used. Even among the 3 banding systems for the Skindex questionnaire, there was substantial disagreement: a given score for the same patient could place them in the lowest band (no effect) in 1 scoring system, the second band (mild effect) in the second system, and the third band (moderate effect) in the third system. For example, a score of 20 on the Skindex questionnaire places that patient in the no-effect category in the Prinsen system, the mild-effect category in the Chen system, and the moderate-effect category in the

Table 6
Comparison of Hongbo and Prinsen systems with severely emotionally impaired patients excluded

Difference	Hongbo (Lower)–Prinsen	Hongbo (Higher)–Prinsen
−3	0	0
−2	5 (2.7)	1 (0.53)
−1	18 (9.6)	5 (2.7)
0	147 (78.6)	88 (47.1)
1	13 (7.0)	76 (40.6)
2	4 (2.1)	13 (7.0)
3	0	4 (2.1)

Nijsten system. Therefore, choosing which study population best matches with each patient or the patient population whereby a particular banding system is being implemented is important. Cultural differences in different patient populations should also be considered; the patients in the Nijsten study were Italian, those in the Prinsen and Hongbo studies were from the United Kingdom, and those in the Chen study were American.

The patient populations for the included studies differ significantly, and these differences can be used to determine the clinical situation in which each banding system might be most appropriate. For example, if inflammatory (acne, psoriasis, seborrheic dermatitis) versus noninflammatory (vitiligo, alopecia, nevi) diagnoses are predominant, this may determine which DLQI assessment tool is most appropriate. More specifically, the Prinsen patient population was dominated by patients with psoriasis (>40%), so this system might be best applied to patients with psoriasis or another inflammatory condition.

The banding system gives a meaning to the absolute scores, which is useful when comparing populations, whether across disease or across demographics. However, there is a need for more studies to look for meaningful changes in scores, especially in the context of an intervention. Do specific interventions cause clinically significant improvements in QOL? Although not discussed in depth in this review, the idea of a minimally important difference, or a score change that is considered by patients to be clinically relevant rather than a score change that might be statistically significant, is another way to measure impact on QOL and the impact of an implemented treatment regimen. A score change of as little as 2.2 to 5.7[43,44] may be considered to be clinically relevant by a patient, but such an improvement does not move a patient from one band to a lower band with less clinical effect. Similarly, an improvement from a score of 18 to a score of 13 still leaves the patient in the category of their skin disease having a very large effect on their QOL when using the Hongbo system.

The utility of QOL assessment tools can be maximized only if there is a way to extract the clinical meaning of the scores derived from the questionnaires. Assigning clinical meaning to scores on QOL questionnaires is not only important for research and patient classification purposes but is even more important for clinical decision making and monitoring clinical improvement as well as cost-effectiveness analysis. As Guyatt and colleagues[22] point out, measures to interpret the clinical meaning of scores on health status questionnaires must be valid, responsive, and interpretable. Without methods of interpretation, the scores are arbitrary numbers and physicians are left to guess at the magnitude of effect or the importance of a change in score in response to treatment. Although no system is perfect, validated systems for assigning clinical meaning are important to make QOL assessment tools applicable and useful in everyday clinical practice.

REFERENCES

1. Division of mental health and prevention of substance abuse world health organization. WHOQOL Measuring Quality of Life; 1997. Available at: http://www.who.int/mental_health/media/68.pdf. Accessed July 18, 2011.
2. Chren MM, Lasek RJ, Quinn LM, et al. Skindex, a quality-of-life measure for patients with skin disease: reliability, validity, and responsiveness. J Invest Dermatol 1996;107(5):707–13.
3. Salek MS, Finlay AY, Luscombe DK, et al. Cyclosporin greatly improves the quality of life of adults with severe atopic dermatitis. A randomized, double-blind, placebo-controlled trial. Br J Dermatol 1993; 129(4):422–30.
4. Motley RJ, Finlay AY. Practical use of a disability index in the routine management of acne. Clin Exp Dermatol 1992;17(1):1–3.
5. Schmitt JM, Ford DE. Work limitations and productivity loss are associated with health-related quality of life but not with clinical severity in patients with psoriasis. Dermatology 2006;213(2):102–10.
6. Finlay AY, Khan GK. Dermatology Life Quality Index (DLQI)–a simple practical measure for routine clinical use. Clin Exp Dermatol 1994;19(3):210–6.
7. Loo WJ, Diba V, Chawla M, et al. Dermatology Life Quality Index: influence of an illustrated version. Br J Dermatol 2003;148(2):279–84.
8. Basra MK, Sue-Ho R, Finlay AY. The Family Dermatology Life Quality Index: measuring the secondary impact of skin disease [Erratum appears in: Br J Dermatol 2007;156(4):791]. Br J Dermatol 2007; 156(3):528–38.
9. Holme SA, Man I, Sharpe JL, et al. The Children's Dermatology Life Quality Index: validation of the cartoon version. Br J Dermatol 2003;148(2):285–90.
10. Basra MK, Fenech R, Gatt RM, et al. The Dermatology Life Quality Index 1994-2007: a comprehensive review of validation data and clinical results. Br J Dermatol 2008;159(5):997–1035.
11. Lewis V, Finlay AY. 10 years experience of the Dermatology Life Quality Index (DLQI) [review]. J Investig Dermatol Symp Proc 2004;9(2):169–80.
12. Hongbo Y, Thomas CL, Harrison MA, et al. Translating the science of quality of life into practice: what do dermatology life quality index scores mean? J Invest Dermatol 2005;125(4):659–64.

13. Evers AW, Duller P, van de Kerkhof PC, et al. The Impact of Chronic Skin Disease on Daily Life (ISDL), 2008 Disease on Daily Life (ISDL): a generic and dermatology-specific health instrument. Br J Dermatol 2008;158(1):101–8.

14. Both H, Essink-Bot ML, Busschbach J, et al. Critical review of generic and dermatology-specific health-related quality of life instruments. J Invest Dermatol 2007;127(12):2726–39.

15. Ware JE Jr. SF-36 health survey update [review]. Spine (Phila Pa 1976) 2000;25(24):3130–9.

16. De Korte J, Mombers FM, Sprangers MA, et al. The suitability of quality-of-life questionnaires for psoriasis research: a systematic literature review [review]. Arch Dermatol 2002;138(9):1221–7 [discussion: 1227].

17. Chren MM, Lasek RJ, Flocke SA, et al. Improved discriminative and evaluative capability of a refined version of Skindex, a quality-of-life instrument for patients with skin diseases. Arch Dermatol 1997; 133(11):1433–40.

18. Chren MM, Lasek RJ, Sahay AP, et al. Measurement properties of Skindex-16: a brief quality-of-life measure for patients with skin diseases. J Cutan Med Surg 2001;5(2):105–10.

19. Nijsten TE, Sampogna F, Chren MM, et al. Testing and reducing skindex-29 using Rasch analysis: Skindex-17. J Invest Dermatol 2006;126(6):1244–50.

20. Jaeschke R, Singer J, Guyatt GH. Measurement of health status. Ascertaining the minimal clinically important difference. Control Clin Trials 1989;10(4): 407–15.

21. Crosby RD, Kolotkin RL, Williams GR. Defining clinically meaningful change in health-related quality of life. J Clin Epidemiol 2003;56(5):395–407.

22. Guyatt GH, Osoba D, Wu AW, et al, Clinical Significance Consensus Meeting Group. Methods to explain the clinical significance of health status measures [review]. Mayo Clin Proc 2002;77(4): 371–83.

23. Finlay AY. Current severe psoriasis and the rule of tens [review]. Br J Dermatol 2005;152(5):861–7.

24. Mrowietz U, Kragballe K, Reich K, et al. Definition of treatment goals for moderate to severe psoriasis: a European consensus. Arch Dermatol Res 2011; 303(1):1–10.

25. Mease PJ, Ory P, Sharp JT, et al. Adalimumab for long-term treatment of psoriatic arthritis: 2-year data from the Adalimumab Effectiveness in Psoriatic Arthritis Trial (ADEPT). Ann Rheum Dis 2009;68(5): 702–9.

26. MacDonald A, Burden AD. Psoriasis: advances in pathophysiology and management [review]. Postgrad Med J 2007;83(985):690–7.

27. Lee RA, Dommasch E, Treat J, et al. A prospective clinical trial of open-label etanercept for the treatment of hidradenitis suppurativa. J Am Acad Dermatol 2009;60(4):565–73.

28. Woods MT, Brown PA, Baig-Lewis SF, et al. Effects of a novel formulation of fluocinonide 0.1% cream on skin barrier function in atopic dermatitis. J Drugs Dermatol 2011;10(2):171–6.

29. Haeck IM, Knol MJ, Ten Berge O, et al. Enteric-coated mycophenolate sodium versus cyclosporin A as long-term treatment in adult patients with severe atopic dermatitis: a randomized controlled trial. J Am Acad Dermatol 2011;64(6):1074–84.

30. Magerl M, Pisarevskaja D, Scheufele R, et al. Effects of a pseudoallergen-free diet on chronic spontaneous urticaria: a prospective trial. Allergy 2010; 65(1):78–83.

31. Rehn LM, Meririnne E, Höök-Nikanne J, et al. Depressive symptoms and suicidal ideation during isotretinoin treatment: a 12-week follow-up study of male Finnish military conscripts. J Eur Acad Dermatol Venereol 2009;23(11):1294–7.

32. Potter PC, Kapp A, Maurer M, et al. Comparison of the efficacy of levocetirizine 5 mg and desloratadine 5 mg in chronic idiopathic urticaria patients. Allergy 2009;64(4):596–604.

33. Szepietowski JC, Balaskas E, Taube KM, et al, Uraemic Xerosis Working Group. Quality of life in patients with uraemic xerosis and pruritus. Acta Derm Venereol 2011;91(3):313–7.

34. Hald M, Agner T, Blands J, et al. Quality of life in a population of patients with hand eczema: a six-month follow-up study. Acta Derm Venereol 2011; 91(4):484–6.

35. Huang YH, Yang CH, Chen YH, et al. Reduction in osmidrosis using a suction-assisted cartilage shaver improves the quality of life. Dermatol Surg 2010; 36(10):1573–7.

36. Stafford R, Farrar MD, Kift R, et al. The impact of photosensitivity disorders on aspects of lifestyle. Br J Dermatol 2010;163(4):817–22.

37. Szepietowski JC, Reich A, Wesołowska-Szepietowska E, et al, for the National Quality of Life in Dermatology Group. Quality of life in patients suffering from seborrheic dermatitis: influence of age, gender and education level. Mycoses 2009; 52(4):357–63.

38. Nijsten T, Sampogna F, Abeni D. Categorization of Skindex-29 scores using mixture analysis. Dermatology 2009;218(2):151–4.

39. Prinsen CA, Lindeboom R, Sprangers MA, et al. Health-related quality of life assessment in dermatology: interpretation of Skindex-29 scores using patient-based anchors. J Invest Dermatol 2010; 130(5):1318–22.

40. Prinsen CA, Lindeboom R, de Korte J. Interpretation of Skindex-29 scores: cutoffs for mild, moderate, and severe impairment of health-related quality of life. J Invest Dermatol 2011;131(9):1945–7.

41. Dunbar S, McCombs K, DeLong LK, et al. Banding and the clinical interpretation of Skindex-29 scores

using an anchor based technique. J Am Acad Dermatol 2010;62(3):AB68.

42. Requena L, Yus ES, Kutzner H. Panniculitis. In: Wolff K, Goldsmith LA, Katz SI, et al, editors. Fitzpatrick's dermatology in general medicine. 7th edition. New York: McGraw-Hill; 2008. Chapter 68. Available at: http://www.accessmedicine.com/content.aspx?aID=2978288. Accessed December 13, 2011.

43. Shikiar R, Willian MK, Okun MM, et al. The validity and responsiveness of three quality of life measures in the assessment of psoriasis patients: results of a phase II study. Health Qual Life Outcomes 2006;4:71.

44. Shikiar R, Harding G, Leahy M, et al. Minimal important difference (MID) of the Dermatology Life Quality Index (DLQI): results from patients with chronic idiopathic urticaria. Health Qual Life Outcomes 2005;3:36.

Future Directions in Dermatology Quality of Life Measures

Laura K. DeLong, MD, MPH[a,b], Suephy C. Chen, MD, MS[b,c],*

KEYWORDS

- Dermatology health status • Clinical significance
- Guidelines • Quality of life

Within the last few decades, outcomes research, and in particular quality of life (QoL) outcomes research, has become integrated into clinical and research practices. This change has transformed medicine from an old model, which had an emphasis on targeting objective measures such as blood pressure, to a new model where subjective measures such as QoL are of importance.[1] Many dermatologic conditions are associated with clinical findings and symptoms that can negatively impact health-related QoL. This change in QoL is often the reason for which care is sought. Furthermore, the experience of health-related QoL is different for each person. This experience may be related to the patient's disease or treatment, and it may incorporate differing cultural and historical experiences. For this reason, treatments are not only targeted to impact objective findings, but also to those that are more subjective such as itch, which is often the most bothersome aspect of the disease to the patient. Said another way, dermatologic diseases carry significant psychosocial burden and morbidity from appearance and impact on symptoms, function, and emotion, with few cases of mortality. Therefore, it is important within dermatology to address and incorporate QoL into clinical and research practices.

Fortunately, much work has been performed in the development and application of different types of QoL measures in dermatology. The paradigm of generic health versus skin-specific versus condition-specific health status instruments has been reviewed extensively elsewhere.[2,3] Similarly, criteria as to how to choose a particular health status QOL instruments have been explored in other well-developed articles.[4,5]

The next generation of dermatology QOL work, in the authors' opinion, should focus not only on validating health status instruments and be rigorously tested for psychometric properties, but also concentrate on methods to assign clinical meaning to these instruments and to explore guidelines for the development of disease-specific measures. Additionally, less work has been performed on health preference measures of QoL (vs health status measures) that can be incorporated into cost-effectiveness analyses. In this atmosphere of limited health care resources, health policymakers will be forced to curtail certain treatments; dermatology needs to be able to join in these discussions by providing quantifiable metrics to incorporate the QoL improvement treatments offer. More specifically, outcomes researchers need to explore approaches to estimate preference-based QoL measures that are not as cumbersome as current

The authors have nothing to disclose.

[a] Department of Dermatology, Emory University School of Medicine, Emory Clinic, Building A, 1365 Clifton Road Northeast Suite 1100, Atlanta, GA 30322, USA
[b] Division of Dermatology, Atlanta Veterans Affairs Medical Center, Decatur, GA 30322, USA
[c] Department of Dermatology, Emory University, 101 Woodruff Circle, Atlanta, GA 30322, USA
* Corresponding author. Department of Dermatology, Emory University, 101 Woodruff Circle, Atlanta, GA 30322.
E-mail address: schen2@emory.edu

Dermatol Clin 30 (2012) 343–347
doi:10.1016/j.det.2011.11.005
0733-8635/12/$ – see front matter © 2012 Published by Elsevier Inc.

methods to maximize available cost-effectiveness analyses.

CLINICAL SIGNIFICANCE OF QoL MEASURES

The principles of evidence-based medicine are used increasingly in dermatology to guide clinical practice and resource allocation. With outcomes research blossoming, more emphasis is being placed on the results of these studies to inform clinical practice. The use of valid and clinically meaningful patient outcomes measures is vitally important to reaching this goal with quality and success. Therefore, there is a need to standardize scoring systems for measuring disease severity and other patient outcomes in the clinical trial setting. Lack of standardization and validity of measures can prohibit the meaningful interpretation of individual studies. Furthermore, wide variations of trial methodology that limit the comparison of data from different sources impact the production of therapy guidelines, compendiums of evidence, and systematic reviews. It has been noted that within the literature, there are almost as many scales as there are trials.[6] Signs and symptoms are frequently mixed up together, and patient-centered outcomes measures, despite the awareness of QoL outcomes, seem to be neglected by an urge to measure objective signs. The clinical meaning of percentage changes in continuous objective scales will always be difficult to interpret and need to be interpreted in conjunction with other outcome measures, as in practice it is the patient who is treated and not the signs of the disease. Despite the known importance, QoL is assessed in a surprising minority of trials.

INTERPRETING RESULTS FROM OUTCOMES DATA

Many health related QoL studies have focused on cross-sectional comparisons between groups, but great interest lies in the assessment of intraindividual change over time. To demonstrate the value and success of various treatments and care protocols, the research needs to show that the observed changes in patients' outcomes are important and clinically substantial. Most studies attempt to assess clinical efficacy of a given intervention compared with another by making group comparisons and evaluating for statistically significant differences. Unfortunately, statistical significance does not in itself provide concise information about a given intervention's clinically meaningful effects.

One approach is to assign clinical meaning to bands of scores of the QoL instrument such that 1 band of scores can be interpreted to have a particular amount of QoL impact. Hongbo and colleagues[7] were among the first to apply this approach in dermatology. By anchoring the QOL scored to a global question of overall impairment to QOL, they were able to assign clinical meaning to bands of scores of the Dermatology Life Quality Index; for example, scores from 0 to 10 represented "no to a small QoL impact." Thus, a change in score from 12 to 8 may represent a clinically meaningful change, while a change from 10 to 6 would not be clinically meaningful even if it were statistically significantly different. Other groups have applied this concept to the Skindex. The authors refer readers to Rogers' article in this issue for a thorough review.

While using clinical bands of scores is a useful first step to interpreting QoL instruments, those methods do not provide information for the minimally important difference (MID), that is the smallest change in QoL scores that the patients perceive is important. This change may be within a clinical band, or may straddle between 2 bands. This determination of the magnitude of intraindividual change necessary to establish clinical relevance remains to be determined for most measures. The methods for linking statistical evaluations and clinically meaningful standards for change are areas of future research. Although there are no agreed upon standards, the question of how to meaningfully interpret changes in QoL scales can be addressed with many existing methods.[8,9] The authors outline several approaches and examples that future investigators may want to explore for existing validated dermatology measures.

Anchor-Based Approach for MID

One approach to establish the MID is to compare with an independent standard or anchor that is itself interpretable and to which the instrument under investigation bears at least a moderate correlation.[10] Possible anchors for dermatology include changes in global ratings by subjects, change from systemic or high-potency topical treatments to low-potency topical maintenance treatments, fewer office visits, fewer missed days from work, or other improved measures of function. In this research, there is a shift from a focus on the mean difference to the difference in the proportion of patients who experience an improvement greater than the MID in the treatment and control groups. Said in another way, if the treatment is effective, more treated than control patients will show an improvement.[10]

Reliable Change Index

The reliable change index (RCI) calculates whether the change in score from before to after treatment is caused by real change or by chance variation. The RCI is calculated using the standard error of measurement (SEM) to estimate the range of chance variation.[11] RCI tables can be generated for the overall and subscales scores of the QoL measure. The RCI alone does not indicate clinical significance; it only expresses the amount of change between before and after treatment scores that would be statistically reliable.

Distribution-Based Methods of Estimating Clinical Significance

Distribution-based strategies estimate clinically significant change by using normative distribution statistics. One main approach involves estimating effect size in change scores, which involves subtracting an individual's baseline scale score from the follow-up score, then dividing those results by the measure's normative sample standard deviation. One weakness with this method is that the standard deviation, used in calculating effect sizes, is sample dependent and therefore not necessarily externally generalizable.

The other main distribution-based method involves using the SEM, because it theoretically does not vary sample to sample, and may be a more stable. The SEM is an estimate of the amount of test error associated with the test taker's true score and is determined by multiplying the standard deviation of the measure by the square root of 1 minus its reliability coefficient. One SEM is then interpreted as the MID in individual patient scores.[12] With this method, a range of true scores can be determined, and scores that fall outside that range would be considered rare scores. Another variant of the distribution approach was based on observations that studies that demonstrated one-half of the standard deviation of a measure represents the upper limit of the MID[13]

Applications in Dermatology

Several of these approaches to determine clinical meaning in QoL scores have been applied in dermatology. The MID concept has been applied using the Dermatology Life Quality Index (DLQI) in chronic idiopathic urticarial.[14] In this work, the authors used data from a phase 2 clinical trial and used both the anchor and distributional approaches for deriving estimates of MID. For the anchoring technique, the authors used a patient-assessed 5-point pruritus score as an anchor. Changes in the DLQI total score that correlated to changes in disease severity, defined as a mean change score in pruritus greater than or equal to 1, were considered the MID. The authors used the SEM method for the distribution-based

approach. They found an estimate of 3.21 and 2.97 using the anchor approach and 2.24 to 3.1 using the distributional approach. They concluded by recommending a range of 2.24 to 3.10 as an MID for the DLQI in interpreting results for patients with chronic idiopathic urticaria.

Shikiar and colleagues[15] estimated MIDs for the DLQI in psoriasis. Since there was no patient-based assessment of the smallest change that they would perceive to be beneficial, the data were used to explore 5 methods to estimate MIDs of the DLQI. The first 3 approaches involved anchor-based methods. They used 2 definitions of significant changes in Psoriasis Area and Severity Index (PASI) scores and compared DLQI change scores. They first defined significant PASI change on the percentage of patients who would perceive (25%) as beneficial and then defined PASI change on what clinicians would deem clinically relevant (50%–74%). The third anchor-based method for estimating MID relied on the association of changes of the DLQI with changes in the Physician's Global Assessment (PGA). A minimal responder was defined as a patient whose PGA improved by either 1 or 2 points from baseline to week 12, whereas a nonresponder would have no difference. The DLQI MID was defined as the difference in the DLQI score between nonresponders and minimal responders.

The last 2 MID estimates were based upon the distributional methods. One used the method using the SEM, while the other estimated the MID using one-half of the standard deviation. Estimates for the DLQI MID ranged from 4.05 (for patient-based PASI difference) to 6.95 (for clinical PASI difference), while the SEM was 2.33, and one-half standard deviation was 3.59. In the conclusion, the authors disclaimed the clinical PASI difference and stated that they believed that it was too conservative for estimating the minimum change that patients will find beneficial. Instead, they modified their estimates and concluded that the MID of the DLQI in psoriasis should be in the range of approximately 2.3 to 5.7.

CHOOSING MEASURES: GUIDELINES WHEN DISEASE-SPECIFIC MEASURES DO NOT EXIST

Many papers have reviewed the psychometric criteria to use when choosing a health status QoL measure to use in clinical trials or clinical setting. However, despite the growth of skin disease and condition-specific QoL measures, there is still a significant gap in many diseases. The questions that arise when no disease-specific measure exists are: should a generic or skin-specific instrument be used, or should researchers develop their own disease-specific measure? Should items be borrowed from various existing instruments, or should researchers add their own items to existing measures?

Outcomes researchers and psychometricians recommend making these decisions based upon information gathered from focus sessions or in-depth interviews with patients with the disease in question.[16] From these interviews, one can then determine whether the conceptual framework describing the issues that are specific to the QoL impact of that particular disease are comprehensively covered in existing, validated instruments. If not, then one should determine whether a subscale from a multidimensional instrument could be used. For instance, the Skindex-29 has 3 subscales: emotion, symptom, and function. Perhaps the emotional subscale would be sufficient to use for the new skin disease being studied, but the symptoms and function subscales are not. One could take an approach where just the emotional subscale, with all of the emotion questions, is used. The disadvantage to this approach is that the entire Skindex profile then cannot be used to compare with other skin diseases. However, the developers of Skindex have argued that the subscale scores have more meaning than does the overall score. Taking this approach 1 step further, using just 1 question from a subscale, would not be advised unless a completely new instrument is being developed and validated. While each individual item has information to convey, a set of items from a variety of sources cannot be summarized in a validated manner; one cannot simply add, average, or take the median of scores from these diversely obtained items.

If subscales from existing instruments are not sufficient, 1 approach would be to develop a new disease-specific measure. The advantage to this endeavor is that the researchers can then ensure that the instrument is comprehensive to the conceptual framework developed from the items elicited from patients, and has been rigorously tested for validity, reliability, and responsiveness. However, the development of a new instrument takes time and great effort. Moreover, federal funding sources tend not to support these efforts.

The final approach represents a compromise of the the previously mentioned approaches. Researchers can take one existing, validated skin-specific instrument, such as the Skindex, and add a disease-specific module. This module would be comprised of items that are relevant to the disease impact, obtained from the focus groups/in-depth interviews, but are not adequately covered in the skin-specific instrument. Scores from the module questions would need to be analyzed individually and could not be integrated into the skin-specific instrument scores unless testing of such an approach was conducted (but then, that effort would be the same as the validation of a brand new instrument). The advantage to this approach would be to have a score from the skin-specific instrument that can then be not only used across time, say before and after intervention, but also be used to compare QoL impact against other skin diseases. The items from the disease-specific module can also be examined across time. While this approach avoids the time-consuming psychometric testing, outcomes researchers advise at a minimum, a pretesting of the module. Between five and 10 nonmedical persons, not necessarily with the disease, should be asked to think aloud and rephrase the items or discuss what each item means to them. This extra effort ensures that the items are understandable and are conveying the researchers' intent.

PREFERENCE-BASED MEASURES

The final proposed focus for the future of QoL research is in developing easier ways to assess utilities, the preference-based QoL measures. As outlined in other papers, the empiric methods of assessing utilities are very time consuming and labor intensive. There has yet to be a validated way to use proxies for utilities in dermatology. Some studies have used population-based estimates such as the EuroQoL where health status measures are used to assess the health status of the subject and then mapped to a population-derived utility estimate for that health state. The issue is that these instruments have not been validated in the dermatology population, and indeed have very real ceiling and possibly floor effects, as illustrated in Seidler and Kini's article in this issue. Thus, future researchers need to test such population-based approaches in dermatology populations before using them.

Another surrogate for measuring utilities is to create mapping strategies. These mapping strategies also use health status measures to describe the health state of the patient, but rather than mapping to a pre-existing table of utilities, they use a mathematical equation, such as a regression model, to transform the health status QoL score into a utility estimate. One such effort using a broad array of dermatologic conditions was made by one of this article's authors (SC), but it was found that the heterogeneity of skin conditions precluded a robust model (S.C. Chen, unpublished data, 2000). Other groups have focused on 1 disease as discussed in Basra's article in this issue concerning the application of the DLQI in chronic hand eczema. However, these efforts need to be validated against empirically obtained utility values.

FUTURE DIRECTIONS FOR OUTCOMES RESEARCH

Addressing the 3 gaps in dermatology QoL, (1) assignment of clinical meaning, (2) quicker methods of developing QoL assessment for specific diseases, and (3) developing proxies for utility assessment, will be vital for the future of outcomes research. The call for assessment of health technology and new therapeutic strategies in terms of efficacy, cost-effectiveness, and net benefit is increasingly loud to determine whether the associated increases in expenditures for health care are justified. This call has altered the culture of clinical practice and health care research by changing how one assesses the end results of health care services. In doing so, it has provided the foundation for measuring the quality of care. The results of dermatology outcomes research can be used by purchasers and consumers to assess the quality of care in health plans. These types of outcomes research also provide policymakers from public programs, such as Medicaid/Medicare, with the tools to monitor and improve quality both in traditional settings and under managed care. In summary, outcomes research is the key to knowing not only what quality of care can be achieved, but how researches, clinicians, and policy makers can achieve it.[17]

REFERENCES

1. Kaplan RM. The significance of quality of life in health care [review]. Qual Life Res 2003;12(Suppl 1):3–16.
2. Chen SC. Dermatology quality of life instruments: sorting out the quagmire. J Invest Dermatol 2007; 127(12):2695–6.
3. Both H, Essink-Bot ML, Busschbach J, et al. Critical review of generic and dermatology-specific health-related quality of life instruments [review]. J Invest Dermatol 2007;127(12):2726–39.
4. Scientific Advisory Committee of the Medical Outcomes Trust. Assessing health status and quality-of-life instruments: attributes and review criteria [review]. Qual Life Res 2002;11(3):193–205.
5. Testa MA, Simonson DC. Assessment of quality-of-life outcomes. N Engl J Med 1996;334(13):835–40.
6. Charman C, Chambers C, Williams H. Measuring atopic dermatitis severity in randomized controlled clinical trials: what exactly are we measuring? J Invest Dermatol 2003;120(6):932–41.
7. Hongbo Y, Thomas CL, Harrison MA, et al. Translating the science of quality of life into practice: what do dermatology life quality index scores mean? J Invest Dermatol 2005;125(4):659–64.
8. Wyrwich KW, Nienaber NA, Tierney WM, et al. Linking clinical relevance and statistical significance in evaluating intra-individual changes in health-related quality of life. Med Care 1999;37(5):469–78.
9. Norman GR, Sloan JA, Wyrwich KW. Interpretation of changes in health-related quality of life: the remarkable universality of half a standard deviation. Med Care 2003;41:582–92.
10. Guyatt G, Schunemann H. How can quality of life researchers make their work more useful to health workers and their patients? Qual Life Res 2007; 16(7):1097–105.
11. Ferguson RJ, Robinson AB, Splaine M. Use of the reliable change index to evaluate clinical significance in SF-36 outcomes. Qual Life Res 2002; 11(6):509–16.
12. Wyrwich KW, Tierney WM, Wolinsky FD. Further evidence supporting an SEM-based criterion for identifying meaningful intraindividual changes in health-related quality of life. J Clin Epidemiol 1999; 52:861–73.
13. Hays RD, Farivar SS, Liu H. Approaches and recommendations for estimating minimally important differences for health-related quality of life measures. COPD 2005;2:63–7.
14. Shikiar R, Harding G, Leahy M, et al. Minimal important difference (MID) of the Dermatology Life Quality Index (DLQI): results from patients with chronic idiopathic urticaria. Health Qual Life Outcomes 2005;3:36.
15. Shikiar R, Willian MK, Okun MM, et al. The validity and responsiveness of three quality of life measures in the assessment of psoriasis patients: results of a phase II study. Health Qual Life Outcomes 2006; 4:71.
16. Swigris JJ, Stewart AL, Gould MK, et al. Patients' perspectives on how idiopathic pulmonary fibrosis affects the quality of their lives. Health Qual Life Outcomes 2005;3:61.
17. Outcomes research. Fact sheet. Rockville (MD): Agency for Healthcare Research and Quality; AHRQ Publication No. 00-P011, March 2000. Available at: http://www.ahrq.gov/clinic/outfact.htm. Accessed September 15, 2011.

Index

Dermatol Clin 30 (2012) 349–354
doi:10.1016/S0733-8635(12)00019-8

Moving?

Make sure your subscription moves with you!

To notify us of your new address, find your **Clinics Account Number** (located on your mailing label above your name), and contact customer service at:

Email: journalscustomerservice-usa@elsevier.com

800-654-2452 (subscribers in the U.S. & Canada)
314-447-8871 (subscribers outside of the U.S. & Canada)

Fax number: 314-447-8029

Elsevier Health Sciences Division
Subscription Customer Service
3251 Riverport Lane
Maryland Heights, MO 63043